Alloimmune disorders of pregnancy

Anaemia, thrombocytopenia and neutropenia in the fetus and newborn

Collectively known as the alloimmune cytopenias, haemolytic disease of the fetus and newborn, alloimmune thrombocytopenia and alloimmune neutropenia are all consequences of maternal immunization to fetal blood cells. The effective prevention, diagnosis and management of these disorders has become a team effort involving haematologists, obstetricians, paediatricians, immunologists, laboratory technicians, midwives and research scientists. This book has been written by experts in their respective fields to bring together the issues of pathogenesis, epidemiology, prevention, diagnosis and clinical management. This comprehensive but accessible account is extensively cross-referenced to emphasize the links between pathogenesis and clinical sequelae, between epidemiology and the rationale for screening programmes, and between diagnosis and therapeutic intervention.

This is an authoritative overview suitable for trainees in obstetrics, maternal and fetal medicine, transfusion medicine and clinical immunology.

Dr Andrew Hadley is Division Manager at the International Blood Group Reference Laboratory and Senior Scientist at the Bristol Institute for Transfusion Sciences, University of Bristol.

Professor Peter Soothill is Professor of Maternal and Fetal Medicine and Head of the Department of Obstetrics and Gynaecology, St Michael's Hospital and University of Bristol.

Alloimmune disorders of pregnancy

Anaemia, thrombocytopenia and neutropenia in the fetus and newborn

Edited by

Andrew G Hadley

International Blood Group Reference Laboratory,
Southmead Road, Bristol

and

Peter Soothill

Department of Maternal and Fetal Medicine,
St Michael's Hospital,
Southwell Street, Bristol

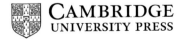

CAMBRIDGE
UNIVERSITY PRESS

CAMBRIDGE UNIVERSITY PRESS
Cambridge, New York, Melbourne, Madrid, Cape Town, Singapore, São Paulo

Cambridge University Press
The Edinburgh Building, Cambridge CB2 2RU, UK

Published in the United States of America by Cambridge University Press, New York

www.cambridge.org
Information on this title: www.cambridge.org/9780521781206

First published 2002
This digitally printed first paperback version 2005

A catalogue record for this publication is available from the British Library

Library of Congress Cataloguing in Publication data

Alloimmune disorders of pregnancy: anaemia, thrombocytopenia, and neutropenia in the fetus and
newborn / [edited by] Andrew G Hadley and Peter Soothill.
 p. cm.
Includes bibliographical references and index.
ISBN 0 521 78120 5 (hardback)
1. Blood diseases in pregnancy. 2. Fetus – Diseases. 3. Pregnancy – Complications. I. Hadley,
Andrew G, 1957– II. Soothill, Peter, 1957–
[DNLM: 1. Anemia, Hemolytic, Autoimmune – Infant, Newborn. 2. Fetal Diseases. 3. Infant,
Newborn, Diseases. 4. Neutropenia – Infant, Newborn. 5. Pregnancy Complications. 6. Prenatal
Diagnosis. 7. Thrombocytopenia – Infant, Newborn. WS 420 A441 2002]
RG572.A456 2002
618.3′261–dc21   2001025639

ISBN-13 978-0-521-78120-6 hardback
ISBN-10 0-521-78120-5 hardback

ISBN-13 978-0-521-01804-3 paperback
ISBN-10 0-521-01804-8 paperback

Contents

3   **Basis and practice of screening for haemolytic disease of the fetus and newborn**   41

Geoff Poole

12   The diagnosis of alloimmune thrombocytopenia   219
Andrew G Hadley

13   The immunological diagnosis of alloimmune neutropenia   235
Geoff Lucas

Contributors

Sherif Abdel-Fattah
Clinical Research Fellow, Fetal Medicine
Research Unit, St Michael's Hospital,
Southwell Street, Bristol, BS2 8EG, UK

David Allen
Head of the Platelet Immunology
Laboratory, National Blood Service, John
Radcliffe Hospital, Oxford, OX3 9DU, UK
dave.allen@nbs.nhs.uk

Neil D Avent
Senior Lecturer, University of the West of
England, Coldharbour Lane, Bristol, BS16
1QY, UK
neil.avent@uwe.ac.uk

Geoff Daniels
Senior Research Fellow, Bristol Institute for
Transfusion Sciences, Southmead Road,
Bristol, BS10 5ND, UK
geoff.daniels@nbs.nhs.uk

Nic Goulden
Consultant Senior Lecturer in Paediatric
Haematology, The Bristol Children's
Hospital, St Michael's Hill, Bristol, BS2 8BJ,
UK

Andrew G Hadley
Divisional Manager, International Blood
Group Reference Laboratory, Southmead
Road, Bristol, BS10 5ND, UK
andrew.hadley@nbs.nhs.uk

Belinda Kumpel
Senior Research Scientist, Bristol Institute
for Transfusion Sciences, Southmead Road,
Bristol, BS10 5ND, UK
belinda.kumpel@nbs.nhs.uk

Geoff Lucas
Head of Platelet and Granulocyte
Immunology, International Blood Group
Reference Laboratory, Bristol, BS10 5ND,
UK
geoff.lucas@nbs.nhs.uk

Kenneth J Moise Jr
Professor of Obstetrics and Gynecology and
Director, Division of Maternal-Fetal
Medicine, University of North Carolina
School of Medicine, Chapel Hill, NC27599-
7570, USA
kmoisejr@med.unc.edu

Michael F Murphy
Consultant Haematologist, National Blood
Service and University of Oxford, John
Radcliffe Hospital, Oxford, OX3 9DU, UK
mike.murphy@nbs.nhs.uk

Geoff Poole
Head of Red Cell Immunohaematology,
National Blood Service, Southmead Road,
Bristol, BS10 5ND, UK
geoff.poole@nbs.nhs.uk

Rachel Rayment
Consultant Haematologist, National Blood
Service, John Radcliffe Hospital, Oxford,
OX3 9DU, UK

David Roberts
Consultant Haematologist, National Blood
Service and University of Oxford, John
Radcliffe Hospital, Oxford, OX3 9DU, UK
david.roberts@nbs.nhs.uk

Glynn Russell
Consultant Neonatal Paediatrician, The
Bristol Children's Hospital, St Michael's Hill,
Bristol, BS2 8BJ, UK

Peter Soothill
Professor of Maternal and Fetal Medicine
and Head of Obstetrics and Gynaecology, St
Michael's Hospital, Southwell Street, Bristol,
BS2 8EG, UK
peter.soothill@bristol.ac.uk

Craig Turner
Research Scientist, Bristol Institute for
Transfusion Sciences, Southmead Road,
Bristol, BS10 5ND, UK
craig.turner@nbs.nhs.uk

Stan Urbaniak
Professor of Transfusion Medicine, Scottish
National Blood Transfusion Service and
University of Aberdeen, Royal National
Infirmary, Foresterhill, Aberdeen, AB9 2ZW,
UK
s.j.urbaniak@abdn.ac.uk

Paul W Whitecar
Fellow, Maternal-Fetal Medicine, Division of
Maternal-Fetal Medicine, University of
North Carolina School of Medicine, Chapel
Hill, NC 27599-7570, USA

Lorna M Williamson
Consultant Haematologist and Senior
Lecturer, National Blood Service and
University of Cambridge, Long Road,
Cambridge, CB2 2PT, UK
lorna.williamson@nbs.nhs.uk

Preface

Definitions and terminology

The alloimmune cytopenias are a group of conditions in which the life span of fetal blood cells or their precursors is shortened by the action of antibodies derived from the mother by placental transfer. Three conditions are recognized: antibodies to fetal red cells, platelets or neutrophils, or their precursors, cause alloimmune anaemia, thrombocytopenia or neutropenia, respectively. Various terms are in common usage for these disorders, many of them inappropriate. For example, alloimmune anaemia is sometimes referred to as Rhesus disease, erythroblastosis fetalis or haemolytic disease of the newborn and all three are misnomers. It is incorrect to use 'Rhesus' to refer to the Rh system, fetal haemolysis may be caused by antibodies outside the Rh system, anaemia is not always associated with erythroblastosis and, finally, the disorder primarily affects the fetus rather than the newborn. Therefore, throughout this book, alloimmune anaemia (perhaps the best term) will be referred to as haemolytic disease of the fetus and newborn (HDFN). For similar reasons, alloimmune thrombocytopenia and alloimmune neutropenia will be used in preference to other terms, such as neonatal alloimmune thrombocytopenia, fetomaternal alloimmune thrombocytopenia and neonatal alloimmune neutropenia, while, at the same time, acknowledging that these terms are also commonly used.

The multidisciplinary approach to the management of the alloimmune cytopenias

The last 10 years of the 20th century saw significant advances in the management of alloimmunized pregnant women; immunologists made progress characterizing the molecular basis of the alloimmune response; molecular biologists solved the genetic basis for all the clinically important blood groups and developed DNA-based fetal typing assays; epidemiologists and health care economists developed a better understanding of the natural history of the alloimmune cytopenias and the cost-effectiveness of preventative programmes; obstetricians and fetal medicine specialists progressed the use of noninvasive fetal monitoring techniques; and haematologists improved the safety and efficacy of the various fetal transfusion therapies. With significant advances being made on so many fronts, the optimal prevention, diagnosis and management of alloimmunized pregnant women has become a team effort involving haematologists, obstetricians, paediatricians, immunologists, laboratory technicians in hospitals and transfusion centres, midwives and research scientists. However, it is rare for the individuals who contribute to this team effort to have a comprehensive overview of all the laboratory and clinical aspects associated with the alloimmune cytopenias.

Our intention in producing this book has been to bring the issues of pathogenesis, epidemiology, prevention, diagnosis and management together in a way which is both comprehensive and relevant to the various professionals involved. To this end, we have tried to avoid subspecialty jargon and to limit the use of abbreviations as far as possible because those used daily by laboratory scientists may be less familiar to clinicians and vice versa.

Andrew G Hadley
Peter Soothill

Foreword

This book is a very good idea. It brings together all the different aspects of the alloimmune cytopenias that are needed to understand them. The two most important are the red cell and the platelet cytopenias and they have features in common as well as characteristics that sharply differentiate them. For each condition, consideration is given to the genetics, the pathophysiology, the evidence for the efficacy and cost-effectiveness of screening and prevention, and to the management of the affected fetus and neonate. To have authoritative chapters on all these topics within the covers of one book is extremely helpful both for those who are new to these clinical problems and for those who, like the author of this foreword, have been grappling with them for over 20 years. The editors and their multidisciplinary team are to be congratulated and thanked for producing this valuable synthesis.

Professor Charles H Rodeck
Department of Obstetrics and Gynaecology
Royal Free and University College London Medical School

Abbreviations

ADCC	Antibody-dependent cell-mediated cytotoxicity
AMIS	Antibody-mediated immune suppression
ARMS	Amplification refractory mutation system
ASPA	Allele-specific primer amplification
C3	Third component of complement
CD	Cluster of differentiation
CLT	Chemiluminescence test
CMV	Cytomegalovirus
CTG	Cardiotocography
DAGT	Direct antiglobulin test
ELISA	Enzyme-linked immunosorbent assay
FBS	Fetal blood sampling
FcγR	Fc gamma receptor (receptor for the Fc domain of IgG)
GAT	Granulocyte agglutination test
GIFT	Granulocyte immunofluorescence test
HbsAg	Hepatitis B surface antigen
HCV	Hepatitis C virus
HIV	Human immunodeficiency virus
HPA	Human platelet antigen
HTLV	Human lymphotropic virus
IAGT	Indirect antiglobulin test
ICH	Intracranial haemorrhage
IL	Interleukin
Ig	Immunoglobulin
im	Intramuscularly
IU	International Units
IUT	Intrauterine transfusion
iv	Intravenously
IVIG	Intravenous immunoglobulin
Hb	Haemoglobin

HDFN	Haemolytic disease of the fetus and newborn
HLA	Human leukocyte antigen or histocompatibility locus antigen
HPA	Human platelet antigen
HNA	Human neutrophil antigen
kD	Kilodalton
LISS	Low ionic strength saline
MAIGA	Monoclonal antibody immobilization of granulocyte antigens assay
MAIPA	Monoclonal antibody immobilization of platelet antigens assay
MMA	Monocyte monolayer assay
ΔOD_{450}	Optical density at a wavelength of 450 nm
PCR	Polymerase chain reaction
PEG	Polyethyleneglycol
PIFT	Platelet immunofluorescence test
RFLP	Restriction fragment length polymorphism
SNP	Single nucleotide polymorphism
TAV	Time-averaged mean velocity
TPH	Transplacental haemorrhage

Pathophysiology of the alloimmune cytopenias

Andrew G Hadley[1] and Craig Turner[2]

[1] International Blood Group Reference Laboratory, Bristol, UK
[2] Bristol Institute for Transfusion Sciences, Bristol, UK

The pathogenesis of the alloimmune cytopenias can be considered in four stages: alloimmunization of the mother, the placental transfer of antibodies to a fetus, the immune destruction of sensitized blood cells and, finally, clinical manifestations which are secondary to the destruction of fetal blood cells such as hydrops, haemorrhage or infection.

1.1 Maternal Alloimmunization

1.1.1 Some key events in the humoral immune response

A comprehensive review of humoral immune responses is outside the scope of this chapter. Nevertheless, a brief consideration of the cells and some of the key processes which result in the production of antibodies is pertinent to several topics covered in this book such as the genetic predisposition to form certain alloantibodies (Section 1.1.3), the mode of action of Rh prophylaxis (Section 5.5), and the basis of new approaches to ameliorate maternal alloimmune responses (Section 14.5). These key steps are shown diagrammatically in Figure 1.1.

Two phases of an immune response are distinguished. The primary response results in very low or undetectable levels of circulating antibody. The second anamnestic response is characterized by much higher concentrations of antibody. The immune response starts with the nonspecific uptake of an antigen by antigen-presenting cells in lymphoid centres such as the spleen and lymph nodes. Internalized antigens are then incorporated into phagolysosomes where they are partially degraded by proteolytic enzymes to peptide fragments. The peptides then associate with HLA class II molecules before being returned to the cell surface and so 'presented' to helper T cells. Interdigitating dendritic cells are particularly efficient at presenting antigen and during a primary immune response they are probably the only cell capable of effective antigen presentation to resting helper T cells. However, B cells can also present antigen and, in secondary immune responses, B

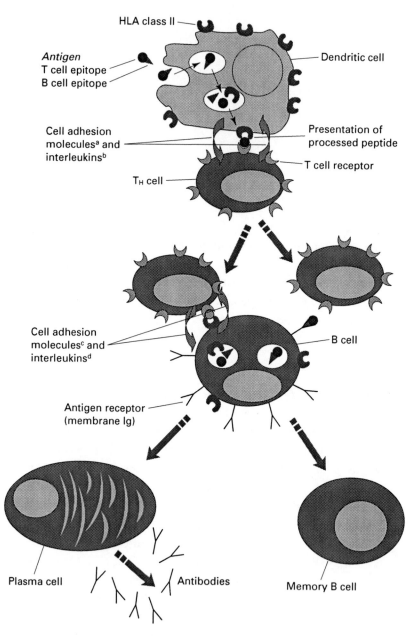

Figure 1.1   Critical steps in the humoral immune response.

Antigens are processed and presented to helper T cells by dendritic cells. In the presence of appropriate secondary signals, helper T cells proliferate and signal antigen-specific B cells to proliferate and secrete antibody.

(a) Co-stimulatory molecules on antigen-presenting cells bind to their ligands on helper T cells; lymphocyte functional antigen 3 (LFA-3) binds to CD2, intercellular adhesion molecule-1 (ICAM-1) binds to LFA-1, CD80/CD86 binds to CD28.

cells with high affinity immunoglobulin antigen receptors may be the most effective antigen-presenting cells.

As mentioned above, peptides are 'seen' by helper T cells when presented as complexes with HLA class II molecules. The binding of peptides to HLA class II molecules depends on complementarity between the peptide and the grove within the HLA molecule. Since the precise topology of the peptide-binding grove of HLA molecules varies according to the HLA allele(s), the ability to bind peptides derived from certain alloantigens is under genetic control. For example, the ability to form antibodies to the human platelet antigen-1a (HPA-1a) is strongly associated with the HLA-DRw3*0101 allele (Section 1.1.3).

Helper T cells express receptors which recognize peptides lodged in the HLA class II groove. It follows that processed peptides contain certain amino acids which contact the HLA class II molecule and a different set of amino acids which contact the T cell receptor. Thus, T cells recognize epitopes made up of linear amino acid sequences (in the HLA grove) rather than the conformational determinants which constitute the epitopes recognized by B cells and the antibodies they secrete. The interaction between antigen-presenting cells and helper T cells is facilitated by a series of cell adhesion and co-stimulatory molecules.[1] Once an antigen has been appropriately presented, helper T cells become activated and secrete cytokines such as interleukin-2 which are necessary for T cells to divide. These in turn release interleukins which cause B cells to differentiate into antibody-secreting clones (Figure 1.1).

In previously primed individuals, B cells can also take up antigen and present it, in the context of HLA class II, to helper T cells. Importantly, antigens displayed on the surface of B cells reflect the repertoire of antigens that B cells can recognize and select via specific membrane-bound antibodies. This means that helper T cells activate those B cells which have bound the antigen responsible for the initial activation of helper T cells (Figure 1.1). Again, the interaction between B cells and

Figure 1.1 (*cont.*)

   (b) Cytokines involved in helper T cell activation include interleukin-1 (IL-1), IL-6, IL-12, IL-15 and tumour necrosis factor α (TNFα). IL-2 is also important in T cell proliferation. Cytokines involved in antigen-presenting cell activation (leading to increased expression of HLA class II and other molecules) include interferon γ (IFNγ), granulocyte–macrophage colony-stimulating factor (GM-CSF), IL-4 and TNFβ.

   (c) Co-stimulatory molecules on activated helper T cells bind to their ligands on B cells; CD28 binds to CD80/CD86, CD40 ligand binds to CD40, LFA-1 binds to ICAM-1 or ICAM-3 and CD2 binds to LFA-3.

   (d) Cytokines involved in B cell activation and differentiation include IL-4 and IL-6, respectively; these are characteristic of helper T cells (T$_H$2). Cytokines involved in the maintenance of T cell activation include IL-1 and IL-6.

helper T cells involves several different receptor–ligand interactions and an exchange of soluble interleukins; HLA class II/peptide complexes and CD40 receptor molecules on B cells are ligated by T cell receptors and CD40 ligand molecules on helper T cells. This signals antigen-specific B cells to proliferate and differentiate into antibody-secreting plasma cells and memory B cells. The latter are responsible for the anamnestic response to rechallenge with antigen. Finally, the antigen-driven process of affinity maturation results in hypermutation of B cells and the secretion of antibody with increased affinity for antigen. Concurrent with the immune response, various mechanisms ensure the regulation of antibody production.[1]

1.1.2 The maternal alloimmune response to fetal red cells

Human red cells express hundreds of different blood group antigens most of which have been reported to elicit a maternal alloimmune response (Chapter 2). Clinically, the most important antigen is D (Section 2.5.1): the antigen is relatively immunogenic, it is well developed early in gestation, a significant proportion of the Caucasian population is D negative, and the antibody is capable of causing fetal haemolysis.

In vitro, the immune response to peptides representing D-specific sequences results in the generation of cytokines characteristic of a helper T cell-dependent response.[2] In vivo, a primary immune response is followed by an anamnestic long-lived secondary immune response associated with the presence of circulating lymphocytes expressing D-specific membrane immunoglobulin.[3] Helper T cells from different D-negative individuals appear to recognize and respond only to a limited number of peptides derived from regions distributed throughout the intracellular, transmembrane and extracellular regions of the D protein.[4]

The likelihood of a D-negative woman becoming immunized depends on several factors and these are reviewed below.

1.1.2.1 Dose of D-positive fetal red cells

Small volumes of fetal red cells enter the maternal circulation during most normal pregnancies and after most normal deliveries (Section 6.4).[5] In the absence of antenatal prophylaxis, anti-D may be detected in sera from less than 1% of D-negative women bearing D-positive fetuses by the end of the third trimester.[6] This implies that, during normal pregnancy, transplacental haemorrhage of sufficient red cells to elicit antibody production is rare.[7] The volume of transplacental haemorrhage detected in the maternal circulation may be significantly greater at delivery, especially when the fetus and mother are ABO compatible. Thus, in the absence of Rh prophylaxis, about 16% of D-negative women become immunized as a result of their first D-positive ABO-compatible pregnancy; about one-half have detectable anti-D by 6 months after delivery and about one-half mount a brisk secondary response during a subsequent D-positive pregnancy indicating that a primary immunization had occurred.[8] The incidence of alloimmunization increases to 31% following transplacental haemorrhage of over 0.1 ml fetal blood.[9]

Transplacental haemorrhage and alloimmunization may follow invasive procedures such as amniocentesis, fetal blood sampling, elective and spontaneous pregnancy loss, and some obstetric manipulations.[10–12] These events and their associated risks of alloimmunization are discussed in more detail (Section 6.4).

1.1.2.2 Rh phenotype of the fetal blood

Red cells with the phenotype R_2r have been found to be more immunogenic than R_1r cells.[13] This may be related to the density of D antigens on these cells; R_2r cells have 14 000–16 000 D antigens and R_1r cells have 9900–14 600 D antigens.[14]

1.1.2.3 ABO incompatibility

The relative rarity with which women become alloimmunized to D when the partner is ABO incompatible was first noted by Levine in 1943.[15] In later studies, it was estimated that blood group A incompatibility between mother and fetus conferred 90% protection against immunization to D; blood group B incompatibility conferred 55% protection.[16] Presumably, the protective effect is due to the ability of anti-A or anti-B to cause rapid intravascular destruction of fetal red cells.

1.1.2.4 Maternal HLA haplotype

Hilden et al. found the HLA-DQB1 allele *0201 in 18% of women with anti-D titres between 16 and 256 and in 85% of women with titres above 512, suggesting an association between this allele and a predisposition to form relatively high levels of anti-D.[17] However, the molecular mechanisms responsible for this association have not been elucidated.

1.1.2.5 Fetal gender

Several studies have reported evidence which suggests that D-positive male fetuses elicit an alloimmune response more frequently than female fetuses. The male to female ratio in three studies was 1.4:1, 1.5:1 and 1.7:1.[9,18,19]

1.1.3 The maternal alloimmune response to fetal platelets

Five of the glycoprotein receptors expressed in the platelet membrane have been shown to be polymorphic in Caucasian populations and so capable of eliciting a maternal alloantibody response leading to thrombocytopenia in the fetus (Section 12.2). Most cases of alloimmune thrombocytopenia are caused by maternal antibodies to the human platelet antigen-1a (HPA-1a). The HPA-1a antigen is caused by the presence of a leucine residue (rather than proline) at position 33 on the β subunit of the fibrinogen receptor (also called glycoprotein IIb/IIIa or CD41/61). In common with the alloimmune response to red cells, maternal anti-HPA antibodies are predominantly IgG1.[20,21]

The pathogenesis of alloimmune thrombocytopenia differs from that of HDFN in that maternal sensitization to fetal platelet antigens often occurs in a first pregnancy, indicating that platelet antigens may be more immunogenic than red cell antigens.[22] For example, transplacental passage of fetal glycoprotein IIIa may occur as early as week 14 of gestation.[23] Moreover, glycoprotein IIIa is found on syncytiotrophoblasts of the placental brush border.[24] Although glycoprotein IIIa is a type I transmembrane protein, its release into the maternal circulation might occur as the cells undergo apoptosis, perhaps during invasion of the endometrium.

The immune response to HPA-1a is under genetic control. Although only 5–10% of HPA-1a-negative women with HPA-1a-positive fetuses produce anti-HPA-1a (Section 4.2.1), the presence of the HLA-DRB3*0101 allele increases the risk of alloimmunization by a factor of 140.[25] Interestingly, the immune response to HPA-1b does not appear to be HLA restricted.[26] This implies that antigen-presenting cells require HLA-DRB3*0101 to present HPA-1a-derived peptides and that leucine at position 33 is involved in peptide binding in the HLA class II groove. This has been substantiated using an in vitro peptide-binding assay to show that leucine does indeed anchor the peptide to the HLA-DRB3*0101 molecule.[27] The proline form did not bind to the HLA-DRB3*0101 molecule which explains the rarity with which anti-HPA-1b antibodies are formed. The alloimmune response to another clinically important platelet antigen, HPA-5b, is also under genetic control.[28]

1.1.4 The maternal alloimmune response to fetal neutrophils

There is a paucity of data on the nature of the maternal immune response to fetal neutrophils. It is well established that immunization may occur in first pregnancies so presumably fetal neutrophils can enter the maternal circulation during normal gestation.[29] The antibodies produced recognize granulocyte-specific antigens expressed on Fcγ receptor III (CD16), the complement receptor 3 (CD11b/CD18) and other, as yet unidentified, glycoproteins.[30,31] Granulocyte antigens are fully expressed at birth and are discussed in detail later (Section 13.3.2).[32]

1.2 Transfer of IgG to the fetus

The second critical step in the pathogenesis of the alloimmune cytopenias is the active transfer of IgG alloantibodies from the mother to the fetus. All four subclasses are actively transferred into the fetus via syncytiotrophoblast cells which express receptors for the Fc domain of IgG.[33,34] These receptors are termed FcRn (Fc receptor neonatal) because they were first demonstrated in neonatal rodents where they transport IgG across the gut. Transfer of IgG across the placenta is slow until around week 24 and so HDFN before this time is rare. The rate of transfer increases exponentially during the second half of gestation until term when IgG levels in the fetus (approximately 15 g/dl) tend to exceed those in the mother (approximately 13 g/dl).[35]

There is great variation between individual pregnancies. The rate of transport may be a major factor determining the severity of cytopenia in the fetus; in HDFN, it may be the rate-limiting step in the reaction between fetal red cells and maternal anti-D.[36,37] There is some evidence that IgG1 is overrepresented in the fetal circulation early in gestation.[38] Also, IgG with relatively high levels of galactose is relatively abundant in the fetal circulation.[39] These forms of IgG may either be transported preferentially or catabolized relatively slowly in the fetus.

Recent studies have elucidated the molecular basis of IgG transport. The key to the process is the ability of FcRn to bind IgG with relatively high affinity at an acidic pH but with negligible affinity at the pH of blood (pH 7.4).[40] The FcRn molecule consists of an α chain which is homologous to HLA class-I molecules associated with β-2-microglobulin. The first step in the process is the nonspecific fluid-phase pinocytosis of IgG (like other plasma proteins) by the syncytiotrophoblasts. The IgG is then trafficked to apical vesicles where the acid pH causes it to bind to FcRn lining the vesicles. FcRn recognizes certain amino acids (isoleucine 253, histidine 310, histidine 435) at the interface between the C_H2 and C_H3 domains of IgG.[41] Each IgG molecule has two heavy chains and may, therefore, bind two FcRn molecules. In this way, IgG binding results in FcRn dimerization which appears to be crucial for IgG trafficking. Bound IgG is then transported across the cells within the vesicles which eventually fuse with the basal cell membrane. This exposes the vesicle contents to neutral pH causing the IgG to dissociate from the FcRn and enter the fetal circulation.

1.3 The immune destruction of blood cells in the fetus

There are very few studies on the action of red cell or platelet antibodies in the fetus. The processes involved in the immune destruction of red cells and platelets have therefore been inferred from observations made in adults and from in vitro experiments. As a result of these studies, it is generally accepted that IgG alloantibodies opsonise blood cells causing their recognition by macrophages which express receptors for the Fc portion of IgG (usually abbreviated FcγR, where γ denotes specificity of the receptor [R] for IgG). Sensitized blood cells may then be destroyed by macrophages via a process termed extravascular lysis.

1.3.1 IgG and Fcγ receptors

The structure and function of IgG has been reviewed extensively[42] and will be discussed only briefly here. IgG molecules are symmetrical, with two identical Fab fragments joined to one Fc fragment via a hinge region. The Fc fragment is comprised of two C_H2 domains and two C_H3 domains. Critical amino acid residues within the Fc region are responsible for interactions with Fcγ receptors on effector cells such as monocytes and macrophages.[42] Four subclasses of IgG have been identified (IgG1, IgG2, IgG3 and IgG4). The subclasses show significant differences in the hinge region length which comprises of 5, 12, 62 and 12 amino acids in IgG1, IgG2, IgG3 and IgG4, respectively. The structure of the hinge region affects the flexibility of IgG. This flexibility, together with other subclass-related differences in amino acids at key positions within the Fc region, determines the relative ability of the IgG subclasses to interact with Fcγ receptors.

Effector cells such as monocytes and macrophages express different receptors for the Fc region of IgG. The structure and function of different Fcγ receptors have been reviewed in detail elsewhere.[43,44] Macrophages express three classes of receptor for the Fc portion of IgG (Fcγ receptor I, Fcγ receptor IIa and Fcγ receptor IIIa). Fcγ receptor I binds human IgG with high affinity. Fcγ receptor IIa has low affinity for human IgG1 and IgG3. Fcγ receptor IIIa has an 'intermediate' affinity for IgG. The function of these Fcγ receptors in relation to red cell and platelet destruction is considered in more detail below.

1.3.2 The immune destruction of fetal red cells

Despite a wealth of in vitro data, it is unclear which of the Fcγ receptors are involved in the immune destruction of sensitized cells. In vitro, in the absence of fluid-phase IgG, Fcγ receptor I mediates the interaction between monocytes or macrophages and IgG anti-D-sensitized red cells.[45] However, a role for Fcγ receptor I in vivo seems unlikely because interactions between anti-D-sensitized red cells and this high affinity receptor are blocked by IgG concentrations several orders of magnitude lower than those found in plasma. Fcγ receptor IIa has a very low affinity for IgG1 and IgG3 and seems unlikely to play a role in the destruction of red cells sensitized with these subclasses.

There is indirect evidence that Fcγ receptor IIIa might play a role in the recognition of IgG-sensitized red cells in vivo. The administration of monoclonal antibodies to Fcγ receptor III increased the lifespan of IgG-sensitized red cells in chimpanzees and caused an increase in the number of circulating platelets in patients with autoimmune thrombocytopenia.[46,47] The adherence of anti-D-sensitized red cells to adult splenic macrophages in cryostat sections is mediated, at least in part, by Fcγ receptor IIIa.[48]

Although the molecular basis for the in utero destruction of IgG-sensitized red

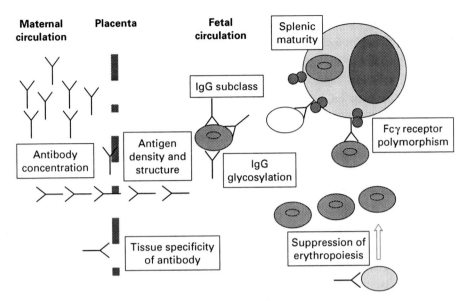

Figure 1.2   Some of the factors which determine the severity of haemolytic disease in the fetus.

cells remains to be fully elucidated, there is evidence to suggest that several factors may influence the extent of red cell destruction and, hence, disease severity. These are shown diagrammatically in Figure 1.2 and are considered below.

1.3.2.1 IgG glycosylation

IgG molecules contain a carbohydrate moiety within the C_H2 domains. The carbohydrate helps to stabilize the tertiary structure of the molecule and is required for IgG to bind to Fcγ receptors. The carbohydrate is heterogeneous and IgG from different individuals may contain different amounts of galactose. In vitro, the amount of incorporated galactose may affect antibody function. For example, monoclonal anti-D secreted under conditions which favour the incorporation of relatively high levels of galactose is more efficient at promoting lymphocyte-mediated lysis of red cells.[49] The relevance of these observations to the pathogenesis of HDFN is not yet established. Nevertheless, IgG galactose levels increase during pregnancy and it has been shown that anti-D in sera from pregnant women promotes lymphocyte-mediated haemolysis with greater efficiency than anti-D in sera from males.[50,51]

1.3.2.2 IgG subclass

Sera from approximately one-third of women with anti-D contain only IgG1 anti-D while sera from most of the remainder contain a mixture of IgG1 and IgG3 anti-D.[52] In vitro experiments using human monoclonal anti-D have shown that the

phagocytosis and lysis of red cells by monocytes are promoted with greater efficiency by IgG3 anti-D than by IgG1 anti-D.[45] The longer hinge region of IgG3 may
confer to the molecule the ability to span the gap between negatively charged red
cells and monocytes with greater efficiency than IgG1. Although an association
between IgG subclass and the extent of haemolysis in utero might be expected,
studies using predominantly serological techniques have generated conflicting
results. Some studies have failed to demonstrate any relationship,[53–55] while others
have reported an association between severe HDFN and IgG1 anti-D alone [56,57] or
the presence of both IgG1 and IgG3.[52,58] The application of quantitative techniques
should resolve these inconsistent results.

1.3.2.3 Antibody concentration

Once immunized, the concentration of antibodies in the mother influences the
severity of haemolysis in the fetus; the concentration of anti-D in the fetal circulation reflects the concentration of anti-D in the maternal circulation.[59] The extent
to which the antibody level determines disease severity and the ability of different
assays to measure antibody concentration are considered in detail elsewhere
(Section 8.3).

1.3.2.4 Antibody specificity

IgG antibodies to most red cell antigens have been reported to cause HDFN. The
relationship between antibody specificity and clinical significance is reviewed in
Chapter 2. However, it is possible to establish criteria which govern the potential of
blood group antibodies to cause haemolysis in utero and these will be discussed
briefly here. First, antibodies with the potential to cause haemolysis in utero recognize antigens which are restricted to the erythroid lineage; antibodies to antigens
with a wider tissue distribution are absorbed by other fetal tissues and hence fail to
localize on fetal red cells. The maturational specificity of blood group antigens may
also affect the pathogenesis of HDFN. Thus, antibodies to antigens of the Kell
system, which are expressed at an early stage of erythroid development, may cause
anaemia by suppressing erythropoiesis or by promoting the immune destruction
of erythroid precursor cells.[60,61] The second criterion is antigen density. Some antigens (for example, Rh antigens) are well expressed early in embryonic development. Other antigens (for example, Lutheran antigens) are poorly expressed on
fetal cells. Antibodies to antigens which are expressed at low density on fetal red
cells are unlikely to cause HDFN.[62] A third criterion may be antigen structure. As
a general rule, antibodies to antigens which are relatively distant from the lipid
bilayer more efficiently promote the recognition of red cells by monocytes.[63] Thus,
IgG anti-K is more effective at promoting the adherence, phagocytosis and lysis of
red cells than IgG anti-D.[54] IgG2 anti-A promotes Fcγ receptor IIa-mediated rec-

ognition of red cells by monocytes whereas IgG2 anti-D does not.[64] However, the implications of these in vitro observations for the pathogenesis of HDFN remain to be elucidated.

1.3.2.5 Antigen density

There is evidence that the density of blood group antigens on fetal red cells may affect the severity of haemolysis. Thus, a D^u-positive fetus (with relatively few D antigens) may have mild HDFN despite the presence of high concentrations of anti-D in the maternal circulation.[65] Moreover, the severity of HDFN due to anti-A or anti-B is partly determined by the number of A or B antigens on the fetal red cells.[66]

1.3.2.6 Function of the fetal spleen

Extravascular haemolysis requires a competent system of phagocytic cells in the fetus. These cells develop at an early gestational age and the presence of macrophages has been demonstrated at 13 weeks' gestation.[67] There are few data on the functional activity of splenic macrophages in the fetus although expression of Fcγ receptors by fetal and neonatal (cord) monocytes is slightly lower than in the adult.[68,69] Nevertheless, fetal macrophages are probably competent to destroy IgG-sensitized red cells by 22–24 weeks' gestation when significant levels of IgG are transported across the placenta.

1.3.2.7 FcγR polymorphisms

Genes encoding several of the Fcγ receptors are polymorphic and these may affect the ability of the receptors to bind IgG. Intuitively then, one might expect these polymorphisms to affect the severity of haemolysis. Seventy per cent of Caucasians express an allotype of Fcγ receptor IIa with an arginine at amino acid position 131 (termed FcγRIIa-R131) rather than a histidine (termed FcγRIIa-H131) and the latter allotype has a relatively high affinity for human IgG2.[70] This might be expected to have implications in the pathogenesis of HDFN due to ABO antibodies which are predominantly IgG2. Indeed, in a relatively small cohort of patients, the Fcγ receptor IIa-H131 allotype was overexpressed in infants with ABO HDFN.[71] This observation awaits further confirmation.

The gene encoding Fcγ receptor IIIa has several polymorphisms. One polymorphism results in the presence of either valine or phenylalanine at amino acid position 158.[72] The gene frequencies are 0.43 and 0.57, respectively. Natural killer cells from individuals who are homozygous for the valine polymorphism bind more monomeric IgG than natural killer cells from individuals who are homozygous for the phenylalanine polymorphism.[73] However, the degree to which this polymorphism influences clinical outcome in HDFN is unknown.

1.3.2.8 Inhibitory antibodies

Occasionally, women with very high levels of anti-D deliver infants with unexpectedly mild HDFN. Sera from the majority of such women contain anti-HLA antibodies which inhibit the interaction between monocytes and anti-D-sensitized red cells.[74,75] It has been proposed that these monocyte-reactive antibodies may cross the placenta and inhibit the destruction of fetal cells by blocking FcγR function on fetal macrophages. The mechanism of inhibition appears to involve the formation of antigen–antibody–FcγR complexes on the macrophage membrane resulting in receptor blockade and inhibition of phagocytosis.[76,77]

1.3.2.9 Fetal gender

Studies into the association between fetal gender and the severity of HDFN have produced conflicting data. Ulm et al. reported that male fetuses were 13 times more likely to develop hydrops than female fetuses, and perinatal mortality was three times higher in male fetuses.[78] In contrast, Ramsey and Sherman did not find that male fetuses were more likely to have severe anaemia.[79]

1.3.3 The immune destruction of fetal platelets

The cellular interactions involved in the alloimmune destruction of platelets in the fetus are less well studied than those involved in red cell destruction. However, studies into autoimmune thrombocytopenia in adults suggest that the mechanism of platelet destruction is analogous to that of red cell destruction in HDFN.

1.3.3.1 Mechanism of antibody-mediated platelet destruction

Early studies showed that autoimmune thrombocytopenia involves the splenic sequestration of platelets in a manner analogous to the extravascular destruction of IgG-sensitized red cells.[80] This suggests that the fetal spleen may be the primary site of platelet destruction in alloimmune thrombocytopenia. There are few data on the effector cells responsible for platelet destruction although peripheral blood monocytes have been shown to respond IgG-sensitized platelets in vitro.[81,82] Data on the role of Fcγ receptors come from both in vivo and in vitro studies. Clarkson et al. showed that administration of a monoclonal antibody to Fcγ receptor III to a patient with autoimmune thrombocytopenia was associated with a rise in platelet count.[47] Studies in transgenic mice have implicated Fcγ receptor IIA in the immune destruction of platelets sensitized with rat IgG2a antiplatelet antibody.[83] However, the extent to which this model reflects platelet destruction in alloimmune thrombocytopenia remains to be established; human IgG1 has a lower affinity for Fcγ receptor IIa than rat IgG2a.

The recognition of sensitized platelets by macrophages probably involves numerous different molecular interactions in that both platelets and macrophages express molecules which mediate their adhesion.[84,85] The initial mediator of this association is P-selectin (CD62P) which is expressed in increased amounts on platelets after activation.[86,87] Ligation of P-selectin by P-selectin glycoprotein ligand-1 on leukocytes results in platelet/leukocyte adhesion.[88] This 'tethering' allows secondary, integrin-mediated adhesion to occur. P-selectin also promotes the secretion by leukocytes of inflammatory cytokines which may, in turn, increase the expression of Fcγ receptors and other adhesion molecules.[89–91]

A role for complement as a mediator of thrombocytopenia has been suggested by experiments using sera containing anti-HPA-1a from patients with posttransfusion purpura. At high concentrations, these antibodies may bind C1q and activate the classical complement cascade resulting in lysis. However, at lower concentrations, they may activate platelets causing the release of serotonin from platelet α granules.[92,93] Increased platelet-bound C3 has also been observed in patients with autoimmune thrombocytopenia.[94] Complement might, therefore, participate in platelet destruction in alloimmune thrombocytopenia by causing cell lysis or by enhancing the recognition of platelets by splenic macrophages via the deposition of C3 fragments or the expression of cell adhesion molecules. However, studies in complement-deficient mice have also shown that thrombocytopenia can develop in the absence of complement proteins.[83] Further studies are required to elucidate the relative importance of these processes in platelet destruction.

In addition to causing the immune destruction of platelets, anti-HPA-1a antibodies from some cases of alloimmune thrombocytopenia are able to inhibit fibrinogen binding to glycoprotein IIb/IIIa; the HPA-1a polymorphism is located near to the 'RGD-binding region' of glycoprotein IIb/IIIa.[95] However, the ability of sera from patients with alloimmune thrombocytopenia to inhibit fibrinogen binding is probably exceptional and is unlikely to be a major risk factor for fetal haemorrhage.[96]

1.3.3.2 Antigen density

The severity of thrombocytopenia may be dependent on antigen density in a manner analogous to red cell destruction. The glycoprotein most densely represented on the platelet membrane is glycoprotein IIb/IIIa, each allelic form being present at approximately 40000 copies per platelet in a heterozygote (Section 12.2.1).[22] Antibodies to antigens expressed on glycoprotein IIb/IIIa, such as HPA-1a, HPA-1b and HPA-3b, have all been associated with severe thrombocytopenia. In contrast, severe thrombocytopenia leading to intracerebral haemorrhage due to anti-HPA-5b is less common and this antigen is expressed in glycoprotein Ia/IIb, which is present at approximately 1500 copies per platelet.[22]

1.3.4 The immune destruction of fetal neutrophils

Several indirect lines of evidence suggest that neutrophil destruction is mediated by macrophages in the fetal spleen; macrophages containing ingested neutrophils have been isolated from the spleens of patients with autoimmune neutropenia and ^{111}In-labelled neutrophils are sequestered in the spleens of patients with circulating antineutrophil antibodies.[97,98] In vitro, neutrophils sensitized with antibodies from women whose infants had alloimmune neutropenia elicit an Fcγ receptor I-mediated metabolic response from human monocytes.[99]

1.4 Conclusions

The alloimmune cytopenias are complex disorders in which the pathophysiology remains to be fully characterized. This is due in part to the inherent difficulty in studying disease processes in the fetus. Nevertheless, future diagnostic and therapeutic advances depend on an improved understanding of the molecular basis of the maternal alloimmune response and the processes involved in the immune destruction of blood cells in the fetus. Progress in these areas should lead to the development of new strategies to modulate maternal immune responses and specifically suppress the destruction of fetal cells. Transgenic animal technology may provide one important means of establishing improved models with which to study these processes and evaluate the potential of new therapies.

1.5 References

1 Roitt I, Brostoff J & Male D (1998). *Immunology*, 5th edn. London: Mosby, pp. 139–53.

2 Hall AM, Stott LM, Vickers MA, Urbaniak SJ & Barker RN (1999). The alloreactive and autoreactive T helper cytokine responses to the RhD protein differ. *Transfusion Medicine*, **9** (suppl 1), 17.

3 Elson CJ & Bradley J (1971). The immunocytoadherence of Rh(D) positive erythrocytes to mononucleated cells from the peripheral blood of Rhesus isoimmunised individuals. *International Archives of Allergy and Applied Immunology*, **40**, 382–97.

4 Stott LM, Hall AM, Wilson DWL, Barker RN & Urbaniak SJ (1999). Helper T cell epitopes on the RhD protein – towards a peptide vaccine for prevention of Rh disease. *Transfusion Medicine*, **9** (suppl 1), 54.

5 Medearis AL, Hensleigh PA, Parks DR & Herzenberg LA (1984). Detection of fetal erythrocytes in maternal blood postpartum with the fluorescence-activated cell sorter. *American Journal of Obsterics and Gynecology*, **148**, 290–5.

6 Mollison PL, Engelfriet CP & Contreras M (1997). *Blood Transfusion in Clinical Medicine*, 9th edn. Oxford: Blackwell Scientific Publications, pp. 390–424.

7 Woodrow JC & Finn R (1966). Transplacental haemorrhage. *British Journal of Haematology*, **12**, 297–307.

8 Bowman JM (1988). The prevention of Rh immunisation. *Transfusion Medicine Reviews*, 2, 129–50.

9 Woodrow JC (1970). Rh immunization and its prevention. *Series Haematologica*, 3, 1–151.

10 Queenan JT (1982). Amniocentesis and isoimmunization. In *Rh Hemolytic Disease. New Strategy for Eradication*, eds. FD Frigoletto, JF Jewette & AA Kongugres. Boston, MA: Hall Medical, pp. 125–34.

11 Grant CJ, Hamblin TJ, Smith DS & Wellstead L (1983). Plasmapheresis in Rh hemolytic disease, the danger of amniocentesis. *International Journal of Artificial Organs*, 6, 83–6.

12 Viëtor HE, Kanhai HHH & Brand A (1994). Induction of additional red cell alloantibodies after intrauterine transfusions. *Transfusion*, 34, 970–4.

13 Murray S (1957). The effect of Rh genotypes on severity in haemolytic disease of the newborn. *British Journal of Haematology*, 3, 143–52.

14 Rochna E & Hughes-Jones NC (1965). The use of purified ^{125}I-labelled anti-γ globulin in the determination of the number of D antigen sites on red cells of different phenotypes. *Vox Sanguinis*, 10, 675–86.

15 Levine P (1943). Serological factors as possible causes in spontaneous abortions. *Journal of Heredity*, 34, 71–80.

16 Murray S, Knox EG & Walker W (1965). Rhesus haemolytic disease of the newborn and the ABO groups. *Vox Sanguinis*, 10, 6–31.

17 Hilden JO, Gottvall T & Lindblom B (1995). HLA phenotypes and severe Rh(D) immunization. *Tissue Antigens*, 46, 3131–315.

18 Renkonen KO & Seppälä M (1962). The sex of the sensitizing Rh-positive child. *Annals of Medicine*, 40, 108–18.

19 Renkonen KO & Timonen S (1967). Factors influencing the immunization of Rh-negative mothers. *Journal of Medical Genetics*, 4, 166–76.

20 Proulx C, Filion M, Goldman M et al. (1994). Analysis of immunoglobulin class, IgG subclass and titre of HPA-1a antibodies in alloimmunized mothers giving birth to babies with or without neonatal alloimmune thrombocytopenia. *British Journal of Haematology*, 87, 813–17.

21 Mawas F, Wiener E, Williamson LM & Rodeck CH (1997). Immunoglobulin G subclasses of anti-human platelet antigen 1a in maternal sera: relation to the severity of neonatal alloimmune thrombocytopenia. *European Journal of Haematology*, 59, 287–92.

22 Newman PJ, McFarland JG & Aster RS (1998). The alloimmune thrombocytopenias. In *Thrombosis and Hemorrhage*, eds. J Loscalzo & AI Schafer. Baltimore, MD: Williams and Wilkins.

23 Morales WJ & Stroup M (1985). Intracranial hemorrhage in utero due to isoimmune neonatal thrombocytopenia. *Obstetrics and Gynecology*, 65, 20S.

24 Vanderpuye OA, Labarrere CA & McIntyre JA (1991). A vitronectin-receptor-related molecule in human placental brush border membranes. *Biochemistry Journal*, 280, 9–17.

25 Williamson LM, Hackett G, Rennie J et al. (1998). The natural history of fetomaternal alloimmunization to the platelet-specific antigen HPA-1a (PL^{A1}, Zw^{a}) as determined by antenatal screening. *Blood*, 92, 2280–7.

26 Kuijpers RWAM, von dem Borne AEG, Kiefel V et al. (1992). Leucine[33]-proline[33] substitution in human platelet glycoprotein IIIa determines HLA-DR52a (Dw24) association of the immune response against HPA-1a (Zw^a/Pl^{A1}) and HPA-1b (Zw^b/Pl^{A2}). *Human Immunology*, 34, 253–356.

27 Wu S, Maslanka K & Gorski J (1997). An integrin polymorphism that defines reactivity with alloantibodies generates an anchor for MHC class II peptide binding: a model for unidirectional alloimmune responses. *Journal of Immunology*, 158, 3221–6.

28 Semana G, Zazoun T, Alizadeh M, Morel Kopp MC, Genetet B & Kaplan C (1996). Genetic susceptibility and anti-human platelet antigen 5b alloimmunization: role of HLA class II and TAP genes. *Human Immunology*, 46, 114–19.

29 Lalezari P & Radel E (1974). Neutrophil-specific antigens, immunology and clinical significance. *Seminars in Hematology*, 11, 281–90.

30 Huizinga TWJ, Kleijer M, Tetteroo PAT, Roos D & von dem Borne AEG Kr (1990). Biallelic neutrophil NA-antigen system is associated with a polymorphism on the phospho-inositol-linked Fcγ receptor III (CD16). *Blood*, 75, 213–17.

31 Bux J (1999). Nomenclature of granulocyte alloantigens. *Transfusion*, 39, 662–3.

32 Madyastha PR, Glassman AB & Levine DH (1984). Incidence of neutrophil antigens on human cord neutrophils. *American Journal of Reproductive Immunology*, 6, 124–7.

33 Morell A, Skvaril F, van Loghem E & Kleemola M (1971). Human IgG subclasses in maternal and fetal serum. *Vox Sanguinis*, 21, 481–92.

34 Story CM, Mikulska JE & Simister NE (1994). A major histocompatibility complex class I-like Fc receptor cloned from human placenta: possible role in transfer of immunoglobulin G from mother to fetus. *Journal of Experimental Medicine*, 180, 2377–81.

35 Kohler PF & Farr RS (1966). Elevation of cord over maternal IgG immunoglobulin: evidence for an active placental IgG transport. *Nature*, 210, 1070–1.

36 Hughes-Jones NC, Ivona M, Ellis J & Walker W (1971). Anti-D concentration in mother and child in haemolytic disease of the newborn. *Vox Sanguinis*, 21, 135–40.

37 Dooren MC & Engelfriet CP (1993). Protection against RhD-haemolytic disease of the newborn by a diminished transport of maternal IgG to the fetus. *Vox Sanguinis*, 65, 59–61.

38 Lubenko A, Contreras M & Rodeck CH (1994). Transplacental IgG subclass concentrations in pregnancies at risk of haemolytic disease of the newborn. *Vox Sanguinis*, 67, 291–8.

39 Williams PJ, Arkwright PD, Rudd P et al. (1995). Selective placental transport of maternal IgG to the fetus. *Placenta*, 16, 749–56.

40 Ghetie V & Ward ES (1997). FcRn, the MHC class I-related receptor that is more than an IgG transporter. *Immunology Today*, 18, 592–8.

41 Kim J-K, Firan M, Radu CG, Kim C-H, Ghetie V & Ward ES (1999). Mapping the site on human IgG for binding of the MHC class I-related receptor, FcRn. *European Journal of Immunology*, 29, 2819–25

42 Jefferis R, Lund J & Pound JD (1998). IgG-Fc-mediated effector functions, molecular definition of interaction sites for effector ligands and the role of glycosylation. *Immunological Reviews*, 163, 59–76.

43 Hulett MD & Hogarth PM (1994). Molecular basis of Fc receptor function. *Advances in Immunology*, 57, 1–127.

44 Deo YM, Graziano RF, Repp R & van de Winkel JGJ (1997). Clinical significance of IgG Fc receptors and FcγR-directed immunotherapies. *Immunology Today*, **18**, 127–35.

45 Kumpel BM & Hadley AG (1990). Functional interactions of red cells sensitised by IgG1 and IgG3 human monoclonal anti-D with enzyme-modified human monocytes and FcR-bearing cell lines. *Molecular Immunology*, **27**, 247–56.

46 Clarkson SB, Kimberley RP, Valinsky JE et al. (1986). Blockade of clearance of immune complexes by an anti-FcR monoclonal antibody. *Journal of Experimental Medicine*, **164**, 474–89.

47 Clarkson SB, Bussel JB, Kimberley RP, Valinsky JE, Nachman RL & Unkeless JC (1986). Treatment of refractory immune thrombocytopenic purpura with an anti-Fcγ-receptor antibody. *New England Journal of Medicine*, **314**, 1236–9.

48 Davenport RD & Kunkel SL (1994). IgG receptor roles in red cell binding to monocytes and macrophages. *Transfusion*, **34**, 79S.

49 Kumpel BM, Rademacher TW, Rook GAW, Williams PJ & Wilson IBH (1994). Galactosylation of human IgG monoclonal anti-D produced by EBV-transformed B-lymphoblastoid lines is dependent on culture method and affects Fcγ receptor-mediated functional activity. *Human Antibodies and Hybridomas*, **5**, 143–51.

50 Rook GAW, Steele J, Brealey R et al. (1991). Changes in IgG glycoform levels are associated with remission of arthritis during pregnancy. *Journal of Autoimmunity*, **4**, 779–89.

51 Urbaniak SJ & Greiss MA (1980). ADCC (K-cell) lysis of human erythrocytes sensitized with Rhesus alloantibodies. III. Comparison of IgG anti-D agglutinating and lytic (ADCC) activity and the role of IgG subclasses. *British Journal of Haematology*, **46**, 447–53.

52 Pollock JM & Bowman JM (1990). Anti-Rh(D) IgG subclasses and severity of Rh hemolytic disease of the newborn. *Vox Sanguinis*, **59**, 176–9.

53 Taslimi MM, Sibai BM, Mason JM & Dacus JV (1986). Immunoglobulin G subclasses and iso-immunized pregnancy outcome. *American Journal of Obstetrics and Gynecology*, **154**, 1327–32.

54 Hadley AG, Kumpel BM, Leader KA, Poole GD & Fraser ID (1991). Correlation of serological, quantitative and cell-mediated functional assays of maternal alloantibodies with the severity of haemolytic disease of the newborn. *British Journal of Haematology*, **77**, 221–8.

55 Garner SF, Weiner E, Contreras M et al. (1992). Mononuclear phagocyte assays, AutoAnalyzer quantitation and IgG subclasses of maternal anti-RhD in the prediction of the severity of haemolytic disease in the fetus before 32 weeks gestation. *British Journal of Haematology*, **80**, 97–101.

56 Parinaud J, Blanc M, Grandjean H et al. (1985). IgG subclasses and Gm allotypes of anti-D antibodies during pregnancy: correlation with the gravity of fetal diease. *American Journal of Obstetrics and Gynecology*, **151**, 1111–15.

57 Nance SJ, Arndt PA & Garratty G (1990). Correlation of IgG subclass with the severity of hemolytic disease of the newborn. *Transfusion*, **30**, 381–2.

58 Zupanska B, Brojer E, Richards Y, Lenkiewics B, Seyfried H & Howell P (1989). Serological and immunological characteristics of maternal anti-Rh(D) antibodies in predicting the severity of haemolytic disease of the newborn. *Vox Sanguinis*, **56**, 247–53.

59 Economides DL, Bowell PJ, Selinger M, Pratt GA & MacKenzie IZ (1993). Anti-D concentrations in fetal and maternal serum and amniotic fluid in rhesus allo-immunised pregnancies. *British Journal of Obstetrics and Gynaecology*, **100**, 923–6.

60 Vaughan JL, Warwick R, Letsky E, Nicoloni U, Rodeck CH & Fisk NM (1994). Erythropoietic suppression in fetal anaemia because of Kell alloimmunization. *American Journal of Obstetrics and Gynecology*, **171**, 247–52.

61 Daniels GL, Hadley AG & Green CA (1999). Fetal anaemia due to anti-K may result from immune destruction of early erythroid progenitors. *Transfusion Medicine*, **9** (suppl 1), 16.

62 Novotny VMJ, Kanhai HHH, Overbeeke MAM, Schlamam-Nijp A, Harvey MS & Brand A (1992). Misleading results in the determination of haemolytic disease of the newborn using antibody titration and ADCC in a woman with anti-Lu^b. *Vox Sanguinis*, **62**, 49–52.

63 Skidmore I & Hadley AG (1996). The effect of specificity on the functional activity of red cell-bound blood group antibodies. *Transfusion Medicine*, **6** (suppl 2), 26.

64 Kumpel BM, van der Winkel JGJ, Westerdaal NAC, Hadley AG & Dugoujon JM (1996). Antigen topography is critical for interaction of IgG2 anti-red-cell antibodies with Fcγ receptors. *British Journal of Haematology*, **94**, 175–83.

65 Dias R, Finney RD, Humphreys D & Graham L (1986). Rhesus D^u incompatibility in a newborn with high levels of anti-D and a benign clinical course. *Vox Sanguinis*, **50**, 52–3.

66 Brouwers HA, Overbeeke MA, Ouwehand WH et al. (1988). Maternal antibodies against fetal blood group antigens A or B, lytic activity of IgG subclasses in monocyte-driven cytotoxicity and correlation with ABO haemolytic disease of the newborn. *British Journal of Haematology*, **70**, 465–9.

67 Billington WD (1992). The normal fetomaternal immune relationship. *Bailliere's Clinics in Obstetrics and Gynaecology*, **6**, 417–38.

68 Mawas F, Wiener E, Ryan G, Soothill PW & Rodeck CH (1994). The expression of IgG Fc receptors on circulating leucocytes in the fetus and new-born. *Transfusion Medicine*, **4**, 25–33.

69 Murphy FJ & Reen DJ (1996). Differential expression of function-related antigens on newborn and adult monocyte subpopulations. *Immunology*, **89**, 587–91.

70 Warmerdam PAM, van der Winkel JGJ, Gosselin EJ & Capel PJA (1990). Molecular basis for a polymorphism of human FcγRII (CD32). *Journal of Experimental Medicine*, **172**, 19–25.

71 Denomme G, Ryan G & Fernandes B (1997). The FcγRIIa-His^{131} allotype is overexpressed in infants with ABO hemolytic disease of the newborn. *Blood*, **90**, 472–3a.

72 Ravetch JV & Perussia B (1989). Alternative membrane forms of FcγRIII (CD16) on human NK cells and neutrophils, cell-type specific expression of two genes which differ in single nucleotide substitutions. *Journal of Experimental Medicine*, **170**, 481–91.

73 Koene HR, Kleijer M, Algra J, Roos D, von dem Borne AEG Kr & de Haas M (1997). FcγRIIIa-158V/F polymorphism influences the binding of IgG by natural killer cell FcγRIIIa, independently of the FcγRIIIa-48L/R/H phenotype. *Blood*, **90**, 1109–14.

74 Dooren MC, Kuijpers RWAM, Joekes EC et al. (1992). Protection against immune haemolytic disease of newborn infants by maternal monocyte-reactive IgG alloantibodies (anti-HLA-DR). *Lancet*, **339**, 1067–70.

75 Shepard SL, Noble AL, Filbey D & Hadley AG (1996). Inhibition of the monocyte chemi-

luminescent response to anti-D sensitized red cells by Fcγ receptor I-blocking antibodies which ameliorate the severity of haemolytic disease of the newborn. *Vox Sanguinis*, **70**, 157–63.

76 Kurlander RJ (1983). Blockade of Fc receptor-mediated binding to U-937 cells by murine monoclonal antibodies directed against a variety of surface antigens. *Journal of Immunology*, **131**, 140–7.

77 Shepard SL & Hadley AG (1997). Monocyte-bound monoclonal antibodies inhibit the FcγRI-mediated phagocytosis of red cells: the efficiency and mechanism of inhibition are determined by the nature of the antigen. *Immunology*, **90**, 314–22.

78 Ulm B, Svolba G, Ulm MR, Bernaschek G & Panzer S (1999). Male fetuses are particularly affected by maternal alloimmunization to D antigen. *Transfusion*, **39**, 169–73.

79 Ramsey G & Sherman LA (1999). Anti-D in pregnancy: value of antibody titres and effect of fetal gender. *Transfusion*, **39**, 105S.

80 McMillan R, Longmire RL, Tavassoli M, Armstrong S & Yelenosky BS (1974). In vitro platelet phagocytosis by splenic leukocytes in idiopathic thrombocytopenic purpura. *New England Journal of Medicine*, **290**, 249–51.

81 Court WS, Christensen AK, Sacks RW & LoBuglio AF (1984). Human monocyte interaction with antibody coated platelets. *American Journal of Hematology*, **17**, 225–36.

82 Lucas GF, Hadley AG & Holburn AM (1987). Anti-platelet opsonic activity in alloimmune and autoimmune thrombocytopenia. *Clinical Laboratory Haematology*, **9**, 59–66.

83 McKenzie SE, Taylor SM, Malladi P et al. (1999). The role of the human Fc receptor FcγRIIA in the immune clearance of platelets: a transgenic mouse model. *Journal of Immunology*, **162**, 4311–18.

84 Jungi TW, Spycher MO, Nydegger UE & Barandun S (1986). Platelet leukocyte interaction: selective binding of thrombin stimulated platelets to human monocytes, polymorphonuclear leukocytes and related cell lines. *Blood*, **67**, 629–36.

85 Rinder HM, Bonan JL, Rinder CS, Ault KA & Smith BR (1991). Dynamics of leukocyte platelet adhesion in whole blood. *Blood*, **78**, 1730–7.

86 de Bruijne-Admiraal LG, Modderman PW, von dem Borne AEG Kr & Sonnenberg A (1992). P-selectin mediates Ca^{2+}-dependent adhesion of activated platelets to many differentiated types of leukocytes: detection by flow cytometry. *Blood*, **80**, 134–42.

87 Kirchhofer D, Riederer MA & Baumgartner HR (1997). Specific accumulation of circulating monocytes and polymorphonuclear leukocytes on platelet thrombi in a vascular injury model. *Blood*, **89**, 1270–8.

88 Lalor P & Nash GB (1995). Adhesion of flowing leucocytes to immobilised platelets. *British Journal of Haematology*, **89**, 725–32.

89 Lorant DE, McEver RP, McIntyre TM, Moore KL, Prescott SM & Zimmerman GA (1995). Activation of polymorphonuclear leukocytes reduces their adhesion to P selectin and causes redistribution of ligands for P selectin on their surfaces. *Journal of Clinical Investigation*, **96**, 171–82.

90 Weyrich AS, McIntyre TM, McEver RP, Prescott SM & Zimmerman GA (1995). Monocyte tethering by P-selectin regulates monocytes chemotactic protein-1 and tumour necrosis factor-alpha secretion. *Journal of Clinical Investigation*, **95**, 2297–303.

91 Weyrich AS, Elstad MR, McEver RP et al. (1996). Activated platelets signal chemokine synthesis by human monocytes. *Journal of Clinical Investigation*, **97**, 1525–34.

92 Schrieber AD, Cines DB, Zmijewski C & Colman RW (1979). Effect of anti-Pl^{A1} antibody on human platelets. II. Mechanism of the complement-dependent release reaction. *Blood*, **53**, 578–87.

93 Cines DB & Schrieber AD (1979). Effect of anti-Pl^{A1} antibody on human platelets. I. The role of complement. *Blood*, **53**, 567–77.

94 Cines DB, Wilson SB, Tomaski A & Schreiber AD (1985). Platelet antibodies of the IgM class in immune thrombocytopenic purpura. *Journal of Clinical Investigation*, **75**, 1183–90.

95 van Leeuwen EF, Leeksma OC, van Mourik JA, Engelfriet CP & von dem Borne AEG Kr (1984). Effect of the binding of anti-Zw^a antibodies on platelet function. *Vox Sanguinis*, **47**, 280–9.

96 Beadling WV, Herman JH, Stuart MJ, Keashen-Schnell M & Miller JL (1995). Fetal bleeding in neonatal alloimmune thrombocytopenia mediated by anti-Pl^{A1} is not associated with inhibition of fibrinogen binding to platelet GPIIb/IIIa. *American Journal of Clinical Pathology*, **103**, 636–41.

97 Blaschke J, Goeken NE, Thompson JS, Dick FR & Gingrich RD (1979). Acquired agranulocytosis with granulocyte-specific cytotoxic autoantibody. *American Journal of Medicine*, **66**, 862–6.

98 McCullough J, Weiblen BJ, Clay ME & Forstorm L (1981). Effect of leukocyte antibodies on the fate *in vivo* of Indium-111-labelled granulocytes. *Blood*, **58**, 164–70.

99 Hadley AG & Holburn AM (1984). The detection of anti-granulocyte antibodies by chemiluminescence. *Clinical and Laboratory Haematology*, **6**, 351–61.

Blood group antibodies in haemolytic disease of the fetus and newborn

Geoff Daniels

Bristol Institute for Transfusion Sciences, Bristol, UK

2.1 Introduction

Human blood groups were discovered in 1900, but the first suspicion that a woman might be immunized by alloantigens on the red cells of her fetus did not appear until 1939, with the discovery of the Rh D antigen.[1] In 1941, Levine et al. showed that blood groups were responsible for a disease associated with stillbirth, hydrops, jaundice and kernicterus.[2] That disease was named erythroblastosis fetalis, although a more appropriate title is haemolytic disease of the fetus and newborn (HDFN).

HDFN is caused by the immune destruction of fetal red cells or their progenitors, facilitated by maternal antibodies. In order for the mother to produce an alloantibody, her red cells must lack the culpable antigen, which the fetus must have inherited from its father. Red cell antigen polymorphism, therefore, is at the root of HDFN. Over 250 well-established blood group specificities have been identified,[3,4] but only a minority of these have been implicated in clinically severe HDFN.

The severity of HDFN varies enormously. At its most extreme, it culminates in fetal or neonatal death, yet in many publications antibodies have been reported to have caused HDFN when the indications have been no more than a positive direct antiglobulin test result with fetal red cells. In this chapter, HDFN will generally only be considered to have occurred when clinical intervention in excess of phototherapy for jaundice, such as intrauterine or neonatal transfusion, was indicated, or when kernicterus or hydrops was reported. Multifarious red cell antigens will be mentioned in this chapter and it is not possible to refer to the original publications describing all of them. The appropriate references can be found in Daniels[5] and Issitt and Anstee.[6]

2.2 Blood group terminology

During the course of the 20th century, several hundred red cell antigens have been identified. The extended time period over which these antigens were discovered has led to a variety of different terminology styles being introduced. In some cases, single capital letters were used; for example, in the ABO system, the letters A and B represent the two main antigens (and the phenotypes in which only those antigens are present) and O is used for the phenotype resulting from homozygosity of a third allele (*O*), which produces neither A nor B. Another approach has been to use a capital letter to represent one antigen and the same letter, in lower case, to represent its allelic antigen (e.g. K and k of the Kell system, S and s of the MNS system). This could be confusing because it implies a dominant–recessive genetic relationship where none exists. Superscripts following a symbol of two letters have also been used to distinguish allelic antigens – for example, Fy^a and Fy^b, as well as Jk^a and Jk^b. With the discovery of further members of some systems, numerical notations were introduced. In the Lutheran system, for example, one pair of allelic antigens is generally called Lu^a and Lu^b, two other pairs are Lu6 and Lu9, and Lu8 and Lu14, and a fourth pair, whose names were established before they were known to belong to the Lutheran system, is Au^a and Au^b. To make matters worse, some antigens were given different names in different laboratories, based on alternative genetic theories – for example D and Rh$_o$ in the Rh system.

The International Society of Blood Transfusion established an internationally agreed numerical terminology for blood group antigens in which most antigens have been assigned to one of 25 blood group systems (Table 2.1).[3,4] A blood group system consists of one or more antigens controlled by a single gene locus or by a complex of two or more very closely linked homologous genes with virtually no recombination occurring between them. Therefore, each blood group system is genetically discrete from every other system. Some systems consist of only one blood group specificity, but Rh, which is the largest, contains 45 (Table 2.1). Each system has a symbol of between one and four upper case letters (e.g. KEL) and a three-digit number (e.g. 006), and each antigen within the system also has a three-digit number. Thus, every antigen has a unique six-digit number. For example, the third antigen of the Kell system, Kp^a, has the number 006003 and the more commonly used alphanumerical symbol, KEL3. Finally, phenotypes are written in the format KEL:−1,2,−3,4 (where minus before the number represents absence of the antigen). Genes are written in the format *KEL 3* and genotypes are written in the format *KEL 1,2/−1,2.*

Insufficient genetic information makes it currently impossible for some blood group antigens to be allocated either to a system or to cause the establishment of a new system. Some of these have been placed into sets of biochemically or serologically related antigens called collections. For example, two antigens with an apparent allelic relationship, Cs^a and Cs^b, have not been shown to be genetically independent of all the existing blood group systems. They cannot, therefore, form a new system and so are termed COST1 (205001) and COST2 (205002) of the Cost

Table 2.1 Human blood group systems and the likelihood of their antibodies to cause HDFN

Antigen no.	Name	Symbol	No. of antigens	Antibodies responsible for HDFN?
001	ABO	ABO	4	Yes, usually mild
002	MNS	MNS	43	Yes, sometimes severe
003	P	P1	1	No
004	Rh	RH	45	Yes, often severe
005	Lutheran	LU	18	No
006	Kell	KEL	26	Yes, often severe
007	Lewis	LE	3	No
008	Duffy	FY	6	Yes, occasionally severe
009	Kidd	JK	3	Very rarely
010	Diego	DI	19	Yes, often severe
011	Yt	YT	2	No
012	Xg	XG	1	No
013	Scianna	SC	3	No
014	Dombrock	DO	5	No
015	Colton	CO	3	Yes, severe
016	Landsteiner–Wiener	LW	3	No
017	Chido/Rodgers	CH/RG	9	No
018	Hh	H	1	Yes
019	Kx	XK	1	Only found in males
020	Gerbich	GE	7	No
021	Cromer	CROM	10	No
022	Knops	KN	5	No
023	Indian	IN	2	No
024	Ok	OK	1	No (potential not known)
025	Raph	RAPH	1	No (potential not known)

(205) collection. In addition, there is a series of low frequency antigens, which have 700 as their first three digits (e.g. By is 700002), and a series of high frequency antigens, with 901 as their first three digits (e.g. Vel is 901001).

Many people working with blood groups prefer to use a more traditional and familiar notation. For example, nobody requests ABO:−1,−2,−3 blood when they want group O. The International Society of Blood Transfusion does not discourage the use of traditional symbols, but recommends that only those symbols listed in the International Society of Blood Transfusion publications be used.[3,4] For example, D antigen of the Rh system should be called RH1 or D, but *not* rhesus, and K antigen of the Kell system should be called KEL1 or K, but *not* Kell or K1.

2.3 The genetics of blood groups

Blood groups are inherited characters. Antigen expression is usually inherited as a dominant character, whereas an antigen-negative phenotype is inherited as a recessive character. If a woman has produced an alloantibody with the potential to cause HDFN, she must have antigen-negative red cells. This usually occurs because she is homozygous either for an allele that does not produce the antigen or for a deletion of that gene. HDFN may result when a fetus inherits the gene encoding the pertinent blood group antigen from its father. If the father is homozygous for the gene encoding the antigen, then the fetus will be antigen positive, but, if he is heterozygous, there is an evens chance that the fetus will be antigen positive. If the father is antigen negative, then the fetus will be antigen negative and not at risk of HDFN (Figure 2.1). This apparently simple situation may be complicated by alleles producing a weak expression of the antigen. For example, if the mother is Rh D negative and has made anti-D, and if the father is heterozygous for a normal *RHD* gene and for *RHD* that produces weak D (D^u), the father's red cells will express normal D antigen, but one-half of his children will have weak D and so be at much reduced risk from HDFN (Figure 2.1).

Anti-Kx is a haemolytic antibody that can be responsible for haemolytic transfusion reactions, but which is unlikely to cause HDFN because of the mode of inheritance of the Kx antigen. Kx is an antigen of high frequency encoded by a gene on the short arm of the X chromosome. Consequently, the rare Kx-negative phenotype almost always occurs as a result of hemizygosity in males for a mutation of the Kx gene on their single X chromosome. Although the Kx-negative phenotype could occur in a female due to homozygosity for the mutation, this would be exceedingly rare.

Most blood group polymorphisms are the result of one or more nucleotide changes encoding amino acid substitutions in an extracellular domain of a red cell surface protein. In null phenotypes, the whole protein is absent from the membrane, usually as a result of a gene deletion or an inactivating mutation. When immunized, women with null phenotypes may make antibodies to a variety of epitopes on the blood group protein and these antibodies often have the ability to cause HDFN.

Carbohydrate antigens, such as those of the ABO system, provide a further complexity to the genetics of red cell surface antigens. Carbohydrate antigens are not encoded directly by the blood group genes that control their expression. Synthesis of oligosaccharide chains is regulated by transferase enzymes, which catalyse the transfer of monosaccharide residues from a nucleotide donor substrate to an acceptor substrate. These transferase enzymes are encoded by the gene that governs antigen expression.

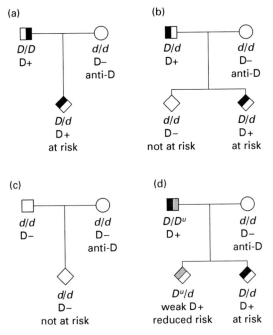

Figure 2.1   Four families demonstrating simple blood group inheritance and its relevance to HDFN, using the Rh D polymorphism as an example. In all four families, the mother has anti-D and so must be homozygous for the D-negative allele, *d*. (a) Father homozygous *D/D*, so all children must be D+ and at risk from HDFN; (b) father heterozygous *D/d*, so half of the children will be D+ and at risk and half will be D− and not at risk; (c) father D− (*d/d*), so all children must be D− and not at risk; and (d) father heterozygous for *D* and a gene for weak D (*Dᵘ*), so all children will be D+, but half will have a weak D and be at reduced risk.

2.4 The effect of antigen expression on the pathogenicity and severity of HDFN

Numerous factors determine whether red cell alloantibodies have the potential to cause HDFN (Section 1.3.2). One important aspect is that the characteristics of particular antigens can determine whether their corresponding antibodies cause HDFN.

Different antigens have very different numbers of molecules on the red cell membrane. Antigens of the ABO and H systems, carbohydrate determinants present on a variety of glycoproteins and glycolipids, are the most abundant, with up to 2×10^6 copies per cell. There are about 10^6 molecules per cell of band 3 (anion exchanger 1), carrying the Diego-system antigens, and of glycophorin A, carrying the MN antigens. The number of antigen sites per cell is substantially less for the other blood groups with $1-2 \times 10^5$ Rh antigen sites and $0.5-2 \times 10^3$ Kell antigen sites per cell.[7] The number of antigens per red cell may be important in influencing whether the antigen is likely to be involved in HDFN, but other factors are more important: ABO, MN and Diego antigens are rarely involved in severe HDFN, whereas the less abundant D and K antigens frequently are.

Some antigens are abundant on the red cells of adults but are present in lower quantity or absent on fetal red cells. One good example is a histo-blood group antigen, I, which is expressed on the internal structure of branched oligosaccharides of red cell glycoproteins and glycolipids. The enzyme responsible for the branching of the oligosaccharides is apparently not active in fetuses and young infants and only linear oligosaccharides are present on their red cells. Occasionally, adults have a rare phenotype in which their red cells lack I and these individuals produce anti-I. Alloanti-I is occasionally active at 37 °C and haemolytic, but cannot cause HDFN due to absence of the corresponding antigen on fetal red cells. Also, reduced antigenic expression on fetal red cells, compared with adult cells, may be one factor responsible for the rare occurrence of severe HDFN caused by ABO antibodies. Other red cell antigens that have substantially reduced expression on fetal red cells compared with those of adults are P1, Lewis, Lutheran, Yt^a, Xg^a, Vel and JMH, and none of these has been involved in severe HDFN.

Many blood group antigens are also present on blood cells other than red cells and in tissues other than blood. This is particularly true of the ubiquitous ABO and H antigens, often called histo-blood group antigens. A and B antigens may also be present on soluble glycoproteins in body fluids. It is likely that any maternal antibody to a histo-blood group antigen crossing the placenta will bind to antigen at numerous locations on the fetus, significantly diluting any haemolytic effect. Similarly, antigens of the Cromer and Lutheran blood group systems are present on placental trophoblast epithelial cells derived from the fetus.[8,9] It is likely that the corresponding antibodies, despite being IgG (predominantly IgG1), are unable to traverse the placenta as they become absorbed by the placenta. Consequently, Lutheran antibodies may appear clinically significant in laboratory functional assays, but do not cause HDFN.[10] Babies of mothers with high-titre antibodies to the high frequency Lutheran antigens Lu^b and Lu6 had the corresponding antigens on their red cells, yet showed no sign of HDFN. Their red cells gave a negative direct antiglobulin test (Section 3.3.1) and no Lutheran antibody was detected in their neonatal sera, suggesting that, despite these antibodies being IgG1, they were unable to cross the placenta.[11] Antigens of the Cromer blood group system are located on a complement-regulatory glycoprotein present on placental trophoblasts (CD55; decay-accelerating factor).[9] Strongly reactive antibodies to Cromer system antigens (Cr^a, Dr^a, WES^b) have become undetectable in the maternal plasma during the second and third trimesters of pregnancy, only to reappear shortly after parturition.[12,13] This phenomenon may result from adsorption of maternal antibodies by the fetally derived placental cells.

Antibodies and antigens of the ABO system are occasionally responsible for HDFN (Section 2.6.1), but incompatibility between fetal A or B antigens and maternal ABO antibodies may also provide some protection against sensitization to the D antigen.[14] The prevalence of anti-D HDFN is reduced where such ABO incompatibility occurs, presumably because enhanced clearance of ABO incompatible D-positive fetal red cells from the maternal blood reduces the frequency of anti-D immunization.

Antigen frequency within a population may also affect the opportunity for an antibody to cause HDFN. If an antigen is rare, it will be an extremely uncommon cause of HDFN, regardless of the haemolytic potential of its corresponding antibody. It is important to remember that absence of any published case of HDFN does not mean that antibodies of a particular rare specificity are incapable of causing HDFN.

2.5 Antibodies that most commonly cause moderate or severe HDFN

2.5.1 Anti-D

Despite the introduction of immunoprophylaxis programmes (Section 6.2) anti-D remains the most common cause of HDFN (Section 6.1.4) in Caucasian populations. Between 12% and 18% of European and North American Caucasian women are D negative, but the incidence of the D-negative phenotype is substantially lower in most other populations. In Africans, 2–5% are D-negative.[15] In Chinese, Japanese and South-East Asians, the D-negative phenotype is rare, often with an incidence of less than three per 1000. A substantial proportion of these women are not truly D negative, but are reported to have very weak D expression (D_{el}) and do not make anti-D.[16,17] Many reviews discussing D frequencies, HDFN due to anti-D and the molecular genetics of Rh address only people of European origin, grossly distorting the world picture.

Antigens of the Rh system are encoded by two closely linked homologous genes, one encoding the D antigen (*RHD*) and the other encoding the CcEe antigens (*RHCE*) (Section 7.3.1). Each gene has a similar genomic organization, consisting of 10 exons of coding sequence. Hydropathy analysis, supported by immunochemical evidence, predicts that the Rh polypeptides cross the red cell membrane 12 times and have internal *N*- and *C*-termini (Figure 2.2). This model provides six extracellular domains which are the putative sites for antibody binding. The extracellular domains consist of between 7 and 22 amino acid residues, with a total of about 80 residues outside the membrane. A maximum of only 10 of these extracellular amino acids differ between the D and CcEe proteins. The Rh proteins are not

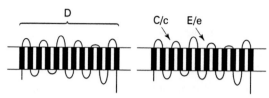

Figure 2.2   Diagrammatic representation of the topology of the RhD and RhCcEe polypeptides in the red cell membrane, showing the 12 membrane-spanning domains, six extracellular loops, and cytoplasmic termini. The RhD polypeptide is absent in D– phenotypes, so D epitopes may be located on any of the extracellular loops. The C/c and E/e polymorphisms represent amino acid substitutions in the second and fourth extracellular loops of the RhCcEe polypeptide, respectively.

glycosylated but are closely associated in the membrane with a glycoprotein, referred to as the Rh-associated glycoprotein, and are probably part of a larger complex of proteins and glycoproteins.[18,19]

The D-negative phenotype results from the absence of the RhD protein from the red cell. In people of European origin, this usually arises from homozygosity for a deletion of the *RHD* gene.[20] In Africans, it usually results from homozygosity for an inactive D gene, the *RHD* pseudogene (*RHDΨ*).[21] The total absence of the RhD protein in the D-negative phenotype explains why no antigen antithetical to D (i.e. 'd') has been found and why D is so immunogenic. The immune system of a D-negative person encountering D-positive red cells is presented with numerous D epitopes on the extracellular regions of the D protein, as opposed to the single amino acid substitution usually associated with a blood group polymorphism.

Although the D-positive/D-negative polymorphism is relatively straightforward, there are numerous complexities involving D antigen expression. In the weak D phenotype (previously called Dᵘ), all epitopes of D are expressed weakly and these individuals do not produce anti-D when transfused with red cells with normal D expression. Weak D red cells are less likely than normal D cells to be responsible for anti-D production and fetuses with weak D are less likely to be severely affected with HDFN.[22] At least some examples of weak D antigens appear to result from amino acid substitutions in the membrane-spanning or intracellular regions of the D protein.[23]

Partial D phenotypes are D-positive phenotypes in which a few or many epitopes of D are not expressed. This loss of epitopes may be due to amino acid substitutions in extracellular domains of the D protein or to the product of hybrid *RHD* genes, in which a segment of the gene is replaced by the homologous segment derived from *RHCE*. When immunized with D-positive red cells, individuals with partial D phenotypes are capable of producing antibodies to those D epitopes absent from their own red cells. Testing of partial D red cells with a profusion of

Table 2.2 Partial D phenotypes

Partial D	LFAs*	Anti-D**
D^{II}		Yes
D^{IIIa}		Yes
D^{IIIb}		Yes
D^{IIIc}		Yes
D^{IVa}	Go^a	Yes
D^{IVb}	Evans	Yes
D^{Va}	D^w	Yes
D^{Vb}		Yes
D^{VI}	BARC	Yes
D^{VII}	Tar	Yes
DFR	FPTT	Yes
DBT	Rh32	Yes
D^{Har}	Rh33, FPTT	Yes
DHMi		Yes
DHMii		No
DNU		No
DHR		Yes
DMH		Yes
DCS		No
DFW		No
DNB		Yes
DAR		Yes
DOL		Yes

Notes:
  * Associated low frequency antigens
 ** Anti-D present in any individual with this phenotype

human monoclonal anti-D has led to the recognition of numerous reaction patterns, often referred to as epitopes. The most recent publication[24] catalogued 37 D epitopes, although the final figure will undoubtedly be higher than this. Over 20 different partial D antigens have been described (Table 2.2), but mostly they are rare. The most common in Caucasians are D^{VI} and D^{VII} and the most common in people of African origin is probably D^{III}.[19,25,26]

Anti-D, when it occurs in women with a partial D antigen, can be responsible for severe HDFN in D-positive fetuses.[5] Adsorption tests have shown that a substantial portion of the anti-D in immunoglobulin preparations does not bind to partial D red cells. It has been asserted that anti-D immunoglobulin should be given to partial D mothers because the anti-D constituent that does not bind to the mother's own cells should be effective in suppressing immunization by the normal D antigen on fetal red cells.[27] This is particularly important in D[VI] mothers, whose red cells lack most D epitopes.

There is little information on the immunogenicity of partial D. A fetus with partial D antigen (D[Va]) stimulated production of anti-D in a D-negative woman as a result of her first pregnancy and this resulted in mild HDFN in her second baby, though the baby also appeared to have the partial D antigen.[28] The mother had received anti-D immunoglobulin after her first pregnancy.

2.5.2 Other antibodies to Rh-system antigens

Rh is the most complex of the human blood group systems, consisting of 45 well-defined antigens. From the phenotyping point of view, the antigens usually considered are D, C, c, E and e.[5] The CcEe determinants, which are located on a separate protein from D, are encoded by *RHCE*, a gene highly homologous to *RHD*. The D and CcEe proteins both consist of 417 amino acids and differ by about 32 residues. The C/c polymorphism is associated with up to four amino acid substitutions, but the defining substitution is in the second extracellular loop with serine at position 103 in C and proline at position 103 in c. The E/e polymorphism results from proline at position 226 in E and alanine in e, in the fourth extracellular loop. Rh epitopes are not, however, linear sequences of amino acids, but also depend on the conformation of the molecule in the membrane. In some cases, the epitopes may be discontinuous, involving interactions between amino acid sequences on more than one extracellular loop. Amino acid substitutions in the membrane-spanning domains of the proteins may affect expression of the CcEe antigens and may even create new specificities.[19]

All antibodies to Rh-system antigens should be considered capable of causing severe HDFN, but the only Rh antibody other than anti-D that regularly causes severe HDFN is anti-c. The c-negative phenotype (common phenotype D Ce, probable genotype *D Ce/Ce*) is present in about 18% of Caucasians and about 50% of Chinese, but it is rare in Africans. In the Oxford region of England, over an 8-year period, 177 (0.06%) of 280 000 pregnancies were complicated by maternal anti-c.[29] Only one was associated with a neonatal death, but a total of 11 babies required exchange transfusion. Forty-one per cent of the sera with anti-c also contained anti-E. In three studies[30–32], between 14% and 21% of c-positive babies born to women with anti-c required exchange transfusion. In England and Wales over the period from 1977 to 1987, 26 babies, representing one in 250 000 births, died from anti-c HDFN. In 1987, despite anti-D prophylaxis, the mortality rate due to anti-c HDFN was still only one-tenth of that due to anti-D.[22]

Anti-C, -E, -e and -G have all caused HDFN but the occurrence of each is rare and the outcome seldom severe. Some Rh antibodies, especially anti-E, react only with protease-treated red cells in serological tests.[33] One 'enzyme-only' anti-E became reactive with untreated red cells during pregnancy and caused HDFN requiring exchange transfusion.[34] Anti-G detects an antigen common to the products of *RHD* and the *C* allele of *RHCE*. Consequently, anti-G reacts with red cells expressing D and/or C. Anti-G may be mistaken for anti-D and may be present together with anti-D. Most molecular methods for predicting fetal phenotype will correctly predict a D-negative C-positive fetus to be D negative, but the fetus could still be at risk if the mother's serum contains anti-G.[35] Anti-C^w is not an uncommon antibody and defines an antigen present on the red cells of about 2–3% of Caucasians. HDFN due to anti-C^w is usually mild but neonatal deaths caused by anti-C^w were reported in the 1940s. Bowman and Pollock[36] consider that these mortalities probably resulted from kernicterus in the absence of exchange transfusion. Other Rh-system antibodies that have been reported to have caused serious HDFN are anti-ce (-f), -Ce, -E^w, -Hr$_0$ (-Rh17), -Hr, -Rh29, -Go^a, -Rh32, -Be^a, -Evans, -Tar and -Rh46.[5]

2.5.3 Anti-K

Since the decline of HDFN caused by anti-D, much more attention has been focussed on HDFN due to anti-K, the original specificity of the Kell blood group system. The K-positive phenotype is present in about 9% of Europeans, but is less common in Africans and extremely rare in Eastern Asia and in native Americans. K achieves its highest level among people of the Arabian and Sinai peninsulas where up to 25% may be K positive.[15] K expression results from a threonine/methionine substitution at position 193 in the Kell glycoprotein, which is a red cell membrane glycoprotein that may function as an endopeptidase and which has the ability to process the biologically active peptide endothelin.[37,38] The amino acid substitution responsible for K expression disrupts a consensus sequence for *N*-glycosylation and the resultant glycosylation change may explain the high immunogenicity of K compared with other Kell system antigens which also result from amino acid substitutions.[37]

In Caucasian populations, anti-K is often the most common immune red cell antibody outside of the ABO and Rh systems.[22] Giblett[39] estimated the relative potency of antigens in stimulating the formation of antibodies and, after ABO and D, K attained the highest score with a relative potency of twice that for c, about 20 times that for Fy^a and over 100 times that for S. Anti-K, like other Kell system antibodies, is generally IgG and, predominantly, IgG1.[38,40]

K antibodies may cause severe fetal anaemia.[5] In one series, maternal anti-K was detected in 127 (0.1%) of 127 076 pregnancies. Thirteen of these pregnancies with maternal anti-K resulted in a K-positive baby, five (38%) of whom were very severely anaemic. Most anti-K appear to be induced by blood transfusion and it is becoming common practice for girls and women of childbearing age to be transfused only with K-negative red cells, although anti-K stimulated by transfusion seems to cause a less severe disease than anti-K stimulated by previous pregnancy.[41]

The pathogenesis of anaemia caused by anti-K differs from that due to anti-D. The severity of the disease due to anti-K is harder to predict than the disease due to anti-D. This is because there is very little correlation between anti-K titre and severity of disease and because HDFN due to anti-K is associated with lower concentrations of amniotic fluid bilirubin than HDFN due to anti-D. Postnatal hyperbilirubinaemia is not prominent in babies with anaemia caused by anti-K. There is also reduced reticulocytosis and erythroblastosis in the anti-K disease, compared with anti-D HDFN. These characteristics suggest that there is less haemolysis in HDFN caused by anti-K, compared with HDFN of comparable severity due to anti-D. This has led to speculation that fetal anaemia due to anti-K results predominantly from a suppression of erythropoiesis.[42,43] Indeed, Kell glycoprotein is one of the first erythroid-specific antigens to appear on erythroid progenitors during erythropoiesis, whereas the Rh proteins appear much later.[44,45] Vaughan et al. found that in vitro proliferation of K-positive erythroid blast-forming units and colony-forming units were specifically inhibited by monoclonal and polyclonal anti-K.[46] They speculated that the Kell glycoprotein might be an endopeptidase involved in regulating the growth and differentiation of erythroid progenitors, possibly by modulating peptide growth factors on the cell surface. Consequently, binding of anti-K could block the enzymatic activity of the Kell glycoprotein and suppress erythropoiesis. This theory, however, does not take into account the K_0 phenotype, in which no Kell glycoprotein is present on the surface of erythroid cells, yet erythropoiesis is apparently normal. It is more likely, therefore, that anti-K suppresses erythropoiesis through the immune destruction of early erythroid progenitors in the fetal liver. Daniels et al. have used a functional assay to demonstrate that K-positive erythroid progenitors cultured from CD34-positive cells derived from a K-positive, Rh D-positive neonate, elicited a strong response from monocytes; no response was obtained with anti-D because Rh antigens do not appear on erythroid cells before they become haemoglobinized erythroblasts.[45]

2.5.4 Other antibodies to Kell-system antigens

The Kell system consists of 23 antigens: four with frequencies between 2% and 16% in at least one major ethnic group, 14 of high frequency and five of low frequency. The Kell system polymorphisms and expression of the low frequency antigens or absence of the high frequency antigens all result from single amino acid substitutions in the large extracellular domain of the Kell glycoprotein.[37] It is likely that antibodies of all Kell-system specificities have the potential to cause HDFN which is usually, but not invariably, mild. HDFN requiring at least fetal transfusion has been reported for anti-k, -Kp^a, -Kp^b, -Js^a, -Js^b, -Ul^a, -Ku and -K22.[5]

2.6 Antibodies that most commonly cause mild HDFN

2.6.1 The ABO system

Anti-A and -B are present in virtually everyone who lacks the corresponding antigen, making ABO different from all other blood group polymorphisms. This characteristic also makes ABO the most important blood group system in transfusion medicine as these antibodies can cause severe haemolytic transfusion reactions. From the HDFN point of view, however, anti-A and -B are less significant.

Taken at its most basic level, there are two ABO antigens, A and B, and four phenotypes, A, B, AB and O (a null phenotype in which neither A nor B is expressed). A and B antigens are oligosaccharide structures on cell surface glycoproteins and glycolipids. The major carriers of A and B on red cells are the anion exchanger (band 3) and the glucose transporter. The *A* and *B* genes do not encode the antigens directly but produce glycosyltransferase enzymes, which catalyse the transfer of immunodominant monosaccharides from a nucleotide donor substrate to an acceptor substrate. The acceptor substrate is an oligosaccharide chain terminating in a fucosylated galactose residue. This precursor structure is referred to as the H antigen and is present on the red cells of almost everyone. The immunodominant sugars of A and B are *N*-acetylgalactosamine and galactose, respectively. The *A* and *B* gene-specified glycosyltransferases differ by four amino acids. The *A* gene product transfers *N*-acetylgalactosamine to H to produce an A-active structure; the *B* gene product transfers galactose to H to produce a B-active structure. The common *O* allele contains a single base deletion, which causes a reading-frame shift and introduces a translation-termination codon, so the *O* allele product has no enzymatic activity and the H structure remains unconverted.[47]

There are many ABO variants but mostly they involve quantitative differences in the activity of the transferases and, consequently, quantitative differences in A or B antigen expression.[5] The most important of these variants is A$_2$ (the common alternative being A$_1$), in which a shift in the position of the translation termination codon of an *A* allele produces a transferase of extended length, with impaired catalytic activity.

ABO frequencies vary in different populations. Typical European (British) frequencies are A 42%, B 8%, AB 3% and O 47%; about 80% of the group A people are A$_1$ and 20% A$_2$. Substantially higher frequencies of O are found in native Americans and in parts of Africa and Australia; higher frequencies of B are found in Central Asia, with B being virtually absent in native Americans and Australians. A_2 is found mainly in Europe and Africa but is very rare or absent in the rest of the world.[15]

Anti-A and anti-B are predominantly IgM but may be IgG. The sera of most group O people contain a cross-reacting antibody, called anti-A,B, that reacts with both A and B antigens and is often partly IgG. ABO HDFN is restricted almost exclusively to the fetuses of group O mothers. The relative clinical significance of anti-A,B compared with anti-A and anti-B is unclear.[48]

About 15% of pregnancies in women of European origin involve a group O mother with a group A or B fetus, yet ABO HDFN requiring clinical intervention is rare, although minor jaundice involving a small degree of red cell destruction may be relatively common. Hydrops due to ABO HDFN is exceedingly rare, but very occasionally exchange transfusion for the prevention of kernicterus is indicated.[22] The main explanation for the low prevalence of clinically significant ABO HDFN is that ABO is a histo-blood group system (Section 2.4). Any antibody crossing the placenta is likely to become bound to placental tissue, reducing the quantity available for destruction of red cells. In addition, A and B red cell antigens are not fully developed in the fetus or even at birth.[5]

About 85% of Caucasians have a gene (*FUT2*) that enables the secretion of soluble A and B antigens in body fluids. There is little evidence, however, that this secretion of A and B antigens plays any role in providing protection from HDFN.[22]

In black people, Arabs and Taiwanese, ABO HDFN has a prevalence 2–6 times higher than in Europeans,[49–51] perhaps because of the stronger expression of A and B antigens in these racial groups. In some populations, parasitic infection may result in higher levels of ABO antibodies, resulting in increased incidence of clinically significant HDFN.

2.7 Antibodies that rarely cause HDFN

Antibodies to red cell antigens from a variety of blood group systems, as well as some antibodies to high and low frequency antigens that do not yet belong to established systems, can also be responsible for causing symptoms of HDFN. In most instances, this entails no more than a positive direct antiglobulin test and slight jaundice, but, occasionally, these antibodies may give rise to HDFN requiring clinical intervention.

2.7.1 MNS system

MNS is a large and complex blood group system. MNS-system antigens are located on one or both of two sialic-rich glycoproteins, glycophorin A and glycophorin B. Most anti-M and -N are not active at 37°C and are usually benign, but severe

HDFN due to anti-M has occurred. Severe HDFN has also been attributed to anti-S, -s and -U. Other MNS antibodies that are reported to have caused HDFN are antibodies to the high frequency antigen En^a and antibodies to the low frequency antigens Mi^a, Vw, Hut, Hil, Mt^a, M^v, Far and s^D.[5]

The MNS red cell phenotype GP.Mur (Mi.III), in which the antigens Mi^a, Hil, MUT and MINY are expressed, is rare in most of the world but is relatively common in South-East Asia with frequencies between 2% and 10%. In Taiwan, antibody to these low frequency antigens (collectively described as anti-'Mi^a') is the most frequent immune blood group antibody, with a prevalence of 0.8% in patients. 'Anti-Mi^a' has caused severe HDFN and, consequently, cell panels for antibody screening in Taiwan include GP.Mur phenotype cells.[51]

2.7.2 Duffy system

The Fy^a/Fy^b polymorphism arises from a single amino acid substitution in the *N*-terminal extracellular domain of the Duffy glycoprotein, a member of the G protein-coupled superfamily of receptors. In a survey of 68 pregnancies in which anti-Fy^a was detected, 10 had indications of mild HDFN and three resulted in severe HDFN, two requiring intrauterine transfusion.[52] The only reported case of HDFN due to anti-Fy^b was treated by postnatal transfusion and phototherapy.[53]

2.7.3 Kidd system

Despite being haemolytic and a common cause of delayed haemolytic transfusion reactions, antibodies to Jk^a and Jk^b, a polymorphism representing an amino acid substitution on a red cell urea transporter, do not usually cause HDFN. One case of HDFN due to anti-Jk^a resulted in kernicterus.[54]

2.7.4 Diego system

The Diego system consists of 21 antigens, each representing an amino acid substitution on band 3 glycoprotein, the red cell anion exchanger.[55] Together with glycophorin A, band 3 is the most abundant red cell surface glycoprotein, with about 10^6 copies per cell. Di^a, the original Diego antigen, is rare in people of European and African origin but is common in native people of the Americas and in China and Japan, with frequencies of around 5% in Japanese rising to over 50% in some native South Americans. In Brazil, four (3.6%) of 112 multitransfused patients had anti-Di^a.[56] Anti-Di^a can cause severe HDFN and, although this is rare in most populations, many examples have been described.[5] HDFN due to anti-Di^b requiring neonatal exchange transfusion has also been reported.[5,57] Anti-Wr^a and anti-ELO, antibodies to two low frequency antigens of the Diego system, have both caused severe HDFN.[5,58]

2.7.5 Colton system

The Co^a/Co^b polymorphism results from a single amino acid substitution in a red cell water channel, aquaporin-1. Anti-Co3 is the antibody which can be produced by the very rare individuals with an aquaporin-1 deficiency. Antibodies to the high frequency antigens Co^a and Co3 have both caused severe HDFN.[59–61]

2.7.6 Other antigens

Only a few of the antibodies to antigens that have not been shown to belong to a blood group system have caused HDFN serious enough to merit consideration of transfusion therapy; of the antibodies to low frequency antigens (700 series), these are anti-Rd, -HJK, -Kg, -REIT, -JFV and -JONES.[5] With the exception of anti-MAM,[62] antibodies to the high frequency antigens (901 series) have not caused severe HDFN.

2.8 Antibodies that do not cause HDFN

The paragloboside and globoside series glycolipid antigens (P1, P [globoside], P^k [CD77], and LKE) have not been implicated in severe HDFN. Red cells of the rare p phenotype lack all these antigens and an antibody, called anti-PP1P^k, is invariably present. Anti-PP1P^k usually contains an IgG3 fraction, but it does not cause HDFN. Anti-PP1P^k is, however, associated with habitual abortion, characteristically in the first trimester. The primary target for the antibodies appears to be the placenta and not the fetus.[63] Anti-P in the rare P^k phenotype has also been associated with habitual abortion.[64] Therapeutic plasmapheresis may be successful in such cases.

Antibodies of the Lutheran system do not cause HDFN, partly because the antigens are expressed only weakly on fetal cells and partly because the antibodies are absorbed by the placenta. Antibodies to the Lewis histo-blood group antigens (Le^a and Le^b) are generally not active at 37 °C and the antigens are not expressed on fetal cells. In addition, antigens of the Yt, Xg, Scianna, Dombrock, LW, Chido/Rodgers, Gerbich, Cromer, Knops, Indian, Kx, Ok and Raph systems and the Cost and Er collections have not been implicated in serious HDFN. Antibody to the high frequency antigen Vel has only caused mild HDFN, probably because anti-Vel is usually IgM and Vel is expressed weakly on fetal cells. Anti-JMH does not cause HDFN because the antigen is not present on fetal cells. Anti-Lan, -At^a and -Jr^a have only caused mild HDFN. Anti-Emm, -AnWj, -Sd^a, -Duclos (only one example known), -PEL and -ABTI have not caused HDFN.[5]

2.9 Conclusions

HDFN due to antibodies with specificities other than D and c of the Rh system and K of the Kell system is rare. It is very important, however, to know the potential of antibodies of other specificities for causing HDFN. This can often be gauged on the basis of previous experience with other examples of the antibody, although this approach is not without hazard. Unexpected haemolysis could result from an unusually potent example of an antibody or a fetus with exceptionally strong expression of the red cell antigen. A more thorough comprehension of the biological reasons why antibodies of some specificities cause HDFN, whereas others do not, would assist in predicting the risk of HDFN in individual pregnancies.

2.10 References

1 Levine P & Stetson RE (1939). An unusual case of intra-group agglutination. *Journal of the American Medical Association*, **113**, 126–7.

2 Levine P, Burnham L, Katzin EM & Vogel P (1941). The role of iso-immunization in the pathogenesis of erythroblastosis fetalis. *American Journal of Obstetrics and Gynecology*, **42**, 925–7.

3 Daniels GL, Anstee DJ, Cartron JP et al. (1995). Blood group terminology 1995. From the ISBT Working Party on Terminology for Red Cell Surface Antigens. *Vox Sanguinis*, **69**, 265–79.

4 Daniels GL, Anstee DJ, Cartron JP et al. (1999). Terminology for red cell surface antigens. ISBT Working Party Oslo report. *Vox Sanguinis*, **77**, 52–7.

5 Daniels G (1995). *Human Blood Groups*. Oxford: Blackwell Science.

6 Issitt PD & Anstee DJ (1998). *Applied Blood Group Serology*, 4th edn. Durham, NC: Montgomery Scientific Publications.

7 Anstee DJ & Cartron J-P (1997). Toward an understanding of the red cell surface. In *Applications of Molecular Biology to Transfusion Medicine*, ed. G. Garratty. Bethesda, MD: American Association of Blood Banks, pp. 17–49.

8 Parsons SF, Mallinson G, Holmes CH et al. (1995). The Lutheran blood group glycoprotein, another member of the immunoglobulin superfamily, is widely expressed in human tissues and is developmentally regulated in human liver. *Proceedings of the National Academy of Sciences USA*, **92**, 5496–500.

9 Holmes CH, Simpson KL, Wainwright SD et al. (1990). Preferential expression of the complement regulatory protein decay accelerating factor at the fetomaternal interface during pregnancy. *Journal of Immunology*, **144**, 3099–105.

10 Novotny VMJ, Kanhai HHH, Overbeeke MAM, Schlaman-Nijp A, Harvey MS & Brand A (1992). Misleading results in the determination of haemolytic disease of the newborn using antibody titration and ADCC in a woman with anti-Lu^b. *Vox Sanguinis*, **62**, 49–52.

11 Herron B, Reynolds W, Northcott M, Herborn A & Boulton FE (1996). Data from two patients providing evidence that the placenta may act as a barrier to the materno-fetal transfer of anti-Lutheran antibodies. *Transfusion Medicine*, **6** (suppl 2), 24 (abstract).

12 Reid ME, Chandrasekaran V, Sausais L, Jeannot P & Bullock R (1996). Disappearance of anti-bodies to Cromer blood group system antigens during mid pregnancy. *Vox Sanguinis*, **71**, 48–50.

13 Poole J, Banks J, Chatfield C, Mallinson G, Slater NG & Kenney A (1998). Disappearance of the Cromer antibody anti-WES[b] during pregnancy. *Transfusion Medicine*, **8** (suppl 1), 16 (abstract).

14 Levine P (1958). The influence of the ABO system on hemolytic disease. *Human Biology*, **30**, 14–28.

15 Mourant AE, Kopec AC & Domaniewska K (1976). *The Distribution of Human Blood Groups and Other Polymorphisms*. London: Oxford University Press.

16 Okubo Y, Yamaguch, H, Tomita T & Nagao N (1984). A D variant, Del? *Transfusion*, **24**, 542.

17 Mak KH, Yan KF, Cheng SS & Yuen MY (1993). Rh phenotypes of Chinese blood donors in Hong Kong, with special reference to weak D antigens. *Transfusion*, **33**, 348–51.

18 Huang C-H (1997). Molecular insights into the Rh protein family and associated antigens. *Current Opinions in Hematology*, **4**, 94–103.

19 Avent ND (1999). The Rhesus blood group system: insights from recent advances in molecular biology. *Transfusion Medicine Reviews*, **13**, 245–66.

20 Colin Y, Chérif-Zahar B, Le Van Kim C, Raynal V, Van Huffel V & Cartron J-P (1991). Genetic basis of the RhD-positive and RhD-negative blood group polymorphism as determined by Southern analysis. *Blood*, **78**, 2747–52.

21 Singleton BK, Green CA, Avent ND et al. (2000). Presence of an RHD pseudogene containing a 37 bp duplication and a nonsense mutation in most Africans with the Rh D-negative blood group phenotype. *Blood*, **95**, 12–18.

22 Mollison PL, Engelfriet CP & Contreras M (1997). *Blood Transfusion in Clinical Medicine*, 10th edn. Oxford: Blackwell Science.

23 Wagner FF, Gassner C, Müller TH, Schönitzer D, Schunter F & Flegel WF (1999). Molecular basis of weak D phenotypes. *Blood*, **93**, 385–93.

24 Scott M (1996). Rh serology – coordinator's report. *Transfusion Clinique et Biologique*, **6**, 333–7.

25 Tippett P, Lomas-Francis C & Wallace M (1996). The Rh antigen D: partial D antigens and associated low incidence antigens. *Vox Sanguinis*, **70**, 123–31.

26 Flegel W, Wagner FF, Müller TH & Gassner C (1998). Rh phenotype prediction by DNA typing and its application to practice. *Transfusion Medicine*, **8**, 281–302.

27 Lubenko A, Contreras M & Habash J (1989). Should anti-Rh immunoglobulin be given to D variant women? *British Journal of Haematology*, **72**, 429–33.

28 Mayne K, Bowell P, Woodward T, Sibley C, Lomas C & Tippett P (1990). Rh immunization by the partial D antigen of category DV[a]. *British Journal of Haematology*, **76**, 537–9.

29 Bowell PJ, Brown SE, Dike AE & Inskip MJ (1986). The significance of anti-c alloimmunization in pregnancy. *British Journal of Obstetrics and Gynaecology*, **93**, 1044–8.

30 Astrup J & Kornstad L (1977). Presence of anti-c in the serum of 42 women giving birth to c positive babies: serological and clinical findings. *Acta Obstetricia et Gynecologica Scandinavica*, **56**, 185–8.

31 Hardy J & Napier JAF (1981). Red cell antibodies detected in antenatal tests on Rhesus posi-

tive women in south and mid Wales, 1948–1978. *British Journal of Obstetrics and Gynaecology*, **88**, 91–100.

32 Kozlowski CL, Lee D, Shwe KH & Love EM (1995). Quantitation of anti-c in haemolytic disease of the newborn. *Transfusion Medicine*, **5**, 37–42.

33 Issitt PD, Combs MR, Bredehoeft SJ et al. (1993). Lack of clinical significance of 'enzyme-only' red cell alloantibodies. *Transfusion*, **33**, 284–93.

34 Garner SF, Devenish A, Barber H & Contreras M (1991). The importance of monitoring 'enzyme-only' red cell antibodies during pregnancy. *Vox Sanguinis*, **61**, 219–20.

35 Hadley AG, Poole GD, Poole J, Anderson NA & Robson M (1996). Haemolytic disease of the newborn due to anti-G. *Vox Sanguinis*, **71**, 108–12.

36 Bowman JM & Pollock J (1993). Maternal C^w alloimmunization. *Vox Sanguinis*, **64**, 226–30.

37 Lee S (1997). Molecular basis of Kell blood group phenotypes. *Vox Sanguinis*, **73**, 1–11.

38 Lee S, Lin M, Mele A et al. (1999). Proteolytic processing of big endothelin-3 by the Kell blood group protein. *Blood*, **94**, 1440–50.

39 Giblett ER (1961). A critique of the theoretical hazard of inter- vs. intra-racial transfusion. *Transfusion*, **1**, 233–8.

40 Hardman JT & Beck ML (1981). Hemagglutination in capillaries: correlation with blood group specificity and IgG subclass. *Transfusion*, **21**, 343–6.

41 Caine ME & Mueller-Heubach E (1986). Kell sensitization in pregnancy. *American Journal of Obstetrics and Gynecology*, **154**, 85–90.

42 Vaughan JI, Warwick R, Letsky E, Nicolini U, Rodeck CH & Fisk NM (1994). Erythropoietic suppression in fetal anemia because of Kell alloimmunization. *American Journal of Obstetrics and Gynecology*, **171**, 247–52.

43 Weiner CP & Widness JA (1996). Decreased fetal erythropoiesis and hemolysis in Kell hemolytic anemia. *American Journal of Obstetrics and Gynecology*, **174**, 547–51.

44 Southcott MJG, Tanner MJA & Anstee DJ (1999). The expression of human blood group antigens during erythropoiesis in a cell culture system. *Blood*, **93**, 4425–35.

45 Daniels GL, Hadley AG & Green CA (1999). Fetal anaemia due to anti-K may result from immune destruction of early erythroid progenitors. *Transfusion Medicine*, **9** (suppl 1), 16 (abstract).

46 Vaughan JI, Manning M, Warwick RM, Letsky EA, Murray NA & Roberts IAG (1998). Inhibition of erythroid progenitor cells by anti-Kell antibodies in fetal alloimmune anemia. *New England Journal of Medicine*, **338**, 798–803.

47 Yamamoto, F, Clausen H, White T, Marken J, Hakomori S (1990). Molecular genetic basis of the histo-blood group ABO system. *Nature*, **345**, 229–33.

48 Issitt, PD & Combs MR (1996). The specificity of antibodies causative of ABO HDN. *Transfusion*, **36** (suppl), 23S (abstract).

49 Kirkman HN (1977). Further evidence for a racial difference in frequency of ABO hemolytic disease. *Journal of Pediatrics*, **90**, 717–21.

50 Al-Jawad ST, Keenan P & Kholeif S (1986). Incidence of ABO haemolytic disease in a mixed Arab population. *Saudi Medical Journal*, **7**, 41–5.

51 Lin M & Broadberry RE (1998). Immunohematology in Taiwan. *Transfusion Medicine Reviews*, **12**, 56–72.

52 Goodrick MJ, Hadley AG & Poole G (1997). Haemolytic disease of the fetus and newborn due to anti-Fy^a and the potential clinical value of Duffy genotyping in pregnancies at risk. *Transfusion Medicine*, 7, 301–4.

53 Carreras Vescio LA, Fariña D, Rogido M & Sóla A (1987). Hemolytic disease of the newborn caused by anti-Fy^b. *Transfusion*, 27, 366.

54 Matson GA, Swanson J & Tobin JD (1959). Severe hemolytic disease of the newborn caused by anti-Jk^a. *Vox Sanguinis*, 4, 144–7.

55 Zelinski T (1998). Erythrocyte band 3 antigens and the Diego blood group system. *Transfusion Medicine Reviews*, 12, 36–45.

56 Zago-Novaretti MC, Soares MOC, Dorlhiac-Llace, PE, Chamone DAF (1992). Anti-Diego in multitransfused patients. *Revista Paulista de Medicina*, 110, IH52 (abstract).

57 Ishimori T, Fukumoto Y, Abe K et al. (1976). Rare Diego blood group phenotype Di(a+b−). I. Anti-Di^b causing hemolytic disease of the newborn. *Vox Sanguinis*, 31, 61–3.

58 Better PJ, Ford DS, Frascarelli A & Stern DA (1993). Confirmation of anti-ELO as a cause of haemolytic disease of the newborn. *Vox Sanguinis*, 65, 70.

59 Simpson WKH (1973). Anti-Co^a and severe haemolytic disease of the newborn. *South African Medical Journal*, 47, 1302–4.

60 Lacey PA, Robinson J, Collins ML et al. (1987). Studies on the blood of a Co(a–b–) proposita and her family. *Transfusion*, 27, 268–71.

61 Savona-Ventura C, Grech ES & Zieba A (1989). Anti-Co3 and severe hemolytic disease of the newborn. *Obstetrics and Gynecology*, 73, 870–2.

62 Montgomery W, Nance S, Kavitsky D et al. (1997). First example of hemolytic disease of the newborn (HDN) due to an antibody to a high incidence antigen present on multiple cell lines (MCL). *Transfusion*, 37 (suppl), 41S (abstract).

63 Lindström K, von dem Borne AEGK, Breimer ME et al. (1992). Glycosphingolipid expression in spontaneously aborted fetuses and placenta from blood group p women. Evidence for placenta being the primary target for anti-Tj^a-antibodies. *Glycoconjugate Journal*, 9, 325–9.

64 Shirey RS, Ness PM, Kickler TS et al. (1987). The association of anti-P and early abortion. *Transfusion*, 27, 189–91.

Basis and practice of screening for haemolytic disease of the fetus and newborn

Geoff Poole

National Blood Service, Bristol, UK

3.1 Introduction

Levine and Stetson in 1939 first discovered an irregular agglutinating antibody in a previously transfused woman who had given birth to a stillborn child.[1] However, it was not until IgG nonagglutinating (or 'incomplete') red cell antibodies could be demonstrated serologically that screening methods for HDFN began to be developed.[2,3] These included the albumin method,[4] the indirect antiglobulin test (IAGT)[5] and the enzyme method.[6] Of these, the albumin method is used less frequently, but the IAGT and, to some extent, the enzyme method remain important in serological screening for HDFN. This chapter reviews these methods and their ability to provide information that is useful for clinicians to identify and manage women at risk of HDFN.

3.2 The basis of screening for HDFN

Adequate and relevant information concerning the presence and nature of red cell alloantibodies in the plasma of pregnant women is essential for the effective management of potential HDFN. The purpose of screening in the laboratory is to provide this information to clinicians. Serological methods are effective in antenatal screening programmes because they are capable of detecting the vast majority of red cell alloantibodies that can cause HDFN (Section 2.5). Furthermore, methods can be chosen which detect IgG antibodies active at 37°C but which do not detect IgM antibodies active at temperatures below 37°C, since these antibodies do not cause HDFN. Serological methods are also used to determine the potency of antibodies (the strength of their reactivity with red cells) (Section 8.2).

Screening work is usually undertaken in blood transfusion laboratories because the techniques used for screening for HDFN are the same as those used in pretransfusion testing. However, there are also some important differences because the clinical relevance of red cell antibodies in the two situations may vary. These differences

Table 3.1 Comparison between the laboratory features of screening for HDFN and pretransfusion testing

	Screening for HDFN	Pretransfusion testing
ABO group	Not important[1]	Critical
Rh D group	Determines frequency of testing and use of prophylactic anti-D	Determines selection of blood
Antibody screen at 37°C	Essential	Essential
Antibody screen below 37°C	Not recommended	Not recommended
Antibody identification	Essential	Essential
Presence of IgG antibody	Relevant	Relevant
Presence of IgM antibody	Not relevant	Relevant
Potency of antibody	Usually valuable	Rarely of value

Notes:
[1] Usually performed, however (see Section 3.3.5).

are summarized in Table 3.1. In practice, screening tests for HDFN and pretransfusion tests are complementary because the presence of a red cell antibody in a pregnant woman may be important not only with respect to HDFN but also with respect to the selection of blood should transfusion be indicated for the mother or fetus. Laboratory protocols are therefore designed to take account of these overlapping requirements. The features of a typical protocol for antenatal testing in the blood transfusion laboratory should include those shown in Table 3.2. Some of the tasks listed require specialist expertise or equipment outside the scope of most laboratories and should be performed in a reference red cell serology laboratory.

3.3 Antenatal screening tests performed in the blood transfusion laboratory

3.3.1 Antiglobulin methods

Coombs et al.[7] are generally credited with the discovery of the indirect antiglobulin test in 1945, although a version of the test had in fact been published over 30 years earlier by Moreschi.[8] One year later, the former workers also described the direct antiglobulin test, which they used to detect in vivo sensitization of red cells in HDFN.[5] Modern laboratories use the indirect antiglobulin test in antenatal and pretransfusion testing, albeit in several different guises, because it remains the simplest way of detecting red cell antibodies of clinical importance. Furthermore, it performs well in respect of two important requirements of a diagnostic test: it has an appropriate level of sensitivity and a high degree of specificity. In the antenatal context, this means that the indirect antiglobulin test is usually positive when a

Table 3.2 Laboratory tasks associated with screening for HDFN

Task	Need	Associated laboratory tests
ABO & D group mother's red cells	Pretransfusion test in case mother needs blood	
Screen mother's plasma for antibody	Determine whether red cell alloantibody is present	Screen mother's plasma for microbiological markers
Identify the specificity of any antibody	Determine whether the antibody has a likely potential to cause HDFN Establish special requirements for blood if needed for mother or fetus	
Assess antibody potency	Assist the obstetrician in clinical management	Assess functional activity of antibody
Phenotype the father's red cells	Determine the probability that the fetal red cells express the antigen against which maternal antibody is directed	
Perform phenotype and direct antiglobulin test on fetus	Establish whether fetal red cells have been sensitized with maternal antibody	Perform amniocentesis to determine bilirubin level in amniotic fluid Perform fetal genotyping of amniocytes Establish haemoglobin level and haematocrit of fetus
Crossmatch blood for fetus	Raise the fetal haemoglobin level	
ABO & D group and direct antiglobulin test on infant's red cells	Pretransfusion test should infant need blood Determine the extent of sensitization of fetal red cells with maternal antibody Determine whether anti-D prophylaxis for the mother is required	Range of haematology/chemistry tests if infant is affected Kleihauer test or flow cytometry if mother is D− and infant is D+
Crossmatch blood for infant	Raise the infant's haemoglobin level Remove bilirubin from the infant's circulation by performing an exchange transfusion	

maternal antibody of potential clinical significance is present, but usually negative in the absence of such an antibody.

The principle of the indirect antiglobulin test is simple. Serum or plasma from the mother is incubated with a panel of screening reagent red cells (Section 3.3.3). If an alloantibody is present, it will bind to antigens expressed on red cells from at least one of the donors. The presence of the bound antibody is detected by addition of an antiglobulin reagent which consists of a nonhuman antibody with specificity for the gamma heavy chain of human IgG. Cell-bound antiglobulin is then demonstrated by liquid-phase agglutination or column agglutination, or in a solid-phase adherence method.[9]

Liquid-phase agglutination methods are generally performed in 75×12 mm glass tubes and require a washing phase (red cells and plasma are diluted with saline, centrifuged and the supernatant removed) in order to remove unbound immunoglobulins before the addition of antiglobulin reagent. Agglutination of reagent red cells indicates the presence of an antibody in the patient's plasma. Tube indirect antiglobulin test methods in the UK generally make use of low ionic strength saline to enhance antibody binding to red cells.[10] Other methods of comparable sensitivity and which are also performed in tubes include the polyethylene glycol indirect antiglobulin test,[11] the manual polybrene test taken through to an indirect antiglobulin test stage[12] and those employing additive reagents from a number of commercial sources. Tube-based indirect antiglobulin test methods require particular attention to the washing and reading stages in order to achieve optimal sensitivity and consistency.[13]

The publication in 1990 of a serological method involving a mixture of Sephadex™ and Sephacryl™ gels has resulted in a very significant change to the performance of the indirect antiglobulin test in many laboratories.[14] The commercial method involves the use of a plastic card containing six channels each with a column of gel admixed with antiglobulin reagent. Plasma or serum and reagent red cells are added to the top of a gel column and, following incubation and carefully controlled centrifugation, red cells coated with antibody are agglutinated and are thus unable to pass through the gel. Positive reactions are therefore distinguished by agglutinates at or near the top of the gel column and negative reactions appear as buttons of red cells at the bottom (Figure 3.1). Since plasma proteins are less dense than the gel, a washing phase is not needed which, together with the relative stability of the reaction endpoint, gives column agglutination methods a degree of simplicity and reliability not achieved by other methods. A similar column agglutination method involving a glass microbead density barrier in place of a gel is also available.[15]

Solid-phase methods based on 96-well plastic microplates provide another alternative to the tube indirect antiglobulin test.[16–18] Although differing in detail, all of these methods achieve a positive reaction endpoint that is characterized by a monolayer of red cells across the bottom of the microplate well. A discrete button of red cells at the bottom of the well indicates a negative reaction (Figure 3.2). Although solid-phase methods are suitable for laboratories undertaking large numbers of antiglobulin tests, they suffer from the disadvantage that they require carefully standardized centrifugation and washing steps.

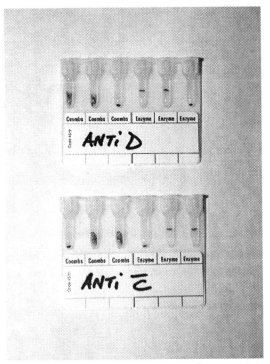

Figure 3.1   Two column agglutination cards showing strong positive, intermediate positive and negative reactions. *Top*: Card contains a weak anti-D in each column tested by an indirect antiglobulin method (columns 1 and 2 using D-positive red cells and column 3 using D-negative red cells) and by an enzyme method (columns 4 and 5 using D-positive red cells and column 6 using D-negative red cells). *Bottom*: Card contains a weak anti-c in each column tested by an indirect antiglobulin method (column 1 using c-negative red cells and columns 2 and 3 using c-positive red cells) and by an enzyme method (column 4 using c-negative red cells and columns 5 and 6 using c-positive red cells).

The enhancement of reactivity of these weak Rh antibodies using an enzyme method is clearly evident.

Reproduced by kind permission of DiaMed-AG, Cressier Sur Morat, Switzerland

When performed correctly, all of the above methods are capable of a degree of sensitivity and specificity adequate for use in a routine blood transfusion laboratory. In general, the solid-phase methods have been found to be rather more sensitive than column agglutination methods, but more prone to unwanted positive reactions.[19] UK guidelines do not mandate that any one particular type of indirect antiglobulin test method should be used for antenatal screening,[20,21] but recommend that the chosen method is carefully validated before introduction into routine use.[22,23]

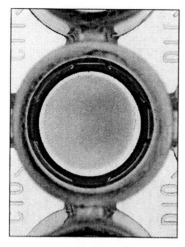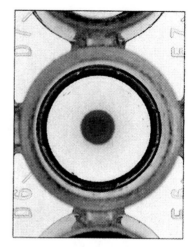

Figure 3.2   Two solid-phase microplate wells showing positive and negative reactions. *Left*:
Monolayer of red cells indicates a positive result. *Right*: Button of red cells indicates
a negative result.
Reproduced by kind permission of Biotest (UK) Ltd, Solihull, UK.

3.3.2 Enzyme methods

Red cells that are treated with a proteinase such as papain or bromelain become
agglutinable by some IgG alloantibodies such as anti-D without the addition of an
antiglobulin reagent.[24,25] Treatment with these proteinases causes cleavage of glycoproteins from the red cell membrane with an associated loss of net negative charge
from the red cells, thereby reducing intercellular repulsive forces. This, and other
mechanisms that may be relevant to the action of enzymes in promoting agglutination of red cells, are reviewed elsewhere.[26]

Enzyme methods are simple to perform because there is no washing phase as in
antiglobulin tests. They also have a very high sensitivity for the detection of antibodies such as anti-D and anti-c, both of which, if present in the mother's plasma,
can cause significant morbidity in the fetus. However, enzyme methods suffer from
two important disadvantages. First, they cannot be used to detect the presence of
an antibody, such as anti-Fy^a, that has a specificity for an antigen that is cleaved
from the red cell surface by a proteolytic enzyme. Thus, an enzyme method should
not be used for antibody screening unless an antiglobulin method is also used.
Second, screening tests using enzyme-treated cells are more likely to be interpreted
as positive in the absence of clinically significant antibody than is the case with antiglobulin methods. This is because positive and negative reactions are more difficult
to distinguish in enzyme methods, and because plasma sometimes contains antibodies which preferentially or only react with enzyme-treated red cells. These
'enzyme-only' antibodies are rarely of clinical significance.

The value of enzyme methods in antenatal screening has been debated. On the one hand, it can be argued that the extra sensitivity of an enzyme method can be useful in detecting antibodies (particularly those with specificity for blood group antigens in the Rh system) that are too weak to be detected by an antiglobulin method. These antibodies may increase in potency during the course of the pregnancy and consequently could give rise to HDFN.[27] On the other hand, a more pragmatic view is that such antibodies are unlikely to give rise to HDFN in the current pregnancy serious enough to cause significant morbidity in the infant.[28] Current UK practice and recommendations in the USA reflect the latter view that laboratories need not use tests using enzyme-treated cells as part of their antibody screening protocols.[29,30] This may be based in part on the recommendation that D-negative pregnant women should have a repeat antibody screen at 28–34 weeks.[20] This is discussed in more detail below (Section 3.3.5).

3.3.3 The choice of red cells for screening tests

Reagent red cells used in screening tests should detect all common, clinically important antibodies. They must, therefore, express the blood group antigens that allow these antibodies to be detected. As a minimum, the following antigens must be represented: C, c, D, E, e, K, k, Fy^a, Fy^b, Jk^a, Jk^b, S, s, M, N, P_1, Le^a and Le^b.[21,31] Furthermore, wherever possible, there should be strong expression of these antigens, so that weak antibodies will be better detected. Anti-D, anti-c and anti-K are alloantibodies that are most likely to cause severe HDFN, and anti-e, anti-Ce, anti-Fy^a, anti-Jk^a and anti-C^w are not uncommon antibodies that are sometimes associated with HDFN (Section 2.5). Therefore, in order to ensure that weak examples of these antibodies are detected during pregnancy, red cells of the Rh phenotype R_1R_1 (probable genotype *D Ce/Ce*) and red cells of the Rh phenotype R_2R_2 (probable genotype *D cE/cE*) should be used in screening tests, and the phenotypes K+, Fy(a+b-) and Jk(a+b-) should also be represented.

As is the case with screening cells used for pretransfusion tests, there is no requirement for the phenotypes Kp(a+) and C^w+ to be represented on red cells used for antenatal screening, notwithstanding the fact that these antibodies are not uncommonly encountered.[21,31] The Kp^a antigen has a frequency of about 2% in Caucasians and the C^w antigen has a frequency of about 4%. As a result of these low frequencies, reagent suppliers find it difficult or impossible to provide a matched set of reagent cells that meet the requirements outlined above and between them express Kp^a and C^w. Anti-Kp^a and anti-C^w are certainly capable of causing HDFN, but it is usually mild and failure to detect these antibodies is unlikely to cause serious problems providing the baby has good general postnatal care.

In practice, the screening cells used in antenatal testing are usually identical to those used in pretransfusion testing, because red cell alloantibodies that may cause

HDFN are usually also capable of reducing the in vivo survival of incompatible red cells following allogeneic transfusion.

3.3.4 Manual *versus* automated methods

Traditional serological methods using glass tubes are capable of achieving very high standards of sensitivity and specificity. However, the pipetting, reading and recording steps of these methods are labour intensive and subject to human error. These disadvantages can be overcome by using a column agglutination or solid-phase microplate method for antibody screening and by employing a semiautomated or automated system. The basic features of automated systems should include: trays or carousels to stack samples; automatic pipetting of samples and reagents; the use of bar codes on samples, and other devices to ensure that positive sample identification is obtained; clot sensor and liquid level alarms; an optical device to record reaction patterns; and comprehensive system management software that interprets reaction patterns and flags discrepant results.

The most flexible option is a robotic liquid-handler that can be adapted to perform pipetting operations for a variety of column agglutination or solid-phase technologies. This is made possible by the use of customized racking systems and by the use of versatile software supplied with the equipment. Similarly, image analysis and colorimetric readers are available which can interpret the reaction patterns obtained using different technologies. In this way, a modular system can be built up which allows antibody screening results to be uploaded into the laboratory's main computer system. However, some operations, such as the transfer of microplates or column agglutination cassettes from the robot to the incubator, must be performed manually.

A second option is to choose a dedicated robotic liquid-handler and reader from a single supplier. The advantage of this is that the introduction of the equipment into the laboratory is likely to be much more straightforward, as it will have been designed for a single technology. The disadvantage is that the user is tied in to this technology for the life of the equipment.

Finally, there are 'walk-away' systems which perform all of the pipetting, incubation and reading stages of antibody screening.[32,33] An example of one such system available in Europe is shown in Figure 3.3. These systems require very little manual intervention and are likely to have a high degree of inbuilt security, thus minimizing the chance of an erroneous result being recorded. However, they may have a lower throughput (because of a longer start to finish time) than a modular system and will of course be more expensive to purchase.

The choice that must be made will therefore be dependent on the throughput volume, the extent of security required and the budget of the laboratory.

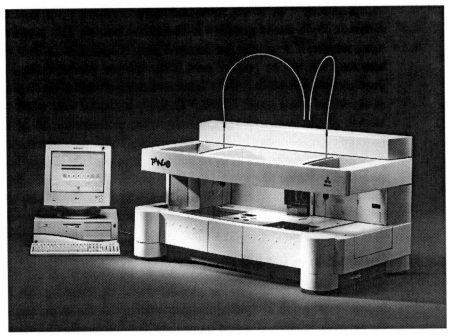

Figure 3.3   PC-operated robotic liquid handling system.
This system can be used for ABO, Rh and K phenotyping, and also for antibody screening/identification, titration and crossmatching. It is claimed that the instrument is capable of performing 25 blood groups or 100 antibody screening tests per hour.
Reproduced by kind permission of Biotest (UK) Ltd, Solihull, UK.

3.3.5 Timing of screening tests

Blood samples for a variety of tests are usually taken from pregnant women during their first routine antenatal assessment (in the UK, termed 'booking'). This usually occurs at 10–16 weeks' gestation. One sample should be sent to the blood transfusion laboratory for ABO and D grouping and for the antibody screen. Depending on the methods in use in the laboratory, clotted or anticoagulated samples may be used, as plasma or serum are generally considered to be equally suitable for antibody detection.[21] Anticoagulated samples will be required by laboratories performing automated ABO and D grouping. The necessity for and timing of a second maternal sample during pregnancy is dependent on the antibody screening test result and on the D status of the mother.

Since anti-D is a frequently encountered antibody, and because it is capable of causing severe HDFN, women who are D negative should have a further blood sample taken at 28–30 weeks' gestation for a further screening test. Prophylactic anti-D should be administered to the mother immediately following venepuncture.[29,34] In the UK, some laboratories routinely perform a third antibody screen at 30–36 weeks' gestation in D-negative women. This practice is discouraged, because if a woman has received prophylactic anti-D, then the antibody screening test will be positive even if she has not produced an alloantibody.[20] Furthermore, it is unlikely that alloimmunization at such a late stage during pregnancy would cause severe HDFN.[20] Opinion is divided over whether D-positive women should have a second antibody screen performed at 28–36 weeks, if the screening test performed at booking is negative. This is no longer recommended in the USA,[29] but continues to be recommended in the UK[20] on the basis that very occasionally during pregnancy D-positive women produce antibodies that pose a potential threat to the fetus.[34,35] It would seem that the discrepancy between these guidelines arises from different views on the cost-effectiveness of repeat testing.[30]

3.4 The identification of red cell alloantibodies

When a red cell alloantibody has been detected using screening cells, further serological investigation is required in order to determine the nature and specificity of the antibody or antibodies that are present. This information is necessary in order for the obstetrician to take a view on the likely clinical significance for the fetus. It will also give the blood bank forewarning of any difficulties that may be encountered in providing blood for the mother, fetus or infant.

3.4.1 Methods

It is essential that an antiglobulin method be used to determine specificity, as activity by indirect antiglobulin test is the best indicator to the laboratory that a clinically significant antibody may be present. Usually, the particular indirect antiglobulin technique that was used for antibody screening will also be suitable for antibody identification. However, because solid-phase methods are more suitable for bulk testing, users of this method for screening often choose to employ an alternative method (e.g. gel or tube indirect antiglobulin test) for antibody identification.

Enzyme methods are generally considered to be more useful for antibody identification than for screening.[21,31] This is because enzyme methods are more sensitive than the indirect antiglobulin test for the detection of Rh antibodies and may, therefore, give clearer reaction patterns if a weakly reactive antibody is present. Furthermore, the use of a second method will improve the likelihood that the presence of more than one antibody specificity will be recognized and may make the resolution of these specificities easier. Finally, the propensity of enzyme methods to give unwanted positive results is less of an irritation with antibody identification work than with antibody screening.

A direct agglutination ('saline') method which detects antibodies capable of agglutinating red cells without the addition of an antiglobulin reagent is often used in antibody identification. However, antibodies that are reactive by this method are most likely to be IgM and, therefore, present no threat to the fetus. The value of the method again lies in the fact that some antibodies which react weakly by indirect antiglobulin test may be better detected by direct agglutination. Moreover, a secondary method may help resolve mixtures of antibody specificities. Workers using a tube indirect antiglobulin method can determine whether red cells are directly agglutinated by examining the red cells before the wash phase of the test is commenced.

3.4.2 The principles of antibody identification

In order to identify the specificity of an alloantibody, the maternal serum or plasma must be tested against a panel of red cells from at least eight individuals. These red cells will have been carefully selected by the supplier to ensure that almost all red cell antibodies, apart from those directed against low frequency antigens, will be reactive against at least one sample from the panel. The panel should also allow the resolution of commonly occurring mixtures of antibodies.[21,31]

When the mother's serum or plasma sample has been incubated with each example of red cells from the identification panel and the test results examined for reactivity, the assignment of results must be compared with the antigen profile of the panel cells. Correlation of positive and negative results with the presence and absence of an antigen on the red cells indicates an antibody of corresponding specificity.

The specificity of the antibody can be assigned with reasonable confidence when it reacts with at least two examples of red cells expressing an antigen and fails to react with at least two examples of red cells lacking the antigen.[21] A slightly more conservative approach is taken in the USA where the general recommendation is that three matching positive and three matching negative reactions should be obtained.[31] The discrepancy between the UK and US guidelines is discussed elsewhere.[36] When the presence of more than one antibody in the patient's plasma is suspected, only results with red cells that possess one or none of the appropriate antigens will be informative, unless the antibodies are detected by different techniques or unless their reaction strengths are very different.

A knowledge of the serological methods by which red cell antibodies of different specificities usually react helps identification. Table 3.3 shows the modes of reactivity and the frequency of occurrence of red cell alloantibodies which are active at 37 °C. Some practical examples of how an identification panel can be used to identify red cell antibodies are shown in Table 3.4. When an antibody has been clearly identified by an indirect antiglobulin method, the presence of other

Table 3.3 Characteristic modes of reactivity of red cell antibodies active at 37°C using three different techniques

System	Antigen	Mode of reactivity of antibody at 37°C			Occurrence at 37°C
		Indirect anti-globulin test	Papain[1]	Direct agglutination	
MNS	M	Some	No	Most	Common
	S	Most	No	Some	Common
	s	Yes	No	Rare	Uncommon
	U	Most	Most	Some	Very uncommon
P	P$_1$	Some	Some	Some	Uncommon
Rh	D	Many	Yes	Some	Very common
	C	Many	Yes	Some	Common
	c	Many	Yes	Rare	Common
	E	Many	Yes	Some	Common
	e	Many	Yes	Rare	Uncommon
	C^w	Many	Yes	Some	Common
Lutheran	Lu^a	Some	No	Some	Uncommon
	Lu^b	Most	No	Rare	Very uncommon
Kell	K	Most	Many	Some	Common
	k	Most	Some	Rare	Uncommon
	Kp^a	Most	Some	Rare	Common
	Kp^b	Most	Some	Rare	Very uncommon
	Js^a	Most	Rare	Rare	Very uncommon
	Js^b	Most	Rare	No	Very uncommon
Lewis	Le^a	Many	Many	Some	Common
	Le^b	Some	Many	Some	Uncommon
Duffy	Fy^a	Yes	No	Rare	Common
	Fy^b	Yes	No	Rare	Uncommon
	Fy3	Yes	Yes	Yes	Very uncommon
Kidd	Jk^a	Most	Some	Rare	Common
	Jk^b	Most	Some	Rare	Uncommon
Diego	Di^a	Most	Some	Some	Very rare
	Di^b	Most	Some	No	Very rare
Yt	Yt^a	Yes	No	No	Very uncommon
	Yt^b	Yes	No	No	Very rare
Xg	Xg^a	Most	No	Some	Very rare
Scianna	Sc1	Yes	No	No	Very rare
	Sc2	Most	Most	Some	Very rare
Dombrock	Do^a	Some	Some	No	Very rare
	Do^b	Yes	No	No	Very rare
Colton	Co^a	Most	Some	No	Very uncommon
	Co^b	Most	Some	No	Very uncommon

Note:

[1] Refers to a direct agglutination method using papain-treated red cells. Some antibodies which are nonreactive by this method will be reactive by a papain-IAGT.

Table 3.4 Three examples of the use of a 10-cell antibody identification panel

ABO	Rh D	C	C^w	c	E	e	MNS M	N	S	s	P P1	Lewis Le^a	Le^b	Kell K	k	Duffy Fy^a	Fy^b	Kidd Jk^a	Jk^b	#1 IAGT	#1 Enz	#2 IAGT	#2 Enz	#3 IAGT	#3 Enz
O ($R_1^wR_1$)	+	+	+	−	−	+	+	+	+	+	+	−	+	−	+	+	+	+	−	4	5	4	0	3	0
O (R_1R_1)	+	+	−	−	−	+	+	−	+	+	+	+	−	+	+	−	+	−	+	4	5	0	0	5	4
O (R_2R_2)	+	−	−	+	+	−	+	+	+	+	−	−	+	+	+	+	+	+	+	4	5	4	0	5	4
O (R_0)	+	−	−	+	−	+	+	+	−	+	−	−	−	−	+	−	−	−	+	4	5	0	0	0	0
O ($r'r$)	−	+	−	+	−	+	−	+	+	+	+	+	−	−	+	+	+	+	−	0	0	4	0	4	0
O ($r''r$)	−	−	−	+	+	+	+	+	+	+	+	−	+	−	+	−	−	+	+	0	0	0	0	3	0
O (rr)	−	−	−	+	−	+	+	+	−	+	+	−	−	+	+	+	+	+	−	0	0	4	0	5	4
O (rr)	−	−	−	+	−	+	−	+	+	+	−	+	−	−	+	+	+	−	+	0	0	4	0	3	0
O (rr)	−	−	−	+	−	+	+	−	−	+	−	−	+	−	+	+	−	+	+	0	0	4	0	0	0
O (rr)	−	−	−	+	−	+	+	+	+	−	−	−	+	−	+	+	−	−	+	0	0	4	0	5	4

Notes:

Key: IAGT = Indirect antiglobulin test; Enz = Enzyme test.

The presence or absence of an antigen on the panel red cells is indicated by a + or − respectively. For clarity, only some blood group antigens are shown. Reaction patterns of plasma samples #1, #2 and #3 with the panel red cells have been graded on a scale from 0 (negative, i.e. no reaction) to 5 (strongly positive), with grades 1, 2, 3 and 4 indicating increasingly strong reactivity.

Plasma sample #1

Reactivity with all D+ cells and lack of reactivity with all D− cells indicates that the sample contains anti-D active by antiglobulin and enzyme methods.

Plasma sample #2

This sample contains anti-Fy^a. Note the lack of reactivity with the enzyme method, because the Fy^a antigen is sited on a membrane glycoprotein that is subject to proteolysis by the enzymes papain, bromelain and ficin, commonly used in serology.

Plasma sample #3

The sample contains anti-K active by the indirect antiglobulin test and enzyme methods, and anti-S active by indirect antiglobulin test only. Note that the anti-S is showing 'dosage': stronger reactions are obtained with K−S+s− red cells than with K−S+s+ cells, because of the greater antigen site density in the former case.

antibodies should be excluded by ensuring that the panel cells that fail to react cover all of the blood group antigens corresponding to other clinically significant antibodies. Other methods, such as the enzyme method, help in this process of confirmation of specificity and exclusion of other antibody specificities. This is illustrated in Table 3.4. Results from samples #1 and #2 show that this process may be straightforward using a single indirect antiglobulin method. Sample #3, however, has given a pattern of reactivity which is more difficult to interpret, and the value of an additional enzyme method is demonstrated by its ability to pick out one specificity (anti-K in this case). Although the requirement of the 'two positive and two negative cells' guideline has been met (at least two of each of K+S−, K−S+ and K−S− red cells in this case), many workers would consider it advisable to test sample #3 against more examples of K−S− red cells, in order to improve the confidence with which antibody specificity has been assigned.

It is good practice to phenotype the mother's red cells using a typing reagent of the same specificity as that assigned to the antibody following identification, because a negative result with this reagent provides some confirmation of the assigned specificity. A positive result with the mother's blood would either indicate that the antibody is an autoantibody rather than an alloantibody, or that the mother's red cells have a variant expression of antigen, or that the assigned specificity is incorrect. Indirect antiglobulin test active autoantibodies are rarely encountered in antenatal serology and generally their presence can be confirmed by performing a direct antiglobulin test on the mother's red cells. Autoantibodies often show no obvious specificity, although autoantibodies with an apparent anti-e specificity are not infrequent. By far the most commonly encountered examples of a variant expression of antigen are the partial D phenotypes (Section 2.5.1).

3.4.3 Difficulties encountered in antibody identification

Sometimes the pattern of reactivity obtained using the identification panel does not show a clear correlation with the profile of one antigen. There are a number of possible explanations for this finding. One of the most likely is that the patient's plasma contains antibodies of more than one specificity. The process by which multiple antibody specificities in a single sample are resolved is similar to that described above, but only occasionally can mixtures of antibodies be resolved using a single identification panel. Usually, a second panel is needed, and sometimes even this is insufficient.

Resolving difficult serological problems is time-consuming and requires care and expertise. However, the time within which a reliable conclusion is arrived at can often be reduced by:

• a knowledge of a pre-existing antibody or antibodies, which will enable the serologist to select red cells that lack the corresponding antigens early on in the investigation, so that other antibodies can be identified or excluded more quickly;

- using other methods, such as the use of papain-treated red cells in the indirect antiglobulin test, which may facilitate the resolution of complex mixtures or the identification of more unusual specificities;
- the careful use of reaction grades (see example #3 in Table 3.4); and
- phenotyping the mother's red cells early on in the investigation, so that likely specificities of alloantibodies can be recognized.

Many red cell alloantibodies show different strengths of reactivity with different examples of antigen-positive red cells and, consequently, may cause extra difficulty in identification. In general, this variability in reactivity is caused by variable antigen expression on the red cell membrane. Antibodies such as anti-c, -e, -M, -S and -Jk^a often show *dosage*, which means that they react more strongly with red cells having homozygous expression of the corresponding gene than with red cells having heterozygous expression (see sample #3 in Table 3.4).

Some antibodies, for example anti-Kn^a and anti-Ch, are particularly difficult to identify, because they show variable reactivity with antigen-positive red cells and because the presence or absence of antigen is not reflected in the antigen profile of the cell panel for antibody identification. Furthermore, antibodies that are directed against high frequency antigens (antigens having a frequency greater than 99% in the general population) can rarely be properly identified without recourse to a special frozen panel of red cells having rare phenotypes. In these situations, the sample should be sent to a reference laboratory that has the resources to undertake more extensive serological investigations.

3.4.4 Implications of detecting a red cell alloantibody during pregnancy

The need for further laboratory work when a red cell alloantibody has been identified depends on the nature and specificity of the antibody detected. It can be assumed that an indirect antiglobulin test-active antibody is likely to be IgG. However, even if the antibody is known to be IgG, it may be of a specificity that is rarely (Section 2.7) or never (Section 2.8) associated with HDFN. Notwithstanding this, as a general rule, the laboratory should determine the potency of an indirect antiglobulin test-active antibody either using a quantitative (Section 8.2) or serological (Section 8.1) assay.

Although it is generally agreed that samples should only be tested when it is likely that results could influence the clinical management of the pregnancy, opinion differs regarding the usefulness of repeat assays of antibody potency during pregnancy. In the USA, there is no clear consensus as to the value of a critical titre below which invasive techniques need not be undertaken.[31] Guidelines in the UK, on the other hand, make specific recommendations concerning the interpretation of anti-D levels (obtained using continuous flow analyzers) and other antibody levels

Table 3.5 Flow chart for red cell antibody testing during pregnancy[1]

	Gestation		
10–16 weeks	17–27 weeks	28–34 weeks	35 weeks–delivery
Anti-D detected	Perform quantitative assay, and check for additional antibodies, at least monthly	Perform quantitative assay, and check for additional antibodies every 2 weeks	Perform quantitative assay, and check for additional antibodies every 2 weeks
Anti-c or Kell-related antibody detected	Perform serological assay, and check for additional antibodies, at least monthly	Perform serological assay, and check for additional antibodies every 2 weeks	Perform serological assay, and check for additional antibodies every 2 weeks
Other antiglobulin test active antibody detected	No testing necessary	Perform serological assay and check for additional antibody	No testing necessary

Note:
[1] Adapted from BCSH guidelines, 1996.[20]

(obtained by serological titration), which will provide the obstetrician with information that may influence clinical management, even when fetal monitoring has begun.[21] A synopsis of the UK British Committee for Standards in Haematology Guidelines is shown in Table 3.5.

3.5 Paternal and fetal phenotyping

In addition to phenotyping red cells from the mother for the reasons described above, it may be useful to establish the phenotypes of red cells from the father and fetus.

3.5.1 Paternal phenotype

If a mother's plasma has been shown to contain a red cell antibody that could affect the fetus, a paternal sample should be requested wherever possible. The paternal red cells can then be phenotyped for the relevant antigen and for its antithetical (alternative) antigen, thus providing information regarding the likelihood of the fetus inheriting the antigen and thereby being exposed to risk of HDFN. In blood group systems such as Kell, where there is a pair of antithetical antigens, interpretation of the phenotype is relatively straightforward. For example, the paternal phenotype K+k+ would indicate that the paternal genotype is *Kk*, and, therefore, that the fetus has an equal (50%) chance of inheriting a paternal *K* gene or a paternal *k* gene. If the maternal alloantibody is anti-K, and the maternal red cells *kk*, the fetus will inherit a maternal *k* gene. There is, therefore, an equal chance that the fetus will

Table 3.6 Estimates of the likelihood of homozygosity for D in Caucasians

Phenotype	Anti-D	Anti-C	Anti-c	Anti-E	Anti-e	Alternative genotypes[1]		Likelihood[2] of homozygosity for D
			Phenotyping reagent					
R_1r	+	+	+	−	+	*DCe/dce*	R^1r	4.8%
						DCe/Dce	R^1R^0	
R_1R_1	+	+	−	−	+	*DCe/DCe*	R^1R^1	97.6%
						DCe/dCe	R^1r'	
R_2r	+	−	+	+	+	*DcE/dce*	R^2r	4.8%
						DcE/Dce	R^2R^0	
R_1R_2	+	+	+	+	+	*DCe/DcE*	R^1R^2	96.7%
						DCe/dcE	R^1r''	
						dCe/DcE	$r'R^2$	
R_2R_2	+	−	+	+	−	*DcE/DcE*	R^2R^2	96.6%
						DcE/dcE	R^2r''	

Notes:

[1] Rare alternative genotypes have not been shown.

[2] Based on Swedish genotype frequencies.[37]

have the genotype *Kk* or *kk*, and therefore an equal chance that the fetus could be affected by the maternal anti-K.

Unfortunately, paternal phenotyping for D is less useful, because there is no antigen antithetical to D. However, linkage disequilibrium between the *D* and *CE* genes means that, if anti-D, -C, -c, -E and -e reagents are used, an estimate of the likely homozygosity for D can be determined (Table 3.6). This approach is reliable for Caucasians, but may be less so for nonCaucasians, because of the differences in gene frequencies in different ethnic groups. For example, the R^0 (*Dce*) haplotype is much more common in some nonCaucasian populations.

3.5.2 Fetal phenotype

This may be determined directly from a pretransfusion fetal blood sample. Care must be taken in interpreting results because both false positive and false negative results may be obtained. Wherever possible, IgM monoclonal phenotyping reagents should be used. A direct antiglobulin test should also be performed on the fetal red cells in order to determine whether the fetal cells have been coated with antibody. The expected findings are either both tests negative (for example, fetus D negative and direct antiglobulin test negative if the maternal antibody is anti-D) or both tests positive (for example, fetus D positive and direct antiglobulin test positive). If the direct antiglobulin test is strongly positive, and phenotyping for the putative implicated antigen gives a negative result using an IgM reagent, 'blocking' of antigen sites by large amounts of maternal antibody should be suspected. A reliable phenotyping result can usually be obtained in these circumstances by removal of the antibody using chloroquine diphosphate[38] or 'ZZAP' reagent.[39] Phenotyping red cells which are direct antiglobulin test positive should not be performed using IgG-specific antiglobulin reagents if at all possible.

Molecular genetic methods provide an alternative to serological methods for typing fetal red cells. These methods are based on the analysis of fetal DNA usually harvested from amniotic fluid and are considered in detail in Chapter 7.

3.6 Laboratory tests immediately following delivery

There is no need for the blood bank to perform laboratory tests on infants of D-positive women unless the infant develops signs suggestive of HDFN or unless the mother is known to have a red cell antibody that may be causative of HDFN. A direct antiglobulin test should then be performed on cord blood cells.

Maternal and cord samples should be taken from D-negative women who have not produced anti-D. The cord sample should be used to determine the infant's D status, thus identifying women who must receive prophylactic anti-D immunoglobulin. A direct antiglobulin test should be performed on cord red cells when the infant is D positive, if the infant develops signs suggestive of HDFN or if the mother is known to have a red cell antibody that may be causative of HDFN.

A positive direct antiglobulin test indicates the potential for a haemolytic process, but the degree of red cell agglutination does not correlate well with the severity of haemolysis. Confirmation of the specificity of the causative antibody can be obtained by testing the plasma or serum of a maternal or cord sample. Elution of antibody from cord red cells may also be helpful.[20,31] If the direct antiglobulin test is positive and tests for red cell alloantibodies are negative, then it is likely that an ABO antibody or an antibody to a low frequency antigen has coated the cord cells. The former can be identified by testing the eluate against A1 and B cells. If an antibody to a low frequency antigen is suspected, then some confirmation may be obtained by testing the eluate against paternal red cells, but determination of the specificity will probably require referral to a reference laboratory.[31]

In addition to these serological tests, a test should also be performed to determine the requirement for anti-D immunoglobulin (Section 6.3). Cord Hb and bilirubin concentrations should also be measured.

3.7 References

1 Levine P & Stetson RE (1939). An unusual case of intra-group agglutination. *Journal of the American Medical Association*, 113, 126–7.

2 Race RR (1944). An 'incomplete' antibody in human serum. *Nature*, **153**, 771–2.

3 Wiener AS (1944). A new test (blocking test) for Rh sensitization. *Proceedings of the Society for Experimental Biology*, **56**, 173.

4 Diamond LK & Denton RL (1945). Rh agglutination in various media with particular references to the value of albumin. *Journal of Laboratory and Clinical Medicine*, **30**, 821.

5 Coombs RRA, Mourant AE & Race RR (1946). In vivo iso-sensitization of red cells in babies with haemolytic disease. *Lancet*, **i**, 264–5.

6 Morton JA & Pickles MM (1947). Use of trypsin in the detection of incomplete anti-Rh antibodies. *Nature*, **159**, 779.

7 Coombs RRA, Mourant AE & Race RR (1945). Detection of weak and 'incomplete' Rh agglutinins: a new test. *Lancet*, **ii**, 15–16.

8 Moreschi C (1908). Neue Tatsachen über die blutkörperchen agglutinationen. *Zentrabl Bakteriol Parasitenk*, **46**, 49, 456.

9 Knight RC & Poole GD (1995). Detection of red cell antibodies: current and future techniques. *British Journal of Biomedical Science*, **52**, 297–305.

10 Moore HC & Mollison PL (1976). Use of a low-ionic-strength medium in manual tests for antibody detection. *Transfusion*, **16**, 291–6.

11 Nance SJ & Garratty G (1987). A new potentiator of red blood cell antigen-antibody reactions. *American Journal of Clinical Pathology*, **87**, 633–5.

12 Lalezari P & Jiang AF (1980). The manual polybrene test: a simple and rapid procedure for detection of red cell antibodies. *Transfusion*, **20**, 206–11.

13 British Committee for Standards in Haematology (1991). Compatibility testing in hospital blood banks. In *Standard Haematology Practice*, ed. B. Roberts. Oxford: Blackwell Scientific, pp. 150–63.

14 Lapierre Y, Rigal D, Adam J et al. (1990). The gel test: a new way to detect red cell antigen-antibody reactions. *Transfusion*, **30**, 109–13.

15 Reis KJ, Chachowski R, Cupido A, Davies D, Jakway J & Setcavage TM (1993). Column agglutination technology: the antiglobulin test. *Transfusion*, **33**, 639–43.

16 Plapp FV, Sinor LT, Rachel JM, Beck ML, Coenen WM & Bayer WL (1984). A solid phase antibody screen. *American Journal of Clinical Pathology*, **82**, 719–21.

17 Rachel JM, Sinor LT, Beck ML & Plapp FV (1985). A solid-phase antiglobulin test. *Transfusion*, **25**, 24–6.

18 Hazenburg CAM, Mulder MB & Beelen JM (1990). Erythrocyte antibody screening in solid-phase: a comparison of two solid-phase microplate assays with the indirect antiglobulin test in polyethylene glycol for the detection of irregular erythrocyte antibodies. *Vox Sanguinis*, **59**, 96–100.

19 Poole GD, Evans RG, Voak D, Scott ML, Chapman JF & Phillips PK (1996). Evaluation of six systems for the detection of red cell antibodies. *MDD Evaluation Report MDA/96/14*. London: HMSO.

20 British Committee for Standards in Haematology (1996). Guidelines for blood grouping and red cell antibody testing during pregnancy. *Transfusion Medicine*, **6**, 71–4.

21 British Committee for Standards in Haematology (1996). Guidelines for pre-transfusion compatibility procedures in blood transfusion laboratories. *Transfusion Medicine*, **6**, 273–83.

22 Voak D (1992). Validation of new technology for antibody detection by antiglobulin tests. *Transfusion Medicine*, 2, 177–9.

23 British Committee for Standards in Haematology (1995). Guidelines for evaluation, validation and implementation of new techniques for blood grouping, antibody screening and crossmatching. *Transfusion Medicine*, 5, 145–50.

24 Löw B (1955). A practical method using papain and incomplete Rh-antibodies in routine Rh blood-grouping. *Vox Sanguinis*, 5, 94–101.

25 Pirofsky B & Mangum MEJ (1959). Use of bromelain to demonstrate erythrocyte antibodies. *Proceedings of the Society for Experimental Biology*, 101, 49–56.

26 Ellisor SE (1982). Action and application of enzymes in immunohematology. In *Seminar on Antigen-Antibody Reactions Revisited*, ed. CA Bell. Arlington, VA: American Association of Blood Banks, pp. 133–74.

27 Garner SF, Devenish A, Barber H & Contreras M (1991). The importance of monitoring 'enzyme-only' red cell antibodies during pregnancy. *Vox Sanguinis*, 61, 219–20.

28 Judd WJ, Steiner EA & Nugent CE (1992). Appropriate serological testing in pregnancy. *Vox Sanguinis*, 63, 293–6.

29 Judd WJ, Luban NLC, Ness PM, Silberstein LE, Stroup M & Widmann FK (1990). Prenatal and perinatal immunohematology: recommendations for serologic management of the fetus, newborn infant, and obstetric patient. *Transfusion*, 30, 175–83.

30 Issitt PD & Anstee DJ (1998). *Applied Blood Group Serology*, 4th edn. Durham, NC: Montgomery Scientific Publications.

31 American Association of Blood Banks (1999). *Technical Manual*, 13th edn, ed. V Vengelen-Tyler. Bethesda, MD: American Association of Blood Banks.

32 Morelati F, Revelli N, Maffei LM et al. (1998). Evaluation of a new automated instrument for pretransfusion testing. *Transfusion*, 38, 959–65.

33 Sandler SG, Langeberg A, Avery N & Mintz PD (2000). A fully automated blood typing system for hospital transfusion services. *Transfusion*, 40, 201–7.

34 British Blood Transfusion Society/Royal College of Obstetricians and Gynaecologists Joint Working Party (1999). Recommendations for the use of anti-D immunoglobulin for Rh prophylaxis. *Transfusion Medicine*, 9, 93–7.

35 Bowell PJ, Allen DL & Entwistle CC (1986). Blood group antibody screening tests during pregnancy. *British Journal of Obstetrics and Gynaecology*, 93, 1038–43.

36 Kanter MH, Poole G & Garratty G (1997). Misinterpretation and misapplication of p values in antibody identification: the lack of value of a p value. *Transfusion*, 37, 816–22.

37 Heiken A & Rasmuson M (1966). Genetical studies on the Rh blood group system. *Hereditas Lund*, 55, 192–212.

38 Edwards JM, Moulds JJ & Judd WJ (1982). Chloroquine diphosphate dissociation of antigen-antibody complexes: a new technique for phenotyping rbcs with a positive direct antiglobulin test. *Transfusion*, 22, 59–61.

39 Branch DR & Petz LD (1982). A new reagent (ZZAP) having multiple applications in immuno-hematology. *American Journal of Clinical Pathology*, 78, 161–7.

Epidemiology and screening for alloimmune thrombocytopenia

Lorna M Williamson[1] and Michael F Murphy[2]

[1] National Blood Service and University of Cambridge, Cambridge, UK
[2] National Blood Service and University of Oxford, Oxford, UK

4.1 Background

Alloimmune thrombocytopenia is the commonest cause of severe neonatal thrombocytopenia. The pathophysiology and diagnosis of the disorder are described elsewhere (Sections 1.1.3, 1.3.3 and Chapter 12). Most cases are diagnosed after birth, hence the commonly used term *neonatal alloimmune thrombocytopenia*. However, there may be severe effects on the fetus in utero, and this, as well as the aetiology, may be emphasized through the use of the alternative term, *alloimmune thrombocytopenia*. In contrast to HDFN, alloimmune thrombocytopenia frequently occurs in first pregnancies.[1,2]

Considerable progress has been made in laboratory aspects of platelet immunology since alloimmune thrombocytopenia was first recognized in the 1950s, allowing more precise diagnosis of the condition (Section 12.4).[3] There have also been advances in fetal and transfusion medicine resulting in improvements in its management, particularly in the antenatal management of women with a previous history of pregnancies affected by alloimmune thrombocytopenia (Section 14.3). These advances in laboratory diagnosis and antenatal management have drawn attention to the fact that the first affected fetus/neonate in a family is only recognized after bleeding has occurred, and this has raised the question of screening for alloimmune thrombocytopenia.

The purpose of this chapter is to review the epidemiology of alloimmune thrombocytopenia and then to consider the case for antenatal screening against the criteria for screening programmes set by the UK's Department of Health National Screening Committee. Finally, areas where knowledge is still lacking, and where research effort should be directed, will be highlighted.

Table 4.1 Alloimmune thrombocytopenia due to HPA-la alloimmunisation during pregnancy

Study (reference)	Number of pregnant women studied	Number of HPA-la-negative women	Number of women with anti-HPA-la	Overall incidence of alloimmune thrombocytopenia
4	1211	26 (2.2%)	2/23 (8.7%)	2 (1:600)
5	5000	81 (1.6%)	3/50 (6%)	1 (1:5000)
6	3473	74 (2.2%)	2/22 (9.1%)	3* (1:1150)
7	24417	618 (2.5%)	46/387 (12%)	22 (1:1100)
9	15471	—	—	10 (1:1500)
10	5362	—	—	5 (1:1126)

Note: * including one twin pregnancy.

4.2 Epidemiology and the natural history of alloimmune thrombocytopenia

4.2.1 The incidence of maternal alloimmunization

Series of cases of alloimmune thrombocytopenia with detectable platelet-specific alloantibodies have implicated anti-HPA-1a in 78–89% of cases; anti-HPA-5b is involved in 6–15% of cases and the remainder are due to other specificities.[1] Thrombocytopenia due to anti-HPA-5b has been reported to be less severe than that due to anti-HPA-1a, but there are few data on the severity of alloimmune thrombocytopenia due to other HPA antibodies.[2]

About 2.5% of pregnant Caucasian women are HPA-1a negative and most of these women will carry HPA-1a-positive fetuses, as 97.5% of individuals are HPA-1a positive. However, only about 10% of HPA-1a-negative women develop anti-HPA-1a (Table 4.1).[4-7] Alloimmunization to HPA-1a appears to be restricted to women with the HLA-DRw52a (HLA-DR3*0101) gene. This is present in only one in three Caucasian women (Section 1.1.3). HPA-1a alloimmunization is rare in women who lack this antigen,[8] with a negative predictive value of the absence of HLA-DR3*0101 for HPA-1a alloimmunization in HPA-1a-negative women of >99%. However, the positive predictive value of its presence for alloimmunization has been estimated to be only 35%,[7] limiting its usefulness in antenatal screening and suggesting that different HLA or some nonHLA genes are also involved. Furthermore, the additional costs of HLA typing would be considerable and these would be much greater than the modest costs of screening all HPA-1a-negative women for HPA-1a antibodies regardless of their HLA type.

4.2.2 The incidence of fetal thrombocytopenia due to maternal alloimmunization

In a large prospective study of 24417 pregnancies in East Anglia, UK, the incidence of severe thrombocytopenia (less than 50×10^9/l) at birth due to alloimmune thrombocytopenia was one in 1100.[7] This is in agreement with previous smaller studies (Table 4.1).[4,6,9,10] It can be estimated that the number of cases of allo-immune thrombocytopenia in the UK is about 400–800 each year (based on 800 000 births in the UK annually and an incidence of alloimmune thrombocyto-penia of one in 1000–2000). It is generally agreed that alloimmune thrombocyto-penia is underdiagnosed in routine clinical practice and this was supported by a recent survey of haematologists in the UK on the recognition and postnatal man-agement of alloimmune thrombocytopenia.[11]

4.2.3 The incidence of intracranial haemorrhage and other sequelae

In considering the frequency of clinical sequelae, care must be taken to differentiate the incidence reported in series of clinically apparent alloimmune thrombocyto-penia from incidence figures derived from screening studies. The incidence of severe thrombocytopenia (one in 1100) in the screening study of Williamson et al. included those cases which would have been diagnosed clinically as well as some asymptomatic cases which would not.[7] The number of asymptomatic cases of alloimmune thrombocytopenia ranges from 10% to 25% of those alloimmu-nized,[1,2,7] and so the incidence of clinically affected cases can be reliably estimated as being in the region of one in 1500 pregnancies.

The long-term outcome in severe cases of alloimmune thrombocytopenia may be devastating, entailing blindness and major physical and mental disability. Intracerebral haemorrhage, which is the major cause of mortality and long-term morbidity in alloimmune thrombocytopenia, occurs in 15–20% of clinically apparent cases. In one study of 137 cases, death due to severe haemorrhage occurred in 7% and there were neurological sequelae in 21%.[2] Although there is a serious risk of severe haemorrhage at the time of delivery, nearly 50% of intracere-bral haemorrhages occur in utero, usually between 30 and 35 weeks of gestation, but sometimes before 20 weeks. There may be more unusual presentations such as isolated fetal hydrocephalus, unexplained fetal anaemia or recurrent miscar-riages.[12] Determination of the long-term clinical effects of alloimmune thrombo-cytopenia in a large cohort of affected children is an area where future research is required.

4.2.4 The influence of obstetric history on clinical outcome

The subsequent pregnancies of HPA-1a alloimmunized women with a history of a previously affected infant are well recognized to be associated with a high risk of recurrence, and a poor outcome.[13] For example, the 10 cases in the report by Burrows and Kelton[9] occurred predominantly in women with a past history of alloimmune thrombocytopenia. All neonates had cord blood platelet counts of less than 50×10^9/l, the majority below 20×10^9/l; three had intracerebral haemorrhages in utero, and one was stillborn. This provides the justification for early antenatal intervention to reduce the risk of morbidity and mortality from severe haemorrhage in families with a past history of an affected infant.

The outcome of pregnancies of women with anti-HPA-1a but no history is different from those with a past history of affected pregnancies. In the prospective study of 24 417 pregnancies by Williamson et al.,[7] of the 26 infants born to women with persistent antibodies in the antenatal period, nine were severely thrombocytopenic (platelet counts less than 50×10^9/l) and 10 had mild thrombocytopenia (platelet counts $50–150 \times 10^9$/l). One had definite evidence of major antenatal intracerebral haemorrhage, and one died due to haemorrhage after fetal blood sampling carried out to investigate unexplained fetal hydrops which itself could have been due to chronic haemorrhage resulting in fetal anaemia. The former infant was found to have a large intracerebral haemorrhage following emergency Caesarean section at 37 weeks' gestation carried out because of an abnormal heart trace during labour; hydrocephalus developed, and the child now has delayed motor development and optic atrophy. From this large study, the incidence of severe antenatal intracerebral haemorrhage appears to be in the range of one in 12 500–25 000 pregnancies.

4.3 Criteria for antenatal screening for alloimmune thrombocytopenia

An important consideration is whether to carry out screening antenatally or postnatally. The advantages of antenatal screening is that alloimmunized women can be identified during the index pregnancy, allowing time for antenatal intervention if this is agreed to be appropriate. Even if no antenatal intervention is undertaken, the mode and timing of delivery could then be planned to ensure minimal trauma to the baby's head and that compatible platelets are made available. Postnatal screening can be achieved by simply carrying out a platelet count on a cord blood sample, but the major drawback of this approach is that the key objective of screening, to prevent morbidity and mortality from intracerebral haemorrhage, is unlikely to be achieved in the first affected pregnancy.

At present in the UK, antenatal screening for alloimmune thrombocytopenia is not routine practice. It is therefore useful to examine the case for screening against the criteria for screening programmes set by the UK's Department of Health Screening Committee. These 10 criteria are considered below in relation to alloimmune thrombocytopenia.

4.3.1 The condition should be an important health problem

The incidence of severe antenatal haemorrhage appears to be in the range of one in 12 500–25 000 pregnancies, equating to 32–64 cases in the UK each year.[7] Assuming that only 50% of fetuses with severe antenatal haemorrhage survive, it can be estimated that there will be 16–32 infants each year in the UK with severe physical and/or mental disability caused by alloimmune thrombocytopenia requiring long-term care with its considerable associated costs.

4.3.2 The epidemiology of the condition should be known

As described above, the epidemiology of the condition is well understood; the incidence of clinically affected cases can be reliably estimated as being in the region of one in 1500 pregnancies.

4.3.3 The natural history of the condition should be understood

The natural history of alloimmune thrombocytopenia is described above. Unfortunately, there is no reliable predictor of severe clinical disease which might be used to select pregnancies for aggressive intervention. In the study of Williamson et al.,[7] a high titre of anti-HPA-1a was predictive of a fetal platelet count of less than $50 \times 10^9/l$, but this observation has yet to be confirmed by other studies using state-of-the-art antibody detection techniques. Furthermore, the limitations of HPA antibody detection and variation in antibody titres were highlighted in a recent quality assessment exercise carried out by platelet serology laboratories.[14] An alternative approach is to examine the biological functions of HPA antibodies. Bioassays such as chemiluminescence and antibody-dependent cell-mediated cytotoxicity have been used in HDFN (Section 8.4) but their role in alloimmune thrombocytopenia has not been established. Some examples of anti-HPA-1a inhibit megakaryocyte precursors in bone marrow cultures.[15] The role of inhibition of erythropoiesis is well established in HDFN due to anti-K (Section 2.5.3),[16] but further work is required to determine if a similar correlation exists in alloimmune thrombocytopenia. The lack of laboratory parameters predictive of severe disease remains a major barrier to routine antenatal screening for alloimmune thrombocytopenia and is an important area for future research.

4.3.4 There should be a recognized latent period or early asymptomatic stage

This could be defined as the presence of maternal anti-HPA antibodies without fetal/neonatal thrombocytopenia, mild thrombocytopenia or even severe thrombocytopenia, but without clinical sequelae. One of the difficulties of antenatal screening for alloimmune thrombocytopenia is that fetal blood sampling is required to differentiate between these degrees of clinical severity in the antenatal period. This has the potential to cause fetal loss from haemorrhage from the cord or to induce premature delivery.[17] There is also the potential to boost antibody levels by causing fetomaternal haemorrhage. Fetal blood sampling for alloimmune thrombocytopenia should be performed at referral centres, where the risk is about 1%. The main problems are most likely with early fetal blood sampling at around 20–22 weeks' gestation when the cord is small and the platelet count may be very low. In the series of Murphy et al.,[18] which extends to nearly 200 fetal blood samplings for alloimmune thrombocytopenia, there were two fetal deaths, one due to bleeding and one due to a cord haematoma.

4.3.5 All the cost-effective primary prevention interventions should have been implemented as far as practicable

There are no available primary prevention interventions for alloimmune thrombocytopenia.

4.3.6 There should be a simple, safe, precise and validated screening test

The first consideration in formulating an approach to screening is to decide whether to type pregnant women for HPA-1a (the antigen) or to test them for anti-HPA-1a (the antibodies). Typing for HPA-1a seems to be the logical first step since 98% of women are HPA-1a positive and can be excluded from further investigation. Reliable assays are available for HPA-1a phenotyping using platelet-rich plasma,[19] platelet-poor plasma[20] or whole blood.[20-22] Genotyping for HPA-1a can be carried out, but it is not yet feasible on a large scale.

Where the father is heterozygous (HPA-1a/1b), it would be advantageous to HPA-1 type the fetus, who has a 50% chance of being HPA-1b/1b (HPA-1a negative) like the mother, and therefore not at risk of alloimmune thrombocytopenia. HPA-1 genotyping can be carried out using chorionic villous or amniotic fluid samples to avoid the risks of fetal blood sampling. In the future, it may be possible to carry out typing for platelet antigens using samples of maternal plasma, as has been described for fetal RhD typing.[23]

Antibody screening can be carried out by a number of different assays. The most commonly used is the monoclonal antibody immobilization of platelet antigens (MAIPA) assay (Section 12.4.2.2) which is both sensitive and specific. However, even reference laboratories do not obtain entirely congruent results and further improvements are required.[14] It is recognized that anti-HPA-1a is undetectable in a small proportion of HPA-1a-negative women with pregnancies affected by alloimmune thrombocytopenia, but the proportion of such cases appears to be decreasing as the testing methods improve.

4.3.7 The distribution of test values in the target population should be known and a suitable cut-off level defined and agreed

HPA-1a typing is generally very reliable, even when used on a large scale, although two HPA-1a negative women were typed incorrectly in a large prospective study of 24417 women[7]; these women had affected infants and were found to be HPA-1a-negative on retesting. A recently developed ELISA method using maternal whole blood and a novel recombinant HPA-1a monoclonal antibody lends itself to large-scale screening as it is suitable for automated sample handling.[22]

Since testing for anti-HPA-1a antibodies is not entirely reliable, it is possible that a small number of affected pregnancies would be missed by a screening algorithm using antibody testing as the first step.

4.3.8 The test should be acceptable to the population

With public concern about the ethical aspects of screening for inherited diseases, it is easy to imagine that screening for alloimmune thrombocytopenia could be perceived as being 'genetic' screening. However, in the large study of Williamson et al.,[7] 74% of HPA-1a-negative women agreed to enrol for further investigation; fetal blood sampling was not part of the protocol but available at a reference centre if requested. All women found to have anti-HPA-1a chose to be managed conservatively, although knowledge of the presence of antibodies increased the rate of Caesarean section to 36% from a baseline level of 15%.

4.3.9 There should be an agreed policy on the further diagnostic investigation of individuals with a positive result and on the choices available to those individuals

There are a number of screening and confirmatory algorithms which could be adopted. A feasible approach to antenatal screening might involve HPA-1a typing at the initial antenatal booking visit to identify HPA-1a-negative women. No additional blood sample would be required, as HPA-1a typing could be carried out on the sample already taken routinely for blood grouping and antibody screening at booking for antenatal care at 10–16 weeks' gestation. As the management protocol discussed below (Section 4.3.10) proposes that no antenatal intervention would be considered until the third trimester, testing for anti-HPA-1a would not be necessary until 28 weeks, when a sample for further red cell antibody testing is routinely taken.[24] Two cohorts of HPA-1a-negative patients would be identified: (1) the non-alloimmunized patients could be considered to be at very low risk for alloimmune thrombocytopenia, and any further intervention (either antenatal or postnatal) would not appear to be justified; and (2) the alloimmunized patients would be considered to be at risk for alloimmune thrombocytopenia. The preferred option for antenatal intervention in women with anti-HPA-1a with no previous history of pregnancies affected by alloimmune thrombocytopenia is not yet clearly identified (Section 4.3.10) and is an area requiring further research.

4.3.10 There should be an effective treatment or intervention for patients identified through early detection

Along with a lack of predictors of severe disease, the lack of consistently effective antenatal therapy for alloimmune thrombocytopenia is a major barrier to routine antenatal screening. There is considerable experience in the antenatal management of alloimmune thrombocytopenia where there has been a previously affected pregnancy, but the optimal management still remains controversial. Therapeutic options are described in detail elsewhere (Section 14.3) and are considered here only briefly. The main options are maternal administration of intravenous immunoglobulin and fetal platelet transfusions; early Caesarean section alone is not considered to be effective in preventing antenatal or perinatal haemorrhage. For both approaches to antenatal management, fetal blood sampling is required for the initial assessment of the fetal platelet count, usually at 20–22 weeks' gestation, and for the monitoring of the effectiveness of treatment.

In one North American study, maternal administration of intravenous immunoglobulin was reported to be successful with no instances of intracerebral haemorrhage and most, but not all, infants achieved a platelet count of greater than 30 $\times 10^9$/l at the end of pregnancy.[13] The addition of steroids did not add to the effect of intravenous immunoglobulin. However, other studies have reported intracerebral haemorrhage during maternal treatment with intravenous immunoglobulin,[25] and a group of European centres treating 37 pregnancies only found success with the use of maternal intravenous immunoglobulin in seven (26%) of 27 cases, and steroids in one (10%) of 10.[26]

It is difficult to understand why there is such an apparent difference in the success of maternal administration of intravenous immunoglobulin between North America and Europe. Relevant factors may include the methods used for assessing the success of treatment and the dose, timing and type of intravenous immunoglobulin used. This is discussed in more detail elsewhere (Section 14.3.2.2). The selection of cases may also be important, and it has been suggested that therapeutic failures occur more frequently in severe cases.[18] The direct injection of IgG to the fetus by cordocentesis was successful in raising the fetal platelet count in one case.[27] However, this method of administering intravenous immunoglobulin has all the risks of fetal blood sampling discussed above, and was not found to be effective by another group.[28]

A number of studies have shown the value of platelet transfusions given by cordocentesis in raising the platelet count, but the platelet count is raised for only a few days. A single predelivery transfusion may protect against bleeding at the time of delivery, but the fetus remains at risk of spontaneous intracerebral haemorrhage earlier in pregnancy. Weekly in utero platelet transfusions have been shown to be effective in preventing intracerebral haemorrhage in severe cases of alloimmune thrombocytopenia.[18] In utero platelet transfusions are described in detail elsewhere (Section 14.3.3).

For pregnancies in HPA-1a-alloimmunized women without a past history of thrombocytopenia, the decision about appropriate antenatal intervention and its timing are problematic. Fetal blood sampling would be required to determine the fetal platelet count and thus the need for treatment. It is likely that a compromise between minimizing the risks of fetal blood sampling and carrying out the procedure early enough to allow effective antenatal treatment in severe cases could be achieved by performing fetal blood sampling at around 30 weeks' gestation.

4.3.11 There should be agreed evidence-based policies covering which individuals should be offered treatment and the appropriate treatment to be offered

As already discussed, there are no evidence-based policies for determining which women with anti-HPA-1a, but without a previous history of affected pregnancies, should be offered treatment, and which should not. Further research is required to identify factors predictive of severe disease and it may be necessary to carry out further large-scale antenatal screening studies to collect the relevant clinical material and to confirm the association of the suspected factor with clinical severity. Likewise, the optimal antenatal treatment is unknown, and further studies are also required in this field.

4.3.12 Clinical management of the condition and patient outcomes should be optimized by all health providers prior to participation in a screening programme

As discussed above, there is as yet no consensus on the optimal treatment for alloimmune thrombocytopenia. Therapeutic options are discussed in detail elsewhere (Section 14.3).

4.4 The cost-effectiveness of a screening programme

There have been no randomized controlled trials to show that antenatal screening for alloimmune thrombocytopenia can reduce morbidity or mortality or that the benefit of the screening programme outweighs the potential for physical and psychological harm. A major problem in the performance of such a trial is the low incidence of intracerebral haemorrhage. An exhaustively large number of women would have to be screened to demonstrate a benefit from intervention. It has been estimated that a randomized study comparing conservative management with invasive therapy with intracerebral haemorrhage as the primary endpoint would require one million pregnancies to be screened (W Murphy, personal communication). Such a study could be carried out as a European initiative and there have been some preliminary discussions about its feasibility between European centres interested in this field. It may well be worth the effort and cost if a definitive answer can be obtained as to whether prevention of intracerebral haemorrhage by screening for alloimmune thrombocytopenia is not only possible, but cost-effective.

4.5 Conclusions

This chapter has reviewed the epidemiology of alloimmune thrombocytopenia and has examined the feasibility of introducing a screening programme against the criteria set by the UK's National Screening Committee. Antenatal haemorrhage due to alloimmune thrombocytopenia can produce devastating clinical effects, but it may be argued that knowledge about alloimmune thrombocytopenia is as yet insufficient to justify the introduction of an antenatal screening programme. Research is required in several areas including the clinical outcome of affected cases, the identification of factors useful for predicting severe disease and the preferred option for antenatal intervention in women with anti-HPA-1a but no previous history of affected pregnancies.

Acknowledgements

The authors acknowledge the contribution of Dr WG Murphy (Dublin), Dr WH Ouwehand (Cambridge) and Professor CH Rodeck (University College, London) in extensive discussions on the subject of antenatal screening for alloimmune thrombocytopenia.

4.6 References

1 Mueller-Eckhardt C, Kiefel V, Grubert A et al. (1989). 348 cases of suspected neonatal alloimmune neonatal thrombocytopenia. *Lancet*, **1**, 363–6.

2 Kaplan C, Morel-Kopp MC, Kroll H et al. (1991). HPA-5b (Br^a) neonatal alloimmune thrombocytopenia: clinical and immunological analysis of 39 cases. *British Journal of Haematology*, **78**, 425–9.

3 Harrington WJ, Sprague CC, Minnich V, Moore CV, Aulvin RC & Dubach R (1953). Immunologic mechanisms in idiopathic and neonatal thrombocytopenic purpura. *Annals of Internal Medicine*, **38**, 433–69.

4 Mueller-Eckhardt C, Mueller-Eckhardt G, Willen-Ohff H et al. (1985). Immunogenicity of and immune response to the human platelet antigen Zw^a is strongly associated with HLA-B8 and DR3. *Tissue Antigens*, **26**, 71–6.

5 Blanchette VS, Chen L, de Friedberg ZS, Hogan VA, Trudel E & Decary F (1990). Alloimmunization to the Pl^{A1} antigen: results of a prospective study. *British Journal of Haematology*, **74**, 209–15.

6 Doughty HA, Murphy MF, Metcalfe P & Waters AH (1995). Antenatal screening for fetal alloimmune thrombocytopenia: the results of a pilot study. *British Journal of Haematology*, **90**, 321–5.

7 Williamson LM, Hackett G, Rennie J et al. (1998). The natural history of fetomaternal alloimmunization to the platelet-specific antigen HPA-1a as determined by antenatal screening. *Blood*, **92**, 2280–7.

8 L'Abbe D, Tremblay L, Goldman M, Decary F & Chartrand P (1992). Alloimmunization to platelet antigen HPA-1a (Zw^a): association with HLA-DRw52a is not 100%. *Transfusion Medicine*, **2**, 251.

9 Burrows RF & Kelton JG (1993). Fetal thrombocytopenia and its relation to maternal thrombocytopenia. *New England Journal of Medicine*, **329**, 1463–6.

10 Dreyfus M, Kaplan C, Verdy E, Schlegel N, Durand-Zaleski I, Tchernia G & the Immune Thrombocytopenia Working Group (1997). Frequency of immune thrombocytopenia in newborns: a prospective study. *Blood*, **89**, 4402–6.

11 Murphy MF, Verjee S & Greaves M (1999). Inadequacies in the postnatal management of fetomaternal alloimmune thrombocytopenia. *British Journal of Haematology*, **105**, 123–6.

12 Murphy MF, Hambley H, Nicolaides K & Waters AH (1996). Severe fetomaternal alloimmune thrombocytopenia presenting with fetal hydrocephalus. *Prenatal Diagnosis*, **16**, 1152–5.

13 Bussel JB, Zabusky MR, Berkowitz RL & McFarland JG (1997). Fetal alloimmune thrombocytopenia. *New England Journal of Medicine*, **337**, 22–6.

14 Metcalfe P, Allen D, Chapman J & Ouwehand WH (1997). Interlaboratory variation in the detection of clinically significant alloantibodies against human platelet alloantigens. *British Journal of Haematology*, **97**, 204–7.

15 Warwick RM, Vaughan J, Murray N, Lubenko A & Roberts I (1994). In vitro culture of colony forming unit-megakaryocyte (CFU-MK) in fetal alloimmune thrombocytopenia. *British Journal of Haematology*, **88**, 874–7.

16 Vaughan JI, Manning M, Warwick RM, Letsky EA, Murray NA & Roberts IAG (1998). Inhibition of erythroid progenitor cells by anti-Kell antibodies in fetal alloimmune anemia. *New England Journal of Medicine*, **338**, 798–803.

17 Paidas MJ, Berkowitz RL, Lynch L et al. (1995). Alloimmune thrombocytopenia: fetal and neonatal losses related to cordocentesis. *American Journal of Obstetrics and Gynecology*, **172**, 475–9.

18 Murphy MF, Waters AH, Doughty HA et al. (1994). Antenatal management of fetal alloimmune thrombocytopenia: report of 15 affected pregnancies. *Transfusion Medicine*, **4**, 281–92.

19 Metcalfe P, Doughty HA, Murphy MF & Waters AH (1994). A simplified method for large-scale HPA-1a phenotyping for antenatal screening. *Transfusion Medicine*, **4**, 21–4.

20 Watkins NA, Armour KL, Smethurst PA et al. (1999). Rapid phenotyping of HPA-1a using either diabody-based hemagglutination or recombinant IgG1-based assays. *Transfusion*, **39**, 781–9.

21 Bessos H, Mirza S, McGill A, Williamson LM, Hadfield R & Murphy WG (1996). A whole blood assay for platelet HPA-1 phenotyping applicable to large scale antenatal screening. *British Journal of Haematology*, **92**, 221–5.

22 Garner SF, Smethurst PA, Merieux Y et al. (2000). A rapid one-stage whole-blood HPA-1a phenotyping assay using a recombinant monoclonal IgG1 anti-HPA-1a. *British Journal of Haematology*, **108**, 440–7.

23 Lo YMD, Hjelm M, Fidler C et al. (1998). Non-invasive prenatal diagnosis of fetal RhD status by molecular analysis of maternal plasma. *New England Journal of Medicine*, **339**, 1734–8.

24 British Committee for Standards in Haematology (1996). Guidelines for blood grouping and red cell antibody testing during pregnancy. *Transfusion Medicine*, **6**, 71–4.

25 Kroll H, Kiefel V, Giers G et al.(1994). Maternal intravenous immunoglobulin treatment does not prevent intracranial haemorrhage in fetal alloimmune thrombocytopenia. *Transfusion Medicine*, **4**, 293–6.

26 Kaplan C, Murphy MF, Kroll H & Waters AH (1998). Fetomaternal alloimmune thrombocytopenia: antenatal therapy with IVIgG and steroids – more questions than answers. *British Journal of Haematology*, **100**, 62–5.

27 Zimmerman R & Huch A (1992). In-utero fetal therapy with immunoglobulin for alloimmune thrombocytopenia. *Lancet*, **340**, 606.

28 Bowman J, Harman C, Mentigolou S & Pollock J (1992). Intravenous fetal transfusion of immunoglobulin for alloimmune thrombocytopenia. *Lancet*, **340**, 1034–5.

5

Principles of antibody-mediated immune suppression and the prevention of maternal RhD alloimmunization

Belinda Kumpel

Bristol Institute for Transfusion Sciences, Bristol, UK

The first evidence that passively administered antibody could suppress the immune response to the corresponding antigen was documented a century ago.[1] Since then, the administration of anti-D to D-negative individuals has become firmly established as an effective measure to prevent alloimmunization to D. Anti-D prophylaxis is the most widespread clinical application of specific antibody-mediated immune suppression. This chapter first reviews the historical background and some of the early experimental and clinical studies on the prevention of RhD alloimmunization. The essential characteristics and possible theories to explain the mechanism of action of prophylactic anti-D are then discussed. Finally, progress made towards the introduction of monoclonal anti-D is reviewed.

5.1 Haemolytic disease of the fetus and newborn due to anti-D

About 50 years ago, there were at least 1000 neonatal deaths a year in England and Wales from HDFN, an incidence of approximately 150 per 100 000 births.[2,3] At a large hospital – Queen Charlotte's in London – between 1946 and 1949, the neonatal death rate was even higher, at 3.2 per 1000.[4] Stillbirths represented an additional 30% of cases. In the early 1940s in Manitoba, Canada, 10% of perinatal deaths were due to HDFN and the death rate of affected babies was 40%.[5] Improved obstetric and neonatal care resulted in a 10-fold reduction in the number of deaths, first as a result of the introduction of neonatal exchange transfusion, then premature delivery and, finally, as a result of intrauterine transfusion, either intraperitoneally or, more recently, by ultrasound-guided delivery into the umbilical cord vessels.

Anti-D is the most frequent cause of HDFN and there are several reasons for this. The D antigen is the most immunogenic blood group, probably because D-negative red cells lack the entire D polypeptide, due to deletion of the *RHD* gene (Section 7.3.1).[6] The RhD and RhCE polypeptides are integral membrane proteins with 12 membrane-spanning regions and six extracellular loops which, unusually, are not glycosylated.[7] The Rh proteins are expressed solely on human erythroid cells,[8] so maternal alloantibodies may localize on fetal red cells. The D antigen is relatively well expressed, with 10000–20000 antigen sites on heterozygous D-positive cells.[9] D is the most common blood group incompatibility with the potential to cause severe HDFN; the gene frequency of *RHD* in Caucasians results in D-negative women carrying D-positive fetuses in about 10% of pregnancies. In addition, the D polypeptide has a 'helper' function for inducing immunity to other blood group antigens.[10]

5.2 Experimental studies on the prevention of RhD immunization

In the 1950s, Chown[11] and Gunson[12] observed the occurrence of fetal cells in maternal blood after the delivery of anaemic infants resulting from massive fetomaternal haemorrhage. They suggested that this might cause the immunization of a D-negative woman by her D-positive fetus. In 1960, in England and the USA, two groups of investigators independently thought that administration of passive anti-D might prevent immunization to D-positive cells. The rationales for their experimental and clinical studies were different.

In Liverpool, Finn et al. suggested that anti-D could be given to D-negative women after delivery to destroy fetal D-positive cells in ABO compatible pregnancies.[13] This approach was taken because it was known that the incidence of D immunization and HDFN was less in ABO incompatible pregnancies.[14] Experimentally, it had been found that 71% of D-negative subjects given 2.5 ml ABO compatible D-positive blood formed anti-D, whereas only 16% became immunized with ABO incompatible D-positive blood.[15] The use of plasma containing mainly IgM anti-D was tested first, to simulate the effect of IgM anti-A and anti-B in protecting against immunization by causing the rapid intravascular destruction of incompatible cells.[13,16] It was observed that the proportion of D-negative subjects who became immunized to D-positive blood was greater in the group given IgM anti-D (eight of 13) compared with the control group (one of 11). The survival of the D-positive cells was somewhat reduced in recipients of the plasma (half-life [$t_{50\%}$], 7 days) compared with the controls ($t_{50\%}$, 25 days). They concluded that IgM anti-D might have enhanced immunization rather than suppressed it.

At that time, it was known that IgG anti-D mediated rapid clearance of D-positive cells to the spleen, whereas ABO incompatible cells accumulated in the liver or were destroyed intravascularly.[17,18] Further, it had been shown that ABO compatible cells coated in vitro with IgG anti-D were not immunogenic, whereas 50% of subjects responded to unsensitized cells, indicating that the passive anti-D had suppressed the anti-D response.[19] In a similar experiment, IgG anti-A was found not to confer protection, so IgG anti-D appeared to be more suppressive than anti-A. These results led to the next experiments in Liverpool. Plasma containing high-titre IgG anti-D was infused after D-positive blood, resulting in reduced survival of the cells; immunization was prevented when 95% of the cells were cleared within 24 hours, but, if insufficient passive anti-D was given then there was neither rapid clearance nor suppression of the anti-D response.[16]

Simultaneously, trials were being undertaken in New York and New Jersey, USA. The rationale for these experiments was that administration of antisera was known to suppress the antibody response to ox red cells injected into rabbits[1] and to diphtheria toxin in guinea pigs.[20] Instead of plasma, anti-D immunoglobulin (Cohn fraction II) was used as it was known not to transmit hepatitis and the processing produced a high concentration of IgG, free of IgM, that could be injected intramuscularly.[21] Two studies demonstrated suppression with these high-titre preparations, either when 5 ml was given 24 hours before 2 ml D-positive cells, repeated at 5-monthly intervals, or when 4 ml was given 72 hours after a single dose of 10 ml D-positive blood. None of four or 14 D-negative subjects was immunized in the two studies, respectively, compared with four of five and six of 13 controls not given anti-D.[21]

At about the same time, Clarke et al. found that 5 ml anti-D immunoglobulin given i.m. cleared D-positive cells more rapidly than 50 ml plasma given i.v., and this group then immediately discontinued the use of plasma.[16] Similar results were reported by German workers.[22] Soon, Hughes-Jones[23] devised a method for assaying the concentration and equilibrium constant of anti-D in the immunoglobulin preparations, which was important for determining the clinical dose.

Immediately after the successful results of these early experiments in male volunteers (using policemen in Liverpool and prisoners in the USA), clinical trials were initiated in the spring of 1964 on women after delivery.

5.3 Clinical studies on the efficacy of RhD prophylaxis

Woodrow et al. observed that one-third of women had a detectable fetomaternal haemorrhage at delivery and that there was an increased incidence of immunization with increasing volume of the haemorrhage.[24] They reasoned that a large fetomaternal haemorrhage at delivery was the most common immunizing event. In order to provide data quickly on the effect of passive anti-D, they selected 'high risk' women for a clinical trial. These women were primiparae (i.e. women not previously immunized by pregnancy) who had delivered ABO compatible D-positive infants and with a fetomaternal haemorrhage in excess of 0.25 ml, as determined by the Kleihauer test (Section 6.3.1).[25] Whereas three of eight women had immune anti-D three months after delivery, none of six injected with 1000 μg anti-D immunoglobulin within 36 hours of delivery was immunized.[24] This study was extended, with similar results; 24% of the control group were immunized at 6 months' post-delivery, but only 4% (three doubtful cases) after treatment.[26]

At the same time, a study in New York on all D-negative women delivering ABO compatible D-positive infants showed that none (of 300) were immunized 6 months' postpartum after treatment with 5000 µg anti-D (RhoGAM), but 8% (19 of 227) of untreated women developed immune anti-D.[27] A larger group was then given 300 µg anti-D, with one of 781 becoming immunized compared with 32 (6%) of 499 untreated patients, which demonstrated the effectiveness of the smaller dose.

In Winnipeg, Canada, 100–300 µg anti-D immunoglobulin given to women either postnatally or antenatally protected them from immunization.[28] In the Netherlands, 333 D-negative women were given 250 µg anti-D within 24 hours of delivery, with only 0.9% of women (all with fetomaternal haemorrhages greater than 50 ml) becoming immunized at 4–6 months, compared with 5% of controls without prophylactic anti-D.[29]

On the basis of these and other trials undertaken during this time, anti-D immunoglobulin was licensed in 1968. RhD prophylaxis was introduced in Australia and Germany in 1967, in the UK for high-risk patients in 1968 and for routine use in 1969.

5.3.1 Dose of anti-D

In the mid 1960s, it was becoming apparent that supplies of anti-D might limit the use of prophylaxis unless an effective small dose could be determined, with or without the use of the Kleihauer test to detect a large fetomaternal haemorrhage which would require a larger dose.[26] Several studies were carried out to determine the optimum dose.

D-negative male volunteers given 2 ml of ABO compatible D-positive cord blood were protected with either 50 µg or 250 µg anti-D, whereas 50% of subjects responded to cells alone.[28] Small doses of anti-D (0–40 µg) were given to D-negative subjects 72 hours after 5 ml of D-positive blood (about 2 ml cells); there was no evidence of suppression with any dose, but there was a greater proportion of responders in the group given 10 µg and, unusually, these subjects initially formed IgM anti-D.[30] Then, in a larger study, the volume of cells was varied, from 11.6 ml to 37.5 ml, with a constant dose of anti-D (267 µg IgG anti-D i.m.) and it was deduced that a dose in the ratio of 20 µg to 1 ml cells would suppress the anti-D response.[31] Thus, although in their first study a ratio of 20:1 was not protective with a 40 µg dose, this ratio was protective with a larger dose in the second study.

In Canada, 145 µg, 290 µg or 435 µg anti-D was given to unselected D-negative women within 72 hours of delivery of ABO compatible D-positive infants, with complete protection at the higher dose and 0.4–0.8% failures at the lower doses. It was noted that no fetal cells were observed in the blood of these unprotected women at delivery, suggesting that antenatal immunization may have occurred in these cases.[32]

'Low-risk' women in Liverpool – those with a fetomaternal haemorrhage after delivery of less than 0.2 ml ABO compatible D-positive blood – were given 200 µg anti-D, with 90% protection when assessed for immune anti-D 6 months after delivery (0.36% versus 3.6% immunization rate in the treated versus control groups) and 82% protection at the end of the subsequent pregnancy (1.8% versus 10.2%, respectively). As above, it was also suggested that failures may have been due to a primary immune response (Section 1.1.1) occurring antenatally, with clearance of fetal cells by the low levels of immune anti-D, which was undetectable serologically.[33]

A study set up by the Medical Research Council in 1967 compared 20 µg, 50 µg, 100 µg and 200 µg anti-D given to almost 2000 D-negative primiparae without immune anti-D within 36 hours of delivery of an ABO compatible D-positive baby.[34] At 6 months, there was a trend towards an increasing frequency of failures as the dose decreased, but failures were similar in all groups at the end of the next pregnancy (1.5%, 1.1%, 1.5% and 2.9% respectively). The overall protection rate was about 90%. The lowest dose was considered suboptimal, and 100 µg (500 IU) has since been used in the UK for routine postnatal prophylaxis (Section 6.2.2. and 6.4).

The dose required to suppress immunization to large fetomaternal haemorrhage (over 100 ml) was less easily defined. Women were not protected at ratios of less than 8.5 µg anti-D per ml fetal cells[35,36] but immunization was prevented with 10 µg per ml,[37] 12 µg per ml,[38] 18 µg per ml[39] or 20 µg per ml.[40,41] Based mainly on the data of Pollack et al., a 'rule of thumb' ratio of 25 µg anti-D per ml fetal cells has been adopted to calculate the extra dose required to protect against immunization by a fetomaternal haemorrhage greater than 4 ml (Section 6.4.6).[31]

5.3.2 The current situation

For the last 30 years in the UK, D-negative women have received anti-D after delivery of a D-positive infant. Thus, 10% of all confinements receive treatment. Over the 15-year period of 1977–1992, the death rate from HDFN due to anti-D in the UK dropped over 10-fold, from 18.4 to 1.3 per 100 000 live births, and it is now a rare disease.[42] The rate of immunization has also dropped, but to a lesser extent, due to some failures of RhD prophylaxis, which are discussed in detail elsewhere (Section 6.2.4). Antenatal prophylaxis is desirable, but has not yet been universally achieved. Over the same period, the death rate due to other alloantibodies (mainly anti-c and anti-K) remained constant, at an average 3.6 per 100 000.[42] Appropriate prophylaxis for these cases is not available.

5.4 Characteristics and requirements of RhD prophylaxis

5.4.1 Ratio of antibody to antigen required for suppression

A review of the data by Mollison[43] concluded that a critical amount of anti-D is required for suppression and that the ratio of the dose of anti-D to volume of red cells may vary. A dose of 10 μg per ml of cells was insufficient for small volumes of cells (0.5 ml) and may even have led to augmentation,[30] but doses using this ratio were suppressive for fetomaternal haemorrhages greater than 50 ml cells. The reason that the effectiveness of a constant ratio of anti-D per volume of cells varies may be that, as the volume of cells and dose of antibody rise, the percentage of D antigen sites bound by anti-D increases. This was calculated to range from 2% (20 μg anti-D and 1 ml cells) to 7.8% (100 μg anti-D and 5 ml cells) to 40% (20 mg anti-D and 1000 ml cells).[10] The percentage of anti-D bound also increases, although only a small proportion of anti-D in the plasma is bound to the cells.[10,44] For example, 18.7% of a 100 μg dose of polyclonal anti-D will be bound to 5 ml cells. It can be estimated from the law of mass action that saturation of D antigen sites with passive anti-D will not occur in clinical practice. In addition to the dose, the equilibrium constant (binding affinity) of the anti-D will determine the amount bound to cells, with high affinity antibodies having enhanced biological effectiveness, especially at low doses.[23] The actual number of molecules of passively administered anti-D bound to cells was determined in a clinical study. Relatively high doses of high affinity monoclonal anti-D were given to D-negative volunteers prior to D-positive cells. On average, about 20% of the D antigen sites were occupied with anti-D at equilibrium, or 1500–10 000 IgG anti-D molecules/cell.[45,46] This suppressed the anti-D immune response.[46] The effectiveness of anti-D-mediated immune suppression may depend on achieving a sufficient density of anti-D molecules bound to the cells. The critical number is about 200–400 IgG anti-D molecules/cell.

5.4.2 Relationship of red cell clearance to antibody-mediated immune suppression

Cells coated with IgG anti-D are rapidly removed from the circulation and sequestered in the spleen.[17,18,47] The rate of clearance is related to the level of red cell coating with anti-D.[46,48,49] With respect to the protective effect afforded by prophylactic anti-D, it appears that small volumes of transfused cells (less than 1 ml) must be completely cleared within 5 days for effective suppression.[43] However, large volumes (over 75 ml of transfused blood[43] or over 10 ml fetomaternal haemorrhage[50]) need not necessarily be entirely removed from the circulation, provided that the majority of cells have been removed by 5–6 days, which requires a sufficient dose of anti-D, as discussed above.

5.4.3 Protection afforded by ABO antibodies

Cells coated with anti-A or anti-B are removed to the liver, if complement-mediated haemolysis does not occur intravascularly.[18] Unlike the spleen, the liver does not participate in immune responses. IgG anti-A or anti-B in group O women appears to be more effective at preventing anti-D immunization than IgM antibodies in group A or B women.[51] ABO incompatibility may prevent a primary but not a secondary anti-D response.[52]

5.4.4 Role of the spleen in RhD prophylaxis

The survival of cells coated with IgG anti-D was prolonged in a splenectomized patient ($t_{50\%}$, 280 minutes) compared with a normal subject ($t_{50\%}$, 30 minutes) and the cells were removed predominantly to the liver in the absence of the spleen.[18] Another splenectomized D-negative patient was given 4 ml D-positive cells and 300 μg anti-D iv, but, despite the large 'suppressive' dose of anti-D, the cells were cleared very slowly ($t_{50\%}$, 14.5 days) and the patient developed immune anti-D by 4 months (study of R Weitzel, reported by Mollison[53]). Thus, the spleen would appear to be involved in anti-D-mediated immune suppression. It is uncertain at which site the anti-D immune response took place in this patient, but the lymph nodes would be the most likely site.

5.4.5 Timing of passive anti-D

In early clinical trials, a time limit of 36 hours after delivery was initially set for administration of anti-D,[26] but 72 hours was later used successfully[54] because this timing was dictated by the prison visiting schedules in the early experiments in the USA.[21] In one study, no suppression was obtained when 100 μg anti-D was given 13 days after 1 ml cells.[55] In another study, prophylactic anti-D was protective when given 7 days before red cells.[56] The rationale for antenatal prophylaxis is to maintain sufficient anti-D in the patient's circulation for at least 6 weeks so that it may mediate clearance of fetal D-positive cells and immune suppression if a fetomaternal haemorrhage occurs. The time limit of 72 hours after delivery has been accepted, although it is also recommended that anti-D should not be withheld if this time limit is exceeded, as it may well still give protection. It may be that passive anti-D should be given before senescent (aged) D-positive cells are removed from the circulation by natural antibodies, i.e. before the D antigen can become immunogenic.[57]

5.4.6 Time of detection of anti-D response

Immune anti-D has not been detected earlier than 4 weeks after injection of D-positive red cells and usually develops 5–20 weeks later.[55,56,58] Normally, only IgG is evident serologically, although IgM is occasionally found, especially after the augmentation caused by administering a small dose of anti-D.[30] The development of anti-D generally precedes that of other blood group antibodies such as anti-C, -E or -K. Antibody levels may vary widely and, in some subjects, when anti-D is not detectable serologically, evidence of immunization is obtained by the brisk development of anti-D 2–4 weeks after challenge with D-positive red cells, suggesting a secondary response (Section 1.1.1).

5.4.7 Effect of passive anti-D on subsequent immunization

There are limited experimental data suggesting that administered anti-D exerts a suppressive effect on D immunization for some months. In male subjects given four injections of D-positive cells each with anti-D im, no subjects were immunized after the first subsequent unprotected 5 ml red cell challenge, although 31% became immunized following a second unprotected challenge of 5 ml blood 7 months later.[26] In a different study, only three of eight individuals given anti-D 2–4 days after two injections of D-positive red cells were immunized by two doses of 10 ml D-positive red cells given 16 and 22 months later; this is about one-half the expected number of responders.[59] A similar effect was observed in male subjects given 5–10 µg anti-D before the first injection of D-positive red cells; only two of six responded to the next unprotected challenge compared with four of five responders in the control group not given anti-D.[56]

5.4.8 Effect of passive anti-D on an established primary response

Clinical studies have shown that antenatal and postnatal RhD prophylaxis is ineffective if anti-D is already present.[32,60] Confirmation that primary RhD immunization cannot be reversed by prophylactic anti-D was obtained by de Silva et al.[61] Volunteers with low levels of immune anti-D were given D-positive cells with or without anti-D, and similar secondary responses were elicited in both groups.

5.4.9 Role of anti-D Fc fragments

$F(ab')_2$ fragments of IgG anti-D did not clear D-positive cells from the circulation of volunteers[62] and, as clearance is required for anti-D mediated immune suppression, $F(ab')_2$ fragments would presumably not be effective for RhD prophylaxis. As IgM anti-D did not mediate immune suppression,[13] the Fc region of IgG is presumably essential.

5.4.10 Epitope specificity

One experiment has been performed to determine the specificity of suppression. D-negative K-negative subjects were given 1 ml D-positive K-positive cells with or without 13–14 µg IgG anti-K, which mediated rapid clearance of the cells to the spleen. One of the 31 treated subjects developed anti-D compared with 11 of the 31 controls, one of whom also produced anti-K.[63] Thus, passive anti-K suppressed the anti-D response, suggesting that the antibody-mediated immune suppression was particle (cell) specific but not epitope specific.

5.5 Theories of the mechanism of action of prophylactic anti-D

Different experimental models have been used to investigate the mechanism of antibody-mediated immune suppression, but none of the animal models currently developed exactly mimics the human situation. Moreover, there may be many different ways by which immune responses are suppressed by the administration of specific antibody, depending on the molecular and cellular events involved in each case.

The exact mechanism by which administered anti-D suppresses the specific anti-D response after exposure to D-positive cells is not known. There are several possibilities, discussed below and illustrated in Figure 5.1. Taking into account the characteristics of RhD prophylaxis and research in other areas of immunology, it would appear that the most likely mode of action involves downregulation of specific B cells, although other mechanisms are conceivable.

5.5.1 Inhibition of B cells by crosslinking heterologous receptors

B cells express specific antigen receptors comprising clonally derived surface immunoglobulin (Section 1.1.1). The cytoplasmic domains of these antigen receptors contain 'immuno-receptor tyrosine-based activation motifs'.[64] Clustering or aggregation of B cell antigen receptors by a multivalent antigen such as D initiates the phosphorylation of tyrosine residues within these signalling motifs. This in turn leads to a cascade of molecular events resulting in B cell activation, proliferation and secretion of antigen-specific antibodies (Figure 5.1a). Many cell surface receptors or their associated subunits with activatory functions contain immunoreceptor tyrosine-based activation motifs. These include the B and T cell antigen receptors and several Fc receptors.[65–67]

Whereas B cell activation, proliferation and antibody secretion may also be stimulated by F(ab')$_2$ anti-Ig, they are inhibited by whole anti-Ig.[68–72] Inhibition requires both that the Fc portions of immunoglobulin bind Fc receptors (Fcγ receptor IIb) on B cells and that the B cell antigen receptors and Fcγ receptor IIb are co-ligated. Crosslinking of Fcγ receptor IIb alone does not inhibit B cell antigen receptor-mediated activation.[69–72] Fcγ receptor IIb has, in common with other inhibitory receptors, a tyrosine-based inhibitory motif in the cytoplasmic tail.[73,74] This has similarities to the tyrosine-based activation motif except that phosphorylation confers an inhibitory signal.[75–77] The inhibitory signals generated by crosslinking Fcγ receptor IIb with the B cell antigen receptors override the activatory signal from B cell antigen receptor aggregation alone[75] and may lead to apoptotic

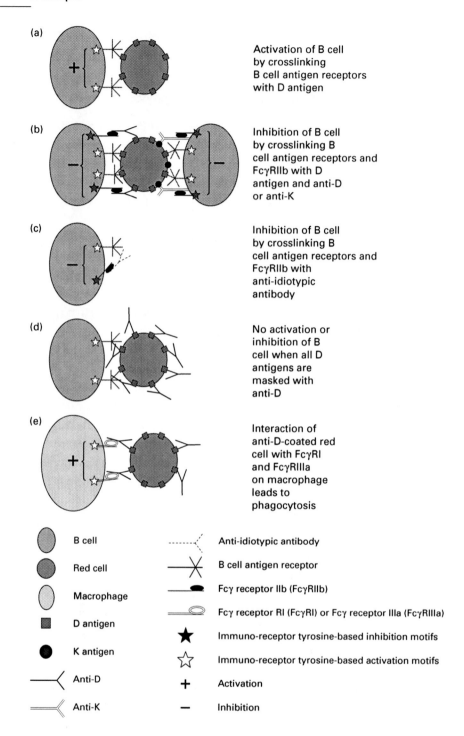

(a) Activation of B cell by crosslinking B cell antigen receptors with D antigen

(b) Inhibition of B cell by crosslinking B cell antigen receptors and FcγRIIb with D antigen and anti-D or anti-K

(c) Inhibition of B cell by crosslinking B cell antigen receptors and FcγRIIb with anti-idiotypic antibody

(d) No activation or inhibition of B cell when all D antigens are masked with anti-D

(e) Interaction of anti-D-coated red cell with FcγRI and FcγRIIIa on macrophage leads to phagocytosis

B cell

Red cell

Macrophage

D antigen

K antigen

Anti-D

Anti-K

Anti-idiotypic antibody

B cell antigen receptor

Fcγ receptor IIb (FcγRIIb)

Fcγ receptor RI (FcγRI) or Fcγ receptor IIIa (FcγRIIIa)

Immuno-receptor tyrosine-based inhibition motifs

Immuno-receptor tyrosine-based activation motifs

+ Activation

− Inhibition

Figure 5.1　Diagrammatic representation of possible mechanisms of antibody-mediated immune suppression.

B cell death.[78] Crosslinking of more than four Fcγ receptor IIb on a B cell may be necessary to generate the inhibitory signal.[79] The molecular events in inhibitory signalling by B cell Fcγ receptor IIb have been reviewed elsewhere.[77,80]

The known characteristics of RhD prophylaxis (Section 5.4) are consistent with inhibition of antigen (D)-specific B cells before an immune response has become established. A diagram of the cellular and molecular interactions (Figure 5.1b) illustrates how Fc (IgG) is required, but that the suppression is cell specific (Section 5.4.10) and not epitope specific. Furthermore, intact red cells are required for the interaction with B cells. It is postulated that co-aggregation of multiple B cell antigen receptors and Fcγ receptor IIb occurs after B cell receptors have bound vacant D antigen sites and Fcγ receptor IIb has ligated anti-D bound to the red cells. It is likely that a certain density of IgG anti-D must be present on the red cells for effective Fcγ receptor IIb–B cell receptor crosslinking to occur; if there is insufficient anti-D, activation of the B cell antigen receptors alone may follow.

In reality, it is possible that this theory will never be adequately tested due to the requirement to study D-reactive immature or primed B cells from the spleen or lymph nodes of a subject in whom anti-D-mediated immunosuppression is taking place. However, none of the other possible mechanisms of action (described below) fulfils all the characteristics of RhD prophylaxis.

5.5.2 Anti-idiotypic antibodies

Anti-idiotypic antibodies are directed against the antigen-binding site of specific antibodies generated during an immune response. It has been postulated that anti-idiotypic antibodies may have a regulatory role in the maintenance of immune responses. If present and directed against anti-D, they could inhibit B cells by cross-linking D-specific B cell antigen receptors and Fcγ receptor IIb in a manner similar to that involved in the downregulation induced by anti-Ig antibodies (Figure 5.1c). However, monovalent anti-idiotypic antibodies probably deliver only weak inhibitory signals. It was found recently that greater co-aggregation (superclustering) of B cell antigen receptors and Fcγ receptor IIb was obtained with anti-idiotypic antibodies together with polyvalent antigen. This combination led to enhanced negative signalling.[81] Thus, D-positive red cells might be required to generate these multiple antigen–B cell receptor interactions for anti-idiotypic antibodies to be suppressive (not shown in Figure 5.1c). There are, however, three observations which mitigate against the theory that anti-idiotypic antibodies are operative in RhD prophylaxis. First, anti-idiotypic antibodies are highly specific,[82 83] and, if present in the anti-D immunoglobulin would be expected to bind the anti-D and form immune complexes, neutralizing the anti-D. This does not occur. Second, anti-idiotypic antibodies are not present in monoclonal anti-D which was found to be suppressive and they also were not detected in serum samples taken subsequently from the subjects given either monoclonal or polyclonal anti-D.[46] Finally, inhibition of anti-D responses by anti-K[63] could not occur via an anti-idiotypic antibody-mediated mechanism.

5.5.3 Masking of antigen sites

This theory supposes that, if sufficient D antigen sites are bound by anti-D, the antigen receptors on D-specific B cells are prevented from interacting with the immunizing antigen (Figure 5.1d). This possibility is unlikely because most of the D antigen sites are not occupied by anti-D.[10,45,46] Moreover, it is unlikely that anti-K could mask all the D antigen sites due to the scarcity of K antigen sites (2500–5000 per cell[84]) compared with D sites (10 000–40 000 per cell[9,85]) and the differing topography of the antigens.[8,86]

5.5.4 Clearance and destruction of D-positive red cells

Small volumes of D-positive cells coated with passive IgG anti-D are rapidly removed from the circulation to the spleen, through interactions with macrophages via their Fcγ receptors (Figure 5.1e). In this situation, sometimes termed antigen deviation, it is suggested that the immunizing antigen is directed away from sites of antigen recognition, resulting in the lack of an anti-D response. Macrophages are relatively poor antigen-presenting cells and are probably only capable of providing a T cell stimulus during a secondary and not a primary immune response (Section 1.1.1). However, after large volumes of D-positive cells are transfused, and if a sufficiently large dose of IgG anti-D is given, immunosuppression does occur even though not all the D-positive cells are rapidly cleared. Thus, there is not a direct relationship between the rate of red cell clearance and suppression of the anti-D response. The spleen and lymph nodes are sites of both antibody formation and cell destruction, so any theory of antigen deviation by passive IgG anti-D must accommodate this dichotomy. The theory of clearance and destruction of antigens on red cells would, however, be compatible with the prevention of anti-D responses by anti-K. With ABO incompatibility, deviation of red cell antigens away from the main immunogenic sites may well occur, as the cells are either lysed intravascularly or phagocytosed by Kupffer cells in the liver, with subsequent lysosomal degradation of the antigen.

5.6 Development of monoclonal anti-D for RhD prophylaxis

The use of human monoclonal anti-D instead of plasma-derived anti-D immunoglobulin offers many attractions. There would be an unlimited supply which could meet the demand for antenatal prophylaxis and, if required, larger doses.

Monoclonal anti-D would be specific, consistent and with a known product profile, which has not always been the case with polyclonal anti-D.[87] In addition, provision of plasma with high-titre anti-D requires the cooperation of D-positive donors to provide accredited D-positive red cells and the availability of D-negative donors who are prepared to be periodically boosted with antigen and plasmapheresed regularly.

5.6.1 Production of monoclonal anti-D

With the advent of hybridoma technology, attempts were first made to produce murine anti-D, but without success. The mouse immune system does not appear to recognize the D antigen. However, since the early 1980s, there have been at least 25 publications documenting the production of human monoclonal anti-D. Usually, the source material was peripheral blood taken from recently immunized donors. B cells were generally immortalized with Epstein–Barr virus[88] to form B-lymphoblastoid cell lines which were then directly cloned or fused with a myeloma cell line before cloning the resultant heterohybridoma. Mouse myelomas have generally been used as fusion partners. In some cases, B cells were fused without immortalization with Epstein–Barr virus. Some workers have selected high affinity anti-D-producing B cell lines by rosetting B cells or B-lymphoblastoid cells with D-positive red cells. The strategies used for producing monoclonal anti-D have been reviewed elsewhere.[89]

Anti-D is almost always restricted to IgG1 and IgG3, with IgG1 predominating in anti-D immunoglobulin.[90–93] Two monoclonal anti-Ds, BRAD-3 (IgG3) and BRAD-5 (IgG1), produced from Epstein–Barr virus-transformed B cell lines in Bristol, England, have been selected for clinical studies on the basis of their high affinity,[46,49] common epitope specificity for the D antigen,[94] high cell growth rate and stable antibody secretion. The glycosylation of these completely human antibodies is similar to that of human serum IgG, although with a slightly greater content of galactose which may be advantageous for their functional activity.[95] Antibodies produced from human–mouse hybridomas may contain nonhuman sugars and sequences.[96]

5.6.2 Half-lives of monoclonal anti-D

In D-negative subjects, BRAD-3 and BRAD-5 had half-lives of 10.2 and 22.2 days, respectively,[97] which were slightly longer than those documented for iodinated myeloma proteins but comparable to other monoclonal IgG1 and IgG3 anti-Ds produced by heterohybridomas.[98,99] The half-life of polyclonal anti-D was 15.6 days.[97] Interaction of IgG with FcRn (Section 1.2) and subsequent protection from lysosomal catabolism is thought to be the mechanism whereby plasma levels of IgG are maintained,[100] as predicted by Brambell et al. in 1964.[101]

5.6.3 In vitro functional activity of monoclonal anti-D

Anti-D-coated red cells are removed from the circulation by the spleen follow-ing interactions with macrophages via their Fcγ receptors (Section 1.3). For RhD prophylaxis to be effective, the fetal D-positive cells must be rapidly cleared. Therefore, the ability of monoclonal anti-D to mediate clearance of D-positive cells was tested in volunteers. First, in vitro assays of the antibody interactions with Fcγ receptor I and Fcγ receptor IIIa (Section 1.3.1) were carried out, as these effector functions are likely to reflect the in vivo activity of anti-D.

Fcγ receptor I-mediated interactions were tested by observing the binding (rosetting) or phagocytosis of monoclonal anti-D-coated red cells by monocytes. A chemiluminescence assay to measure monocyte metabolism during phagocyto-sis (Section 8.4.4), as well as an antibody-dependent cell-mediated cytotoxicity assay to measure the extracellular lysis of red cells (Section 8.4.2), was also used. In general, IgG3 anti-D was more active than IgG1 anti-D.[102–105] A synergistic effect was observed in the monocyte chemiluminescence test with blends of IgG1 and IgG3 anti-D.[104] IgG2 anti-D was inactive.[106]

In contrast, assays utilizing Fcγ receptor IIIa on natural killer cells demonstrated that, whereas some antibodies mediated both adherence and haemolysis of red cells, others were far less effective.[107,108] Considerable variation was observed between the ability of different monoclonal anti-Ds to mediate haemolysis by natural killer cells, which could not be explained by epitope specificity or Gm allo-type.[107,109] A correlation was observed between the ability of monoclonal antibod-ies to mediate haemolysis in natural killer cell-mediated assays and their ability to promote binding of red cells to macrophages within spleen sections, interactions mediated solely by Fcγ receptor IIIa.[110] In studies of 45 monoclonal anti-D's pro-duced in different laboratories, only BRAD-5 was particularly effective in these assays[109,111,112] and this antibody was nearly as haemolytic as polyclonal anti-D.[92]

5.6.4 In vivo red cell clearance mediated by monoclonal anti-D

Some monoclonal anti-Ds have been tested in vivo for their ability to promote the accelerated clearance of D-positive red cells. In some studies, autologous cells have been coated in vitro with anti-D prior to injection and, in others, D-positive cells have been injected into D-negative subjects before or after injection of anti-D. The latter more closely mimics the situation in RhD prophylaxis. Data from six studies, comparing antibody characteristics with their in vitro functional activity and their ability to clear red cells, are presented in Table 5.1.

BRAD-3 was the only monoclonal anti-D which promoted sequestration of pre-sensitized autologous D-positive cells at a rate comparable to polyclonal anti-D.[49] With one exception (an antibody called UCHD4), all monoclonals exhibited some activity in this type of study. Experimental conditions and coating levels of the

Table 5.1 Summary of in vivo red cell clearance studies with monoclonal anti-D

Reference	Anti-D	IgG subclass (cell line)	In vitro functional activity		Study	Dose of anti-D	Red cell clearance	$t_{50\%}$ (h)
			FcγRI	FcγRIIa				
114	UCH D4	IgG1 (h)	Low	Low	D+ → D+		None	
	UCH D4	IgG1 (h)	Low	Low	D+ → D−	(150 µg im)	None	624
49	FOG-1	IgG1 (hm)	Medium	Low	D+ → D+		↑↑	
	BRAD-3	IgG3 (h)	High	Low	D+ → D+		↑↑↑	
	(Polyclonal)	(IgG1,3)	Medium/high	High	D+ → D+		↑↑↑	
115	190/31	IgG1 (hm)	Medium	Low	D+ → D− (chimp)	(400 µg iv)	↑↑	1.5
	P3x229	IgG3 (hm)	High	Low	D+ → D− (chimp)	(400 µg iv)	↑	4.8
46	BRAD-3	IgG3 (h)	High	Low	D+ → D−	(300 µg im)	↑↑	12.7
	BRAD-5	IgG1 (h)	Medium	High	D+ → D−	(300 µg im)	↑↑↑	5.9
	Polyclonal	IgG1,3	Medium/high	High	D+ → D−	(100 µg im)	↑↑	5.0
116	G12	IgG1 (hm)	Medium	Low	D+ → D+		↑↑	
	G12	IgG1 (hm)	Medium	Low	D+ → D−	(300 µg iv)	↑	
	Polyclonal	IgG1,3	Medium/high	High	D+ → D−		↑↑↑	48–72
117	THERAD 19	IgG1 (hm)	Medium	Low	D+ → D+	(150 µg iv)	↑↑	
	THERAD 27	IgG3 (hm)	High	Low	D+ → D+		↑	~3
	Polyclonal	IgG1,3	Medium/high	High	D+ → D+		↑↑↑	

Notes:

h = human B cell line; hm = heterohybridoma cell line; chimp = chimpanzee.

antibodies varied between different studies, but, for individual antibodies, clearance rates were related to the amount of anti-D on the red cells.

In D-negative subjects, only BRAD-5 mediated red cell clearance at a comparable rate to polyclonal anti-D.[46] The half-lives of cells were calculated from the time of injection of cells or antibody. The in vivo results reflected the ability of the antibodies to promote red cell lysis by natural killer cells: of the monoclonal antibodies tested in vivo, BRAD-5 was the only antibody to mediate strong Fcγ receptor IIIa interactions, as discussed above.

5.6.5 Suppression of the anti-D response by monoclonal anti-D

Notwithstanding the requirement to promote accelerated red cell clearance, the most important function of prophylactic anti-D is the ability to suppress the immune response to D-positive red cells. There has been only one report of the suppression of RhD immunization by monoclonal anti-D. In the red cell clearance study[46] described above, D-negative male subjects given monoclonal anti-D 2 days before ^{51}Cr-labelled red cells did not become immunized. Subsequently, they were challenged 6 and 9 months later with D-positive cells, and blood samples were taken every 2 weeks and tested for anti-D. Two subjects seroconverted at 10 and 14 weeks after the first unprotected challenge, and three further individuals produced anti-D at 2–4 weeks after the second unprotected challenge. Three had been given BRAD-3 (100 μg or 300 μg), one BRAD-5 (300 μg) and one polyclonal anti-D (100 μg, 500 IU). The slow anti-D response after the first challenge was consistent with a primary anti-D response and the brisk formation of anti-D following the second challenge indicated a secondary response following a primary response with antibody levels below the limits of detection.[46] Although accelerated red cell clearance had been observed with all subjects in this study, one volunteer did not become sensitized following 100 μg BRAD-3 despite a slow rate ($t_{50\%}$ of 41 hours) of red cell removal. The responder rate (21%) was rather low. The simultaneous administration of anti-D with the initial dose of red cells may have induced some form of tolerance[113] as discussed earlier (Section 5.4.7). These findings were confirmed in a large multicentre study when 95 D-negative male subjects were given 400 μg of a 1:3 blend of BRAD-3:BRAD-5 24 hours after injection of 5 ml D-positive cells.[118] Further clinical trials with BRAD-3 and BRAD-5 are in progress.

5.7 References

1 Von Dungern F (1900). Beiträge zur immunitätslehr. *Munch Med Wochenschr*, 47, 677–80.
2 Urbaniak SJ (1985). Rh(D) haemolytic disease of the newborn: the changing scene. *British Medical Journal*, 291, 4–6.
3 Tovey LAD (1992). Towards the conquest of Rh haemolytic disease: Britain's contribution and the role of serendipity. *Transfusion Medicine*, 2, 99–109.

4 Tovey LAD (1990). Haemolytic disease of the newborn and its prevention. *British Medical Journal*, **300**, 313–16.

5 Bowman JM (1998). RhD hemolytic disease of the newborn. *New England Journal of Medicine*, **339**, 1775–7.

6 Colin Y, Chérif-Zahar B, Le Van Kim C, Raynal V, Van Huffel V & Cartron J-P (1991). Genetic basis of the RhD-positive and RhD-negative blood group polymorphism as determined by Southern analysis. *Blood*, **78**, 2747–52.

7 Avent ND & Reid ME (2000). The Rh blood group system: a review. *Blood*, **95**, 375–87.

8 Avent ND (1999). The Rhesus blood group system: insights from recent advances in molecular biology. *Transfusion Medicine Reviews*, **13**, 245–66.

9 Rochna E & Hughes-Jones NC (1965). The use of purified ^{125}I-labelled anti-γ globulin in the determination of the number of D antigen sites on red cells of different phenotypes. *Vox Sanguinis*, **10**, 675–86.

10 Pollack W (1984). Mechanisms of Rh immune suppression by Rh immune globulin. In *Haemolytic Disease of the Newborn*, ed. G. Garratty, pp. 53–66. Arlington, VA: American Association of Blood Banks,

11 Chown B (1954). Anaemia from bleeding of the fetus into the mother's circulation. *Lancet*, **1**, 1213–15.

12 Gunson HH (1957). Neonatal anemia due to fetal hemorrhage into the maternal circulation. *Pediatrics*, **20**, 3–6.

13 Finn R, Clarke CA, Donohue WTA et al. (1961). Experimental studies on the prevention of Rh haemolytic disease. *British Medical Journal*, **1**, 1486–90.

14 Nevanlinna HR & Vainio T (1956). The influence of mother-child ABO incompatibility on Rh immunization. *Vox Sanguinis*, **1**, 26–36.

15 Stern K, Davidsohn I & Masaitis L (1956). Experimental studies on Rh immunization. *American Journal of Clinical Pathology*, **26**, 833–43.

16 Clarke CA, Donohue WTA, McConnell RB et al. (1963). Further experimental studies on the prevention of Rh haemolytic disease. *British Medical Journal*, **1**, 979–84.

17 Hughes-Jones NC, Mollison PL & Veall N (1957). Removal of incompatible red cells by the spleen. *British Journal of Haematology*, **3**, 125–33.

18 Jandl JH, Jones AR & Castle WB (1957). The destruction of red cells by antibodies in man. I. Observations on the sequestration and lysis of red cells altered by immune mechanisms. *Journal of Clinical Investigation*, **36**, 1428–59.

19 Stern K, Goodman HS & Berger M (1961). Experimental isoimmunization to hemoantigens in man. *Journal of Immunology*, **87**, 189–97.

20 Smith T (1909). Active immunity produced by so-called balanced or neutral mixtures of diphtheria toxin and antitoxin. *Journal of Experimental Medicine*, **11**, 241–56.

21 Freda VJ, Gorman JG & Pollack W (1964). Successful prevention of experimental Rh sensitization in man with an anti-Rh gamma2-globulin antibody preparation. A preliminary report. *Transfusion*, **4**, 26–32.

22 von Schneider J & Preisler O (1965). Untersuchungen zur serologischen prophylaxe der Rh-sensibilisierung. *Blut*, **12**, 4–7.

23 Hughes-Jones NC (1967). The estimation of the concentration and equilibrium constant of anti-D. *Immunology*, 12, 565–71.

24 Woodrow JC, Clarke CA, Donohue WTA et al. (1965). Prevention of Rh-haemolytic disease: a third report. *British Medical Journal*, 1, 279–83.

25 Kleihauer E, Braun H & Betke K (1957). Demonstration von fetalem hamoglobin in den erythrocyten eines blutausstrichs. *Klin Wochenscr*, 35, 637–8.

26 Combined Study (1966). Prevention of Rh-haemolytic disease: results of the clinical trial. A combined study from centres in England and Baltimore. *British Medical Journal*, 2, 907–14.

27 Pollack W, Gorman JG, Freda VJ, Ascari WQ, Allen AE & Baker WJ (1968). Results of clinical trials of RhoGAM in women. *Transfusion*, 8, 151–3.

28 Zipursky A & Israels LG (1967). The pathogenesis and prevention of Rh immunization. *Canadian Medical Association Journal*, 97, 1245–57.

29 de Wit DC, Borst-Eilers E, van der Weerdt ChM & Kloosterman GJ (1968). Prevention of Rhesus immunization. A controlled clinical trial with a comparatively low dose of anti-D immunoglobulin. *British Medical Journal*, 4, 477–9.

30 Pollack W, Gorman JG, Hager HJ, Freda VJ & Tripodi D (1968). Antibody-mediated immune suppression to the Rh factor: animal models suggesting mechanism of action. *Transfusion*, 8, 134–45.

31 Pollack W, Ascari WQ, Kochesky RJ, O'Connor RR, Ho TY & Tripodi D (1971). Studies on Rh prophylaxis. I. Relationship between doses of anti-Rh and size of antigenic stimulus. *Transfusion*, 11, 333–9.

32 Buchanan DI, Bell RE, Beck RP & Taylor WC (1969). Use of different doses of anti-Rh IgG in the prevention of Rh isoimmunization. *Lancet*, 2, 288–90.

33 Woodrow JC, Clarke CA, McConnell RB, Towers SH & Donohue WTA (1971). Prevention of Rh-haemolytic disease: results of the Liverpool 'low-risk' clinical trial. *British Medical Journal*, 2, 610–12.

34 Report of MRC Anti-D Working Party (1974). Controlled trial of various anti-D dosages in suppression of Rh sensitization following pregnancy. *British Medical Journal*, 2, 75–80.

35 Hughes-Jones NC & Mollison PL (1968). Failure of a relatively small dose of passively administered anti-Rh to suppress primary immunization by a relatively large dose of Rh-positive red cells. *British Medical Journal*, 1, 150–1.

36 de Wit DC & Borst-Eilers E (1968). Failure of anti-D immunoglobulin injection to protect against Rhesus immunization after massive foeto-maternal haemorrhage. Report of 4 cases. *British Medical Journal*, 1, 152–4.

37 Bowman JM & Chown B (1968). Prevention of Rh immunization after massive Rh-positive transfusion. *Canadian Medical Association Journal*, 99, 385–8.

38 Woodrow JC, Bowley CC, Gilliver BE & Strong SJ (1968). Prevention of Rh immunization due to large volumes of Rh-positive blood. *British Medical Journal*, 1, 148–50.

39 Keith L, Cuva A, Houser K & Webster A (1970). Suppression of primary Rh-immunization by anti-Rh. *Transfusion*, 10, 142–7.

40 Pollack W, Ascari WQ, Crispen JF, O'Connor RR & Ho TY (1971). Studies on Rh prophylaxis. II. Rh immune prophylaxis after transfusion with Rh-positive blood. *Transfusion*, 11, 340–4.

41 Bowman HS, Mohn JF & Lambert RM (1972). Prevention of maternal Rh immunization after accidental transfusion of D (Rh0)-positive blood. *Vox Sanguinis*, 22, 385–96.

42 Clarke C & Hussey RM (1994). Decline in deaths from Rhesus haemolytic disease of the newborn. *Journal of the Royal College of Physicians*, 28, 310–11.

43 Mollison PL (1984). Some aspects of Rh haemolytic disease and its prevention. In *Haemolytic Disease of the Newborn*, ed. G Garratty, pp. 1–32. Arlington, VA: American Association of Blood Banks.

44 Chapman GE (1996). A pharmacokinetic/pharmacodynamic model for the action of anti-D immunoglobulin in effecting circulatory clearance of D+ red cells. *Transfusion Medicine*, 6, 227–33.

45 Kumpel BM & Judson PA (1995). Quantification of IgG anti-D bound to D-positive red cells infused into D-negative subjects after intramuscular injection of monoclonal anti-D. *Transfusion Medicine*, 5, 105–12.

46 Kumpel BM, Goodrick MJ, Pamphilon DH et al. (1995). Human RhD monoclonal antibodies (BRAD-3 and BRAD-5) cause accelerated clearance of RhD+ red blood cells and suppression of RhD immunization in RhD− volunteers. *Blood*, 86, 1701–9.

47 Mollison PL, Hughes-Jones NC, Lindsay M & Wessely J (1969). Suppression of primary Rh immunization by passively-administered antibody. Experiments in volunteers. *Vox Sanguinis*, 16, 421–39.

48 Mollison PL & Hughes-Jones NC (1967). Clearance of Rh positive cells by low concentration of Rh antibody. *Immunology*, 12, 63–73.

49 Thomson A, Contreras M, Gorick B et al. (1990). Clearance of RhD-positive red cells with monoclonal anti-D. *Lancet*, 336, 1147–50.

50 Lubenko A, Williams M, Johnson A, Pluck J, Armstrong D & MacLennan S (1999). Monitoring the clearance of fetal RhD-positive red cells in FMH following immunoglobulin administration. *Transfusion Medicine*, 9, 331–5.

51 Ascari WQ, Levine P & Pollack W (1969). Incidence of maternal Rh immunization by ABO compatible and incompatible pregnancies. *British Medical Journal*, 1, 399–401.

52 Bowman JM (1986). Fetomaternal ABO incompatibility and erythroblastosis fetalis. *Vox Sanguinis*, 50, 104–6.

53 Mollison PL (1975). Rh and isoimmunization. Summary of workshop held at the 2nd International Congress of Immunology at Brighton, England, in July 1974. *Vox Sanguinis*, 28, 406–8.

54 Freda VJ, Gorman JG & Pollack W (1977). Prevention of Rh-hemolytic disease with Rh-immune globulin. *American Journal of Obstetrics and Gynecology*, 128, 456–60.

55 Samson D & Mollison PL (1975). Effect on primary Rh immunization of delayed administration of anti-Rh. *Immunology*, 28, 349–57.

56 Gunson HH, Stratton F & Phillips PK (1976). The primary Rh0(D) immune response in male volunteers. *British Journal of Haematology*, 32, 317–29.

57 Kay MMB, Marchalonis JJ, Schluter SF & Bosman G (1991). Human erythrocyte aging: cellular and molecular biology. *Transfusion Medicine Reviews*, 5, 173–95.

58 Contreras M & Mollison PL (1981). Failure to augment primary Rh immunization using a small dose of 'passive' IgG anti-Rh. *British Journal of Haematology*, 49, 371–81.

59 Freda VJ, Gorman JG, Pollack W, Robertson JG, Jennings ER & Sullivan JF (1967). Prevention of Rh isoimmunization. Progress report of the clinical trial in mothers. *Journal of the American Medical Association*, 199, 390–4.

60 Bowman JM & Pollock JM (1984). Reversal of Rh alloimmunization. Fact or fancy? *Vox Sanguinis*, 47, 209–15.

61 de Silva M, Contreras M & Mollison PL (1985). Failure of passively administered anti-Rh to prevent secondary responses. *Vox Sanguinis*, 48, 178–80.

62 von dem Borne AEG Kr, Beckers D & Engelfriet CP (1977). Mechanisms of red cell destruction mediated by non-complement binding IgG antibodies: the essential role in vivo of the Fc part of IgG. *British Journal of Haematology*, 36, 485–93.

63 Woodrow JC, Clarke CA, Donohue WTA et al. (1975). Mechanism of Rh prophylaxis: an experimental study on specificity of suppression. *British Medical Journal*, 2, 57–9.

64 Cambier JC (1995). New nomenclature for the Reth motif (or ARH1/TAM/ARAM/YXXL). *Immunology Today*, 16, 110.

65 Cambier JC (1995). Antigen and Fc receptor signaling. The awesome power of the immunoreceptor tyrosine-based activation motif (ITAM). *Journal of Immunology*, 155, 3281–5.

66 Deo YM, Graziano RF, Repp R & van de Winkel JGJ (1997). Clinical significance of IgG Fc receptors and FcγR-directed immunotherapies. *Immunology Today*, 18, 127–35.

67 Reth M (1989). Antigen receptor tail clue. *Nature*, 338, 383–4.

68 Elson CJ, Singh J & Taylor RB (1973). The effect of capping by anti-immunoglobulin antibody on the expression of cell surface immunoglobulin and on lymphocyte activation. *Scandinavian Journal of Immunology*, 2, 143–9.

69 Sidman CL & Unanue ER (1976). Control of B-lymphocyte function. I. Inactivation of mitogenesis by interactions with surface immunoglobulin and Fc-receptor molecules. *Journal of Experimental Medicine*, 144, 882–96.

70 Phillips NE & Parker DC (1983). Fc-dependent inhibition of mouse B cell activation by whole anti-μ antibodies. *Journal of Immunology*, 130, 602–6.

71 Phillips NE & Parker DC (1984). Cross-linking of B lymphocyte Fcγ receptors and membrane immunoglobulin inhibits anti-immunoglobulin-induced blastogenesis. *Journal of Immunology*, 132, 627–32.

72 Bijsterbosch MK & Klaus GGB (1985). Crosslinking of surface immunoglobulin and Fc receptors on B lymphocytes inhibits stimulation of inositol phospholipid breakdown via the antigen receptors. *Journal of Experimental Medicine*, 162, 1825–36.

73 Cambier JC (1997). Inhibitory receptors abound? *Proceedings of the National Academy of Science*, 94, 5993–5.

74 Unkeless JC & Jin J (1997). Inhibitory receptors, ITIM sequences and phosphatases. *Current Opinions in Immunology*, 9, 338–43.

75 Muta T, Kurosaki T, Misulovin Z, Sanchez M, Nussenzweig MC & Ravetch JV (1994). A 13-amino-acid motif in the cytoplasmic domain of FcγRIIb modulates B-cell receptor signalling. *Nature*, 368, 70–3.

76 Van den Herik-Oudijk IE, Capel PJA, van der Bruggen T & Van de Winkel JGJ (1995). Identification of signaling motifs within human FcγRIIa and FcγRIIb isoforms. *Blood*, 85, 2202–11.

77 Coggeshall KM (1998). Inhibitory signaling by B cell FcγRIIb. *Current Opinions in Immunology*, **10**, 306–12.

78 Ashman RF, Peckham D & Stunz LL (1996). Fc receptor off-signal in the B cell involves apoptosis. *Journal of Immunology*, **157**, 5–11.

79 Dickler HB & Kubicek MT (1988). Effects of various forms of monoclonal anti-FcγR II (2.4G2) on B lymphocyte responses. *Molecular Immunology*, **25**, 1169–74.

80 Anderson CC & Sinclair NR StC (1998). FcR-mediated inhibition of cell activation and other forms of coinhibition. *Critical Reviews in Immunology*, **18**, 525–44.

81 Sato K & Ochi A (1998). Superclustering of B cell receptor and FcγRIIb1 activates Src homology 2-containing protein tyrosine phosphatase-1. *Journal of Immunology*, **161**, 2716–22.

82 Natvig JB, Kunkel HG, Rosenfield RE, Dalton JF & Kochwa S (1976). Idiotypic specificities of anti-Rh antibodies. *Journal of Immunology*, **116**, 1536–8.

83 Walker RY, Andrew S, Kumpel BM & Austin EB (2000). Murine monoclonal antibodies reactive with a human monoclonal anti-RhD antibody (BRAD-5). *Transfusion Medicine*, **10**, 225–31.

84 Jaber A, Blanchard D, Goossens D et al. (1989). Characterization of the blood group Kell (K1) antigen with a human monoclonal antibody. *Blood*, **73**, 1597–602.

85 Hughes-Jones NC, Gardner B & Lincoln PJ (1971). Observations on the number of available c, D, and E antigen sites on red cells. *Vox Sanguinis*, **21**, 210–16.

86 Lee S, Zambas ED, Marsh WL & Redman CM (1991). Molecular cloning and primary structure of Kell blood group protein. *Proceedings of the National Academy of Sciences USA*, **88**, 6353–7.

87 Lawlor E, Power J, Garson JA et al. (1999). Transmission rates of hepatitis C virus by different batches of a contaminated anti-D immunoglobulin preparation. *Vox Sanguinis*, **76**, 138–43.

88 Miller G (1984). Epstein-Barr virus – immortalization and replication. *New England Journal of Medicine*, **310**, 1255–6.

89 Fletcher A & Thomson A (1995). The introduction of human monoclonal anti-D for therapeutic use. *Transfusion Medicine Reviews*, **9**, 314–26.

90 Mattila PS, Seppala IJT, Eklund J & Makela O (1985). Quantitation of immunoglobulin classes and subclasses in anti-Rh(D) antibodies. *Vox Sanguinis*, **48**, 350–6.

91 Gorick BD & Hughes-Jones NC (1991). Relative functional binding activity of IgG1 and IgG3 anti-D in IgG preparations. *Vox Sanguinis*, **61**, 251–4.

92 Kumpel BM (1997). In vitro functional activity of IgG1 and IgG3 polyclonal and monoclonal anti-D. *Vox Sanguinis*, **72**, 45–51.

93 Ahaded A, Debbia M, Beolet M, Le Pennec PY & Lambin P (1999). Evaluation by enzyme-linked immunosorbent assay of IgG anti-D and IgG subclass concentrations in immunoglobulin preparations. *Transfusion*, **39**, 515–21.

94 Jones JW, Lloyd-Evans P & Kumpel BM (1996). Quantitation of RhD antigen sites on weak D and D variant red cells by flow cytometry. *Vox Sanguinis*, **71**, 176–83.

95 Kumpel BM, Rademacher TW, Rook GAW, Williams PJ & Wilson IBH (1994). Galactosylation of human IgG monoclonal anti-D produced by EBV-transformed B-lym-

phoblastoid cell lines is dependent on culture method and affects Fc receptor-mediated functional activity. *Human Antibodies and Hybridomas*, **5**, 143–51.

96 Montaño RF & Romano EL (1994). Human monoclonal anti-Rh antibodies produced by human-mouse heterohybridomas express the Gal α1-3 Gal epitope. *Human Antibodies and Hybridomas*, **5**, 152–6.

97 Goodrick J, Kumpel B, Pamphilon D et al. (1994). Plasma half-lives and bioavailability of human monoclonal RhD antibodies BRAD-3 and BRAD-5 following intramuscular injection into RhD-negative volunteers. *Clinical and Experimental Immunology*, **98**, 17–20.

98 Callaghan TA, Fleetwood P, Contreras M, Mollison PL & Scherrmann J-M (1993). Human monoclonal anti-D with a normal half-life. *Transfusion*, **33**, 784–5.

99 Wallny H-J, Kluth S, Struff W, Rohm D & Kloft M (1997). Quantification of human anti-D monoclonal antibodies for clinical phase I trials using a highly sensitive flow-cytometric assay. *Biotest Bulletin*, **5**, 515–21.

100 Ghetie V & Ward ES (1997). FcRn: the MHC class I-related receptor that is more than an IgG transporter. *Immunology Today*, **18**, 592–8.

101 Brambell FWR, Hemmings WA & Morris IG (1964). A theoretical model of γ-globulin catabolism. *Nature*, **203**, 1352–5.

102 Wiener E, Jolliffe VM, Scott HCF et al. (1988). Differences between the activities of human monoclonal IgG1 and IgG3 anti-D antibodies of the Rh blood group system in their abilities to mediate effector functions of monocytes. *Immunology*, **65**, 159–63.

103 Hadley AG, Kumpel BM & Merry AH (1988). The chemiluminescent response of human monocytes to red cells sensitized with monoclonal anti-Rh(D) antibodies. *Clinical and Laboratory Haematology*, **10**, 377–84.

104 Hadley AG & Kumpel BM (1989). Synergistic effect of blending IgG1 and IgG3 monoclonal anti-D in promoting the metabolic response of monocytes to sensitized red cells. *Immunology*, **67**, 550–2.

105 Kumpel BM & Hadley AG (1990). Functional interactions of red cells sensitized by IgG1 and IgG3 human monoclonal anti-D with enzyme-modified human monocytes and FcR-bearing cell lines. *Molecular Immunology*, **27**, 247–56.

106 Kumpel BM, van de Winkel JGJ, Westerdaal NAC, Hadley AG, Dugoujon JM & Blancher A (1996). Antigen topography is critical for interaction of IgG2 anti-red cell antibodies with Fcγ receptors. *British Journal of Haematology*, **94**, 175–83.

107 Kumpel BM, Leader KA, Merry AH et al. (1989). Heterogeneity in the ability of IgG1 monoclonal anti-D to promote lymphocyte-mediated red cell lysis. *European Journal of Immunology*, **19**, 2283–8.

108 Hadley AG, Zupanska B, Kumpel BM & Leader KA (1992). The functional activity of FcγRII and FcγRIII on subsets of human lymphocytes. *Immunology*, **76**, 446–51.

109 Kumpel BM & Jackson DJ (1996). Characterization and functional activity of human Rh monoclonal antibodies. *Transfusion Clinique et Biologique*, **6**, 453–458.

110 Kumpel BM & Davenport RD (1996). Comparison of two FcγRIII-mediated assays of anti-D functional activity, using spleen and K cells. *Transfusion Medicine*, **6** (suppl 2), 20.

111 Dangu C, Patereau CI, Goosens D & Brossard Y (1996). Interest of three ADCC assays for the functional study of IgG anti-D. *Transfusion Clinique et Biologique*, **3**, 23s.

112 Kumpel BM (1996). Coordinator's report: An assessment of the functional activity of human Rh monoclonal antibodies after their evaluation by nine laboratories. *Transfusion Clinique et Biologique*, 6, 439–52.

113 Mollison PL, Frame M & Ross ME (1970). Differences between Rh(D) negative subjects in response to Rh(D) antigen. *British Journal of Haematology*, 19, 257–66.

114 Crawford DH, Azim T, Daniels GL & Huehns ER (1988). Monoclonal antibodies to the D antigen. In: *Progress in Transfusion Medicine*, ed. JD Cash, pp. 175–97. Edinburgh: Churchill Livingstone.

115 Blancher A, Socha WW, Roubinet F et al. (1993). Human monoclonal anti-D-induced clearance of human D-positive red cells in a chimpanzee model. *Vox Sanguinis*, 65, 47–54.

116 Belkina EV, Nikolaeva TL & Olovnikova NI (1996). Monoclonal immunoglobulin anti-D for prevention of hemolytic disease of the new-born. *Transfusion Clinique et Biologique*, 3, 28s.

117 Urbaniak SJ, Greiss MA, Perera WS et al. (1998). Assessment of in vivo function of IgG1 and IgG3 monoclonal anti-D by clearance of Tc99 labelled autologous Rhesus D positive red blood cells. *Transfusion*, 38 (suppl) 33s.

118 Smith N, Ala FA, Lee D et al. (2000). A multi-centre trial of monoclonal anti-D in the prevention of immunisation of RhD− male volunteers by RhD+ red cells. *Transfusion Medicine*, 10 (Suppl 1), 8.

The clinical application of anti-D prophylaxis

Stan Urbaniak

Scottish National Blood Transfusion Service and University of Aberdeen, Aberdeen, UK

6.1 Epidemiology

6.1.1 Causes and incidence of alloimmunization

Anti-D is still the commonest cause of moderate and severe haemolytic disease of the fetus and newborn (HDFN) in the developed world. Alloimmunization after pregnancy with a D-positive baby is not as frequent as might be expected from the predicted incidence of D incompatibility between father and mother (60% of D-negative pregnant women carry a D-positive fetus). There are a number of reasons for this. First, the volume of fetal cells crossing the placenta may be too small to initiate a response. Second, ABO incompatibility between mother and fetus offers some protection. Third, the Rh phenotype of the fetus affects antigenicity. Fourth, some women appear to be better responders to a small antigenic stimulus than others.[1] About 17% of at-risk unprotected women are immunized by an ABO compatible pregnancy. Only 8% develop anti-D in the 6 months following a first pregnancy, but a further 9% develop anti-D early in a subsequent pregnancy, indicating that they had been 'sensitized' by the earlier pregnancy.[2]

6.1.2 Ethnic groups

About 15–17% of the UK white population is D negative, and a similar approximation can be made for the Caucasian populations of North America, Europe, Australia and New Zealand. The incidence of D negatives is about 10% in Arabs, about 5% in ethnic blacks, 4–10% in Asian Indians and less than 1% in ethnic Chinese.[3] HDFN associated with anti-D is therefore largely a disease affecting Caucasians, and Caucasians thus form a target for cost-effective preventive prophylaxis programmes. In many parts of the developing world, prophylaxis is incomplete or nonexistent due to the higher priorities placed on other healthcare programmes.

6.1.3 Use of D-negative transfusions for young women

About 90% of D-negative persons will make anti-D if exposed to a sufficient dose of D-positive red cells by transfusion.[4,5] It is, therefore, best practice to transfuse only D-negative blood into D-negative recipients, particularly those of child-bearing years. Because of the severe consequences of immunization, young women should be given priority in times of shortage of D-negative blood. In cases of accidental transfusion with D-positive blood, steps should be taken to prevent immunization (Section 6.2.8).

6.1.4 Relative importance of anti-D before and after the introduction of anti-D prophylaxis programmes

Prior to the availability of specific measures to manage affected fetuses, HDFN due to anti-D resulted in about one death per 2180 births.[6] After the introduction of exchange transfusion, amniocentesis, intrauterine transfusion, controlled early delivery and anti-D prophylaxis, mortality was reduced to one death per 62 500 births, although the latter is an underestimate due to the failure to register deaths before 28 weeks' gestation.[7,8] The introduction of anti-D immunoglobulin prophylaxis resulted in a 90% reduction in alloimmunization, and in a reduction in babies affected by HDFN. As a consequence, other significant alloantibodies such as anti-c or anti-K are seen relatively more frequently; however, in absolute terms, anti-D is still the commonest cause of severe HDFN.[1]

6.2 Prophylaxis programmes

6.2.1 Suppression of the immune response

Although the 'Rh antigen' was discovered in 1940 by Landsteiner and Weiner,[9] and the association between HDFN and the presence of anti-Rh (anti-D) was then made, it was not until 1954 that Chown[10] reported that mothers were sensitized by a fetomaternal haemorrhage, and the association was made between fetal red cells and the stimulation of maternal antibodies. This association, and the observation that ABO incompatibility gave partial protection, led to efforts to suppress the immune response by passive administration with plasma containing IgM anti-D. This was not successful and later studies with IgG anti-D immunoglobulin fractionated from plasma showed suppression of the immune response in volunteers deliberately injected with D-positive red cells (Section 5.2). Since fetomaternal haemorrhage had been shown to occur mainly at delivery, two groups in the UK and USA were able to demonstrate in clinical trials that immunization in D-negative women could be suppressed when concentrated anti-D immunoglobulin was given im soon after delivery.[11,12] In male volunteers, complete suppression could be shown if anti-D was administered up to 72 hours after exposure to D-positive red cells, although partial protection can be shown for some days later. Following on from these initial studies, prophylaxis programmes were introduced in many countries with a standard dose of anti-D immunoglobulin being given, preferably, immediately at the time of delivery of a D-positive baby, and no later than 72 hours afterwards. Early trials showed that 100 μg of anti-D (500 IU) given i.m. was as effective as larger doses,[13] and dosage studies indicated that 20 μg of anti-D (100 IU) will suppress the immune response to 1 ml of D-positive red cells (packed cells, *not* whole blood). To give a margin of safety, due to inherent inaccuracies in quantifying anti-D and the size of fetomaternal haemorrhage, the World Health Organisation recommended 25 μg of anti-D (125 IU) per ml of D-positive red cells.[14]

A full review of the clinical trials involving anti-D immunoglobulin after childbirth is given in Chapter 5.

6.2.2 Recommendations and guidelines

Many countries have some form of professional guidelines which summarize the occasions on which anti-D immunoglobulin is recommended. In the UK, current practice has been reviewed and two recent guidelines have been published, with essentially the same recommendations.[15-17] Different doses are conventionally used in different countries for historical reasons. For example, a dose of 300 μg (1500 IU) is commonly used in North America, 100 μg (500 IU) in the UK, 125 μg in Australia and 200–250 μg (1000–1250 IU) in Europe and elsewhere.

The clinical situations in which anti-D immunoglobulin is recommended are detailed in Tables 6.1, 6.2 and 6.3 and consist of all those events during which fetomaternal haemorrhage might occur, and result in alloimmunization. In the UK, the standard prophylaxis regimen is to administer 500 IU anti-D immunoglobulin after the birth of a D-positive child, and after significant events during pregnancy after 20 weeks' gestation. Before 20 weeks, a smaller dose of 250 IU is recommended. In some countries (for example, the USA and Australia), the cut-off for the full size dose for events during pregnancy is 12 weeks' gestation. For all events after 20 weeks, and at delivery, a Kleihauer test (or equivalent) to measure fetal cells should be performed on the maternal blood (Section 6.3), and, if the fetomaternal haemorrhage is more than 4 ml, a larger dose of anti-D immunoglobulin should be given (125 IU per 1 ml of fetal red cells). Ideally, anti-D immunoglobulin should be given as soon as possible and not later than 72 hours after the event. If, inadvertently, it has not been given earlier, some protection may be provided up to 13 days after exposure.[18]

A detailed discussion of prophylaxis for bleeding during pregnancy is given elsewhere (Section 6.4 and Table 6.3). In the event of intermittent bleeding during pregnancy, it is important to repeat therapy at 6-weekly intervals as very low levels of passively administered anti-D may enhance antibody formation in the presence of an antigenic stimulus.[1]

Anti-D immunoglobulin cannot reverse the immune response once alloanti-D

Table 6.1 Events following which anti-D immunoglobulin must be given to all D-negative women with no anti-D and/or with antibodies other than anti-D

• Delivery of a D-positive infant* (including by Caesarian section)	• Antepartum haemorrhage
	• External version of the fetus
• Abortion	• Closed abdominal injury
• Invasive prenatal diagnosis:	• Ectopic pregnancy
– amniocentesis	• Intrauterine death
– chorionic villus sampling	• Stillbirth
– fetal blood sampling	
• Other intrauterine procedures:	
– insertion of shunts	
– embryo reduction	

Dose: before 20 weeks' gestation→250 IU (50 µg)
            after 20 weeks' gestation**→500 IU (100 µg)

Timing: as soon as possible, but not later than 72 hours after the event.

Notes:

* also if the D type of the infant has not been determined or is in doubt, and the mother is to be discharged early.

** in conjunction with a Kleihauer or equivalent test to assess the size of any fetomaternal haemorrhage.

Table 6.2 Prophylactic anti-D immunoglobulin should be given following abortions to all D-negative women with no anti-D and/or with antibodies other than anti-D

• Therapeutic termination of pregnancy

• Spontaneous abortion followed by instrumentation

• Spontaneous complete or incomplete abortion after 12 weeks' gestation

• Threatened abortion *before 12 weeks*
   – when bleeding is heavy or repeated or is associated with abdominal pain; in particular, if these events occur as gestation approaches 12 weeks

• Threatened abortion *after 12 weeks*
   – all women are eligible; in addition, when bleeding continues intermittently after 12 weeks' gestation, anti-D immunoglobulin should be given at approximately 6-weekly intervals, and the size of fetomaternal haemorrhage assessed.

Table 6.3 Follow-up of large fetomaternal haemorrhage

Estimation of haemorrhage	Serum/plasma	Action
No fetal cells	Free anti-D	No further action
No fetal cells	No free anti-D	Give further dose of anti-D. Retest for free anti-D in 48 hours
Fetal cells present	Free anti-D	Repeat fetomaternal haemorrhage test in 48 hours
Fetal cells present	No free anti-D	Quantify and give further anti-D Repeat fetomaternal haemorrhage test in 48 hours

Source: Adapted from British Committee for Standards in Haematology Guidelines.[38]

has been produced (Section 5.4.8), but in some cases residual activity from antenatal prophylactic anti-D (see below) may be present in the maternal serum, or weak 'enzyme only' naturally occurring anti-D may be detected. Since these cannot be readily distinguished from immune anti-D, where weak anti-D is detected at delivery, anti-D immunoglobulin should still be administered unless it is clearly demonstrated that the mother is already immunized.

Anti-D immunoglobulin is required in appropriate cases where other alloantibodies (such as anti-c or anti-K) have already been detected during pregnancy.

Current UK guidelines also recommend the use of routine antenatal prophylaxis, with 500 IU to be administered at 28 and 34 weeks' gestation. The standard post-delivery dose of 500 IU is always required, in addition, if the baby is D positive.

6.2.3 Effectiveness in Caucasian populations

The failure rate of postnatal prophylaxis is remarkably consistent worldwide at 1–2% despite different doses being used, ranging from 500 IU in the UK to 1500 IU in the USA.[19] The failure rate in the UK has remained relatively constant since the introduction of routine prophylaxis in the early 1970s.[20]

6.2.4 Reasons for continued failures

Despite explicit updated guidelines having been in place in the UK for many years,[21] a number of avoidable cases of failure to protect occur each year and several clinical audits have shown that there is room for improvement with current protocols. As many as one-third of the cases of alloimmunization might have been prevented if anti-D immunoglobulin had been given when it should have been.[15] There are various reasons for failure: first, failure to give additional anti-D for larger fetomaternal haemorrhages; second, failure to give anti-D for recognized events leading to

Table 6.4 The effect of duration of pregnancy on the occurrence of anti-D

	Time of anti-D detection during pregnancy		
Up to 28 weeks	29 – 36 weeks	37 weeks – term	Reference
14%	38%	48%	19
8%	16%	76%	25
5%	37%	58%	26

fetomaternal haemorrhage; third, injection into fatty tissue rather than muscle (delay in absorption); fourth, delayed administration (over 72 hours); and, fifth, antepartum immunization in the absence of overt causes. The two major causes of failure to protect are an unrecognized large fetomaternal haemorrhage at delivery and an unrecognized fetomaternal haemorrhage which may occur without any obvious cause.

6.2.5 Anti-D immunization during pregnancy

Since as little as 0.1 ml of red cells may initiate an immune response in a good responder,[22] there is ample opportunity for anti-D to appear during pregnancy before delivery, even in the absence of an observed precipitating event. The overall incidence during uneventful first pregnancies reported worldwide is approximately 0.87%.[19] As might be expected from the natural history of spontaneous fetomaternal haemorrhage, anti-D tends to appear towards the end of pregnancy, as a result of repeated challenges of larger volumes of D-positive red cells (Table 6.4).

Analysis of the time when anti-D is first detected in primigravidae clearly shows that, on average, less than 10% of intrapartum alloimmunizations are detectable before 28 weeks' gestation. The major risk occurs after 28 weeks, with most alloimmunizations detected in the last trimester, when the fetus is fully developed and the fetoplacental volume is greatest. Even these data underestimate the true rate of alloimmunization since some women do not have detectable anti-D in their blood until early in a second pregnancy. The incidence of spontaneous fetomaternal haemorrhage during pregnancy is discussed elsewhere (Section 6.4.3).

As a result of such findings, several workers, but particularly Bowman and colleagues in Canada,[23] have advocated the use of additional anti-D during the course of pregnancy in an attempt to reduce alloimmunization to a minimum.

6.2.6 Antenatal administration of anti-D immunoglobulin

A number of uncontrolled trials have shown that administration of anti-D immunoglobulin during the later stages of pregnancy, starting at 28 weeks' gestation, can reduce alloimmunization rates, particularly in first pregnancies. While the weight of evidence is considerable in demonstrating a reduction in alloimmunization to about 0.2%, there is only one controlled clinical trial meeting the requirements of the Cochrane review process.[15,24]

6.2.6.1 Dose and timing of anti-D administration

Based on observations of the incidence of fetomaternal haemorrhage and anti-D alloimmunization during pregnancy, an adequate dose of antepartum anti-D at 28 weeks should prevent the 90% of intrapartum sensitization that occurs as a result of occult fetomaternal haemorrhage after 28 weeks' gestation. A single dose of 300 µg anti-D, as used in North America, would in theory result in approximately 20 µg remaining in the mother at the time of delivery 12 weeks later, assuming a circulating half-life of 21 days for anti-D immunoglobulin. This would be sufficient to neutralize up to 1 ml of fetal red cells, but the 1% of women with a fetomaternal haemorrhage of over 1 ml at 30–39 weeks would not be protected.[25] Some women have no detectable anti-D at delivery, probably due to interaction with, and clearance of, fetal red cells from the circulation and Bowman's current practice is to give additional anti-D to those women who do not have residual anti-D late in pregnancy.

In theory, it is more effective to administer anti-D in divided doses; administration of 500 IU at 28 and 34 weeks would result in a slightly higher residual anti-D at term. Evidence for the efficacy for this protocol has been obtained in a study in Yorkshire, England, and in a French randomized controlled study.[26,27] The administration of two doses of 1500 IU (at 28 and 34 weeks) did not appear to be more efficacious than a single dose at 28 weeks.[28] A lower dose of 250 IU at 28 and 34 weeks was not as effective as 500 IU and was not recommended.[29]

Two protocols for antenatal prophylaxis have therefore been shown to be efficacious – a single dose of 1500 IU at 28 weeks' gestation, or a dose of 500 IU at 28 weeks and a second dose at 34 weeks. In practice, the observed failure rates of either programme are similar; the divided dose schedule requires less anti-D, but incurs greater costs of administration. In the UK, the two 500 IU dose protocol is recommended for women who are not already immunized.[16,17] Although more cost-effective if restricted to primigravidae (Section 6.5), the view of a Consensus Panel on anti-D prophylaxis was that there was no ethical or economic justification for this, and that antenatal prophylaxis should be offered to all eligible D-negative women if sufficient anti-D was available.[15]

6.2.6.2 Safety to the fetus

Although up to 10% of anti-D immunoglobulin injected into a pregnant woman may cross the placenta,[30] and may cause fetal anaemia, even with the largest dose of 1500 IU no ill effects have been demonstrated other than a transient positive direct antiglobulin test on fetal cells at delivery.[25,31] Anaemia or jaundice have not been demonstrated in several studies.[26,31–33] Concern about transmission of infectious disease is unfounded, and is considered elsewhere (Section 6.5.2).

6.2.7 Anti-D immunoglobulin use on women with weak D or partial D

The D^u or 'weak D' phenotype in most individuals differs from normal D only in having fewer antigenic sites per red cell, and these cells react weakly or variably with different sera containing anti-D (Section 2.5.1). Molecular analysis of weak D phenotypes shows that the majority have altered D proteins resulting in diminished expression of the D antigen.[34] Such individuals do not make anti-D, and therefore do not require antenatal or postnatal prophylaxis with anti-D immunoglobulin. On the other hand, when a baby is identified as weak D positive, the mother should receive prophylaxis, at the standard dose. Nevertheless, the risk of immunization by weak D in the absence of prophylaxis is very small since current blood grouping reagents identify all but the weakest of partial Ds as D positive. Some weak D phenotypes are, in fact, partial D variants and these individuals can be immunized to form anti-D; however, this is unlikely to be of any clinical significance.

The partial D phenotypes arise from genomic rearrangements of the *RHD* and *RHCE* genes (Section 7.3.1) and result in a lack of expression of some of the D epitopes at the surface of the variant red blood cells;[35] these individuals can make anti-D (which is restricted to reactivity against the missing epitopes); although this must happen rarely given the number of occasions when such 'incompatible' transfusions would occur by chance. The commonest partial D phenotype is category D^{VI}. It is common practice to use reagents which identify partial D^{VI} women as D negative and therefore eligible for anti-D immunoglobulin prophylaxis in the standard doses, at the usual times. In theory, a partial D^{VI} baby typed as D negative could immunize a D-negative mother, but this must be an extremely rare event.

6.2.8 Anti-D immunoglobulin use after the accidental transfusion of D-positive red cells
6.2.8.1 Red cell transfusions

Inadvertent transfusion of D-positive blood into a D-negative individual will result in anti-D being detected in more than 70% of cases after infusion of a full donation, with an additional 15–20% being sensitized and capable of producing anti-D after a further challenge.[4,5] Anti-D immunoglobulin should be given in sufficient doses, calculated on the amount of red cells transfused, on the basis that 500 IU of anti-D immunoglobulin given im will protect against 4 ml of D-positive red cells.[16,17] The standard 500 IU vial size may be used for up to 15 ml red cells (four vials), but, for larger volumes, it is more convenient and less painful for the patient to use the larger vial sizes (2500 IU or 5000 IU). If a whole donation has been accidentally transfused, anti-D immunoglobulin prepared for intravenous use (e.g. WinRho-SD) would be the preparation of choice, being almost twice as effective, unit for unit, as the intramuscular preparation and achieving immediate high plasma levels of anti-D. If only im product is available, it should be given at more than one site in divided doses, and possibly over 2 or 3 days, depending on the volume to be given. Large volumes of circulating D-positive red cells are most accurately determined by flow cytometry (Section 6.3.2) and should be measured every 48 hours. Further anti-D should be given, based on the residual red cell volume, until all D-positive red cells have disappeared from the circulation. With the administration of such large amounts of anti-D, the patient may experience the symptoms of a mild haemolytic transfusion reaction; not more than 10000 IU per day is recommended to avoid reactions. If 2 or more units of incompatible blood have been transfused, consideration should be given to exchange transfusion to reduce the amount of D-positive red cells and the amount of anti-D required (a single volume exchange will achieve a 63% reduction). In such circumstances, protection is not guaranteed despite administration of apparently adequate amounts of anti-D immunoglobulin.

6.2.8.2 Platelet transfusions

When platelet transfusions are given to D-negative women of childbearing years by choice, they should be D negative. Although the immune system may be suppressed by chemotherapy in the majority of haematological patients, cases of alloimmunization to D have been described.[36] If D-positive platelets have to be used in fertile women, anti-D immunoglobulin should be given to prevent immunization by the small amount of red cells that may be present in the platelet concentrates.[17] Quality standards (in the UK) require that a concentrate prepared from a single donation of red cells should contain less than 0.1 ml of red cells. A dose of 250 IU will be sufficient to protect against three adult doses of platelets (18 donations).[37] The injection may be given subcutaneously if there is concern about tissue bleeding with intramuscular injection.

6.2.8.3 Granulocyte transfusions

Granulocyte preparations for transfusion may be contaminated with as much as 30 ml red cells. Although undesirable, it may be necessary to transfuse granulocytes from D-positive donors to D-negative female patients and the appropriate dose of anti-D immunoglobulin should be given based on the calculated volume of red cells transfused.

6.3 Detection of fetal red cells in the maternal circulation

D-negative pregnant women are at risk of alloimmunization whether or not fetal cells are detectable in the maternal circulation. The requirement for a test of fetomaternal haemorrhage is to determine the need for *additional* anti-D if the volume of fetal cells detected is greater than that which the standard dose of anti-D immuno-globulin will protect against.[38,39] Countries vary in their approach to the need for a test of fetomaternal haemorrhage. A test is recommended, for example, in the UK, USA, Canada, Ireland, France and Australia, but not in most European Union countries.

6.3.1 The Kleihauer–Betke acid-elution test

The Kleihauer–Betke acid-elution test was the first test to be introduced for the detection of fetomaternal haemorrhage. The test depends on the fact that fetal red cells contain fetal haemoglobin (HbF) which is insoluble at acid pH (pH 3.3). The test is useful as a screening assay. Blood films are made from maternal blood, treated with an acid buffer solution to elute adult Hb, then stained to identify HbF-containing fetal cells. Adult red cells appear as 'ghosts', while fetal red cells are visible as deep pink-stained refractile cells which can then be counted and expressed as a proportion of adult cells. Clearly, this test has inaccuracies because red cell volume varies between women, maternal HbF-containing cells are known to increase during pregnancy and there are some conditions associated with high HbF levels such as hereditary persistent HbF, sickle cell anaemia, thalassaemia and aplastic anaemia. In these cases, there will be an overestimate of the size of feto-maternal haemorrhage, which will waste anti-D, but not put women at risk of immunization.[39]

Accurate assessment of fetomaternal haemorrhage by the Kleihauer test requires attention to detail, accuracy in making films, calibration of microscopes, the use of controls and the accurate identification and counting of fetal cells. The use of a graticule can assist in accuracy. Detailed technical recommendations are published,[38] and a National External Quality Assessment Scheme is available in the UK. This has shown that lack of attention to technical detail and errors in calculation are the major reasons for 'wrong results'.

6.3.2 Flow cytometry

The estimation of fetomaternal haemorrhage by flow cytometry depends on the identification of D-positive red cells in the presence of D-negative red cells. Fluorochrome-labelled anti-D is used in the direct test, and fluorochrome-labelled anti-IgG after incubation with anti-D in an indirect version of the test. Availability of monoclonal reagents allows the standardization of the assay. Rigorous attention to detail in calibration, selection of settings and performance of calculations, as well as the requirement for an expensive flow cytometer, means that this test is largely restricted to reference laboratories. Some general technical considerations have been published.[38] The limit of sensitivity for accurate counting is one in 1000 (about 2 ml fetomaternal haemorrhage), although sensitivity down to 1:10 000 has been reported. [40,41] Accuracy and reproducibility falls with fetomaternal haemorrhages below 2 ml, but accuracy is better than the Kleihauer test with bigger fetomaternal haemorrhages because a larger number of cells are counted. Flow cytometry is of value in assessing the need for additional anti-D immunoglobulin in large fetomaternal haemorrhages and where the D group of the fetus is unknown, but suspected to be D negative; large unnecessary doses can be avoided in these cases. It is also of value in conditions where maternal HbF is high and would falsely increase the Kleihauer estimate.

6.3.3 Serological tests of fetomaternal haemorrhage

Serological techniques to screen for D-positive cells in maternal blood include the rosette test and the gel column test. These tests are only useful as screening tests and cannot accurately assess the size of fetomaternal haemorrhage. The microscopic weak D test is not recommended, because it is too insensitive and gives too many false negative results. The rosette test is performed by adding anti-D to maternal blood to coat any D-positive red cells present. Unabsorbed anti-D is removed by washing, and D-positive enzyme-treated indicator red cells are then added. These indicator cells cluster around any anti-D-coated fetal cells to form rosettes, which are then counted, and the size of fetomaternal haemorrhage estimated from a standard curve. The test is useful for detecting larger bleeds, above 4 ml. In these cases, the exact size of the fetomaternal haemorrhage needs to be determined accurately so that the requirement for additional anti-D can be calculated. The rosette test is commonly used in the USA as a screening test.[42] The gel test can identify fetal D-positive cells to a level of 0.2% (equivalent to a 4.8 ml fetomaternal haemorrhage) and could be used to screen for larger bleeds requiring additional anti-D immunoglobulin.[43]

6.3.4 Calculating the size of fetomaternal haemorrhage

Various formulae can be used to derive the size of fetomaternal haemorrhage. With the Kleihauer test, Mollison's formula is recommended.[1] This assumes an average maternal red cell volume of 1800 ml, that fetal cells are 22% larger than maternal cells and that only 92% of fetal cells stain darkly. This results in the formula:

Fetomaternal haemorrhage (in ml) = ratio of fetal/adult cells × 2400
e.g. six fetal cells per 6000 adult cells = fetal/maternal ratio of 1/1000
estimate of fetomaternal haemorrhage = 1/1000 × 2400 i.e. 2.4 ml fetal red cells.

With flow cytometry, red cells are recorded as individual events, and registered as D positive or D negative; the same maternal red cell volume (1800 ml) is assumed, and an allowance made for fetal red cell volume.

e.g. 2000 D-positive cells counted per 200000 D-negative cells

fetal/maternal ratio $= 1/100$

estimate of fetomaternal haemorrhage $= 1/100 \times 1800 \times 1.22 = 22$ ml fetal red cells.

When the size of a fetomaternal haemorrhage calculated by the Kleihauer test is compared with the estimate by flow cytometry, the Kleihauer test seems to overestimate the size of haemorrhage in some cases, particularly the higher volumes, at least in part due to false-positive maternal HbF cells. This would tend to suggest that anti-D immunoglobulin is being overprescribed in many cases.

6.4 Fetomaternal haemorrhage and dose of anti-D immunoglobulin

6.4.1 Fetomaternal haemorrhage at delivery

Fetomaternal haemorrhage has been shown to occur most consistently at delivery, at the time of separation of the placenta. There is a clear association between the volume of the haemorrhage and the likelihood of immunization, as was demonstrated in studies before the availability of anti-D immunoglobulin. If no fetomaternal haemorrhage was observed at delivery, 3% became immunized; with a haemorrhage above 0.1 ml, 31% became immunized. Fetomaternal haemorrhage over 4 ml occurs in about 1% of deliveries, and haemorrhage over 12 ml in 2–3 deliveries per 1000.[1] Hence, it is important to retain tests which identify these larger haemorrhages so that additional anti-D immunoglobulin can be given after delivery. However, it is also important to bear in mind that immunization can, and does, occur in the absence of a demonstrable fetomaternal haemorrhage, since the single sample used to determine haemorrhage may not coincide with the appearance of fetal red cells in the maternal circulation. Thus, anti-D immunoglobulin should be given for recognized events (described below) whether or not fetal cells are detected in the maternal circulation. In rare cases, the fetomaternal haemorrhage can be so large as to cause a D-negative mother to test as weak D positive, with a considerable risk of alloimmunization unless recognized and extra anti-D given.

6.4.2 Bleeding during pregnancy

Vaginal bleeding before 28 weeks' gestation may be associated with spontaneous, threatened, complete or incomplete miscarriage (abortion). After 24 weeks, bleeding is classified as antepartum haemorrhage. In theory, each of these events may be associated with fetomaternal haemorrhage and require prophylactic anti-D immunoglobulin (see Tables 6.1, 6.2 and 6.3).

In spontaneous abortion, up to 35% of women may have small-volume fetomaternal haemorrhage (up to 0.05 ml).[1] The risk of immunization is about 1.5–2%.[44] Where instrumentation is used to remove retained products of conception after spontaneous abortion, larger fetomaternal haemorrhage is more likely due to breach of the chorio-decidual space and anti-D immunoglobulin should always be given.[45]

The situation is more complex with threatened abortion, where the pregnancy continues.[46] Bleeding in early pregnancy is common – about 21% of pregnancies have some form of bleeding before 20 weeks and not all women who bleed will need anti-D immunoglobulin.[47] Before 12 weeks, vaginal bleeding is more likely to be uterine rather than fetal because the chorio-decidual space has not been breached. Any fetomaternal haemorrhage is likely to be less than 0.1 ml and up to 3% of women may become immunized by this dose.[48] In practice, this seems to be a rare event before 12 weeks' gestation, affecting about one in 100 alloimmunized women (CR Whitfield, personal communication). It is possible that fetomaternal haemorrhage is more likely (but not proven) if associated with painful or heavy bleeding which continues, and it is considered prudent to give anti-D immuno-globulin in these circumstances. Asymptomatic women with threatened miscar-riage before 12 weeks do not require anti-D. After 12 weeks' gestation, there is a consensus that all women should be given anti-D immunoglobulin due to the greater likelihood of larger fetomaternal haemorrhage and opportunity for alloimmunization.

Antepartum haemorrhage, occurring later in pregnancy, is more commonly associated with fetomaternal haemorrhage. It may also be associated with abrup-tion, when massive fetomaternal haemorrhage which threatens fetal viability may occur, but this can also happen without vaginal bleeding. A test of fetomaternal haemorrhage is required in these circumstances, so that the appropriate dose of anti-D immunoglobulin can be given.

Women who continue to bleed during pregnancy will require additional anti-D immunoglobulin. A pragmatic approach is to administer the standard dose of anti-D at 6-weekly intervals, and to monitor each episode with a test for fetomaternal haemorrhage to check for the need for a larger dose.

6.4.3 Spontaneous fetomaternal haemorrhage during first, second and third trimesters

A number of studies have shown that 'occult' fetomaternal haemorrhage occurs in the absence of any identified precipitating event. The D antigen is well devel-oped by 6 weeks' gestation, although the risk of fetomaternal haemorrhage in the first trimester is limited by the small amount of fetal red cells. The fetoplacental blood volume increases from 25 ml at 19 weeks to 150 ml at 31 weeks and so, as expected, spontaneous fetomaternal haemorrhages occur with increasing fre-quency and volume during the course of pregnancy. There are some difficulties in the accurate assessment of very small fetomaternal haemorrhages due to per-sistent HbF or the increase in F-cells above the normal limit (0.9%) between 8 and

32 weeks' gestation in 25% of normal pregnancies. The incidence of very small spontaneous fetomaternal haemorrhages in the first trimester is therefore uncertain. Using a standardized sensitive test capable of detecting a 0.01 ml haemorrhage, and testing prospectively every 2 weeks during pregnancy, Bowman et al. detected fetomaternal haemorrhages in 3% of women during the first trimester, in 12.1% of women during the second trimester and in 45.4% of women during the third trimester.[49] In this series, only one woman (3%) had a fetomaternal haemorrhage over 5 ml.

Routine monitoring using the Kleihauer test during trials of antenatal anti-D gives an indication of spontaneous fetomaternal haemorrhage at 28 and 34 weeks' gestation, when the women attend for anti-D prophylaxis. The prevalence and size of fetomaternal haemorrhages increase at the end of pregnancy. Large haemorrhages (over 5 ml fetal red cells) in the last trimester were observed in 0.5% women;[27] haemorrhage of over 10 ml was reported in 0.27% of women.[49] These analyses from only two samples taken during each pregnancy almost certainly underestimate the true incidence during pregnancy, especially in the third trimester, when prophylactic anti-D would be expected to result in clearance of some D-positive fetal red cells from the maternal circulation.

6.4.4 Other significant events during pregnancy

Abdominal trauma late in pregnancy due to vehicular seat belt accidents or blows to the abdomen may precipitate a large fetomaternal haemorrhage (over 25 ml). Women with such injuries usually present to Accident and Emergency Units, rather than Obstetric Units, and the need for anti-D immunoglobulin and a Kleihauer test is often overlooked.[50]

Ectopic pregnancy, intrauterine death and stillbirth may also result in fetomaternal haemorrhage, and larger doses of anti-D immunoglobulin should be given as based on a test to measure the size of the haemorrhage.

6.4.5 Fetomaternal haemorrhage due to medical procedures

6.4.5.1 During pregnancy

Iatrogenic fetomaternal haemorrhages can occur as a result of diagnostic procedures carried out on pregnant women. Amniocentesis and chorionic villous sampling are commonly carried out for the detection of chromosomal disorders and have been shown to induce fetomaternal haemorrhage. Prior to ultrasonography, about 3% of women undergoing amniocentesis were shown to have fetomaternal haemorrhages over 0.1 ml, with 1.6% having haemorrhages of over 1 ml.[51] Therefore, prophylactic anti-D immunoglobulin is recommended at amniocentesis in D-negative women. Chorionic villous sampling can be carried out earlier than amniocentesis, at about 11 weeks' gestation, and, although fetomaternal haemorrhages have not been reported, rises in alpha-fetoprotein after chorionic villous sampling have been taken as indirect evidence of fetomaternal leak, and prophylactic anti-D immunoglobulin is recommended. [52,53]

Fetal blood sampling carries a risk of a leak of red cells, which may, on occasion, be life-threatening to the fetus, either as a result of cord tamponade or exsanguination. In women not already immunized to D, such as those being managed for alloimmune thrombocytopenia (Section 14.3.1), anti-D immunoglobulin is advised.

Other intrauterine procedures such as embryo reduction and insertion of shunts present a potential for accidental fetomaternal haemorrhage, although they have not formally been shown to cause alloimmunization, and anti-D immunoglobulin is recommended.

6.4.5.2 Termination of pregnancy

Therapeutic abortion is a clear risk factor for alloimmunization, particularly with instrumentation. About 4% of women have a fetomaternal haemorrhage of over 0.2 ml fetal blood and about 4–5% become immunized.[44] Prophylactic anti-D immunoglobulin is therefore indicated, according to the gestational age (see Table 6.2). After 20 weeks' gestation, a test for fetomaternal haemorrhage is required to determine the need for larger doses of anti-D.

6.4.5.3 At induced delivery

Delivery by Caesarean section and removal of the placenta manually is associated with a 23.5% incidence of fetomaternal haemorrhage compared with 5.2% for normal vaginal delivery; the volume of haemorrhage is also often greater.[1] External cephalic version is also associated with larger haemorrhages.[54] It is therefore essential that a test for fetomaternal haemorrhage is carried out to assess the need for additional anti-D immunoglobulin. It should be noted that fetal cells may not appear in the maternal circulation until some days later if spilt into the abdominal cavity.

6.4.6 Calculation of the required dose of anti-D

The requirement for *additional* anti-D immunoglobulin is based on the estimation of fetomaternal haemorrhage and will depend on the standard dose used. With the 500 IU dose, the threshold is 4 ml, and the 1500 IU dose is assumed to protect against 15 ml of fetal D-positive red cells. Any additional dose of anti-D immunoglobulin should be given immediately, calculated as 125 IU per 1 ml of fetal red cells to the nearest vial, rounding up. A repeat test of fetomaternal haemorrhage is required 48 hours later, together with a test for the presence of free anti-D in the serum/plasma.[16,17,38] Further follow-up is as shown in Table 6.3.

6.5 Procurement of hyperimmune anti-D

6.5.1 Identification, recruitment, boosting and accreditation of donors

When anti-D immunoglobulin was first produced for clinical trials and early routine postpartum prophylaxis, the only sources of anti-D-containing plasma for fractionation were women who had already been immunized by pregnancies affected by HDFN, or men and women who had been immunized by blood transfusion. After the US and Medical Research Council (UK) trials were reported, it soon became apparent that donor programmes would be needed in order to maintain sufficient supplies of anti-D for universal routine use. These programmes required individuals to be deliberately injected with D-positive red cells in order to boost anti-D levels. Initially, the programmes relied heavily on selected individual red cell donors, preferentially of R_2R_2 phenotype. Since there was no matching of other phenotypes, unwanted nonD antibodies were raised in some individuals.[55] There was also the risk of transmitting viral infections prior to the introduction of screening, although potential red cell donors were excluded on history and examination. As soon as screening tests became available, both red cell donors and plasma donors were tested due to the potential risks involved to both boosted recipient, and the mothers (and their babies) receiving pooled immunoglobulin products. As the prophylaxis programmes became more successful, fewer immunized women were available to source anti-D plasma, and programmes were introduced whereby D-negative male volunteers (and nonfertile women) were deliberately immunized with red blood cells to produce a primary response, followed by the boosting of anti-D to high levels.

It is obviously more cost-effective to recruit suitable individuals who have already been immunized 'naturally' since only a few injections of red cells are likely to elicit high levels of anti-D. Various primary immunizing schedules may be used in new donors – either repeated monthly injections of red cells or a larger initial dose, followed by a booster injection.[5,56] In practice, either approach works satisfactorily in attaining high levels of anti-D.

For donors of anti-D, the highest standards of safety are required, with the use of accredited red cell donations which have been quarantine frozen in liquid nitrogen for 1 year while the donor is followed postdonation. It is also important to ensure matching for nonD clinically important antigens to avoid raising unwanted antibodies which will make providing emergency transfusions for the immunized donor more difficult, and also contaminate the anti-D immunoglobulin.[57] The details are summarized in Tables 6.5 and 6.6.

Because of ethical concerns about immunizing volunteers deliberately, and the resources required to set up accredited panels of red cells, many countries have opted not to produce their own anti-D or have, in recent years, abandoned their

Table 6.5 Accreditation of red cells for immunizing donors

- Regular red cell donors recruited
- Informed consent obtained
- Full phenotype for Rh, Ss, Kell, Duffy, Kidd antigens
- Negative mandatory microbiology markers
- Red cell donors enter 6-month accreditation period
- Leukodepleted donation taken and stored frozen for 6 months in quarantine
- Release donation from quarantine after repeat microbiology screen of donor tests are negative

Table 6.6 Anti-D plasma donor selection

- Donors/patients with pre-existing immune anti-D preferred for boosting
- For primary immunization, regular (apheresis) donors preferred
- If female, must be sterile/postmenopausal
- Counselling session (with partner) to discuss programme
- Medical examination including mandatory microbiology markers
- Informed written consent obtained
- General practitioner and Life Assurance Office informed.

programmes due to increasing public concerns about the transmission of (unknown) infections. As a result, the majority of the anti-D plasma is produced in the USA from paid donors. Nevertheless, until the advent of new variant Creutzfeldt–Jacob disease, the UK was essentially self-sufficient in anti-D immunoglobulin for postpartum use due to successful immunization programmes which had commenced shortly after the introduction of prophylaxis. The prophylaxis programmes will determine the amount of anti-D immunoglobulin required. A standard postnatal prophylaxis programme requires about 1 million IU anti-D immunoglobulin per million of population (about 52 million IU in the UK); extension to routine antepartum prophylaxis to all women increases the amount to about 4 million IU anti-D immunoglobulin per million of (Caucasian) population.[46] Because the current yield of anti-D immunoglobulin from plasma by Cohn fractionation is in the region of 20%, the amount of anti-D plasma required from donors is about five times higher.

6.5.2 Manufacture of anti-D immunoglobulin and safety considerations

Plasma containing anti-D is converted into vials of immunoglobulin by fractionation in an appropriate licensed manufacturing establishment. The process most widely used to produce anti-D immunoglobulin for intramuscular use is some variation of the cold ethanol fractionation of Cohn. These products have been used worldwide for over 35 years with an excellent safety record – no anti-D immuno-globulin produced in this way has transmitted hepatitis B virus, human immuno-deficiency virus or hepatitis C virus.[58,59] This is partly because of the screening procedures to select and accredit red cells and plasma donors, but largely due to the fact that the cold ethanol fractionation process itself renders infected plasma virus safe by partitioning and, possibly, by virucidal action. Anti-D immunoglobulin for im use, therefore, has one of the best safety records of any fractionated product. Additional virucidal steps, such as treatment by solvent detergent or by pepsin at pH 4, are now being included by the various manufacturers at the request of the regulatory authorities.

Anti-D produced for intravenous use requires a different manufacturing process, usually some variation of ion exchange chromatography, and it is known that such processes are inherently less safe than cold ethanol fractionation and, in the absence of virucidal steps, have transmitted hepatitis C infection.[58,60] Manufacturers are now also required to demonstrate that the plasma pools used for fractionation are negative for hepatitis C virus by nucleic acid testing for viral genome. The current generation of anti-D immunoglobulins produced for im and iv use have additional virucidal steps included, and nucleic acid testing for human immunodeficiency virus and hepatitis B virus is also under consideration by the regulatory authorities.

The UK has an additional problem associated with bovine spongiform enceph-alopathy and new variant Creutzfeldt–Jacob disease, and theoretical concerns that abnormal prions might be transmitted by blood and plasma products.[61] As a result, all anti-D currently used in the UK is manufactured in the UK from anti-D plasma sourced from US donors.

6.6 Economics of prophylaxis programmes

6.6.1 Cost-effectiveness of antenatal versus postnatal prophylaxis

The standard postpartum prophylaxis programme which reduces alloimmuniza-tion by 90% is highly cost-effective in populations that have significant numbers of D-negative women and has been a major factor in contributing to the reduction in HDFN mortality and morbidity.[19] On the other hand, the addition of antenatal treatment to this programme was found to be much less cost-effective.[62] In the presence of limited supplies of anti-D, it was concluded that countries should implement the former, and then carry out cost-effective analyses to determine whether or not to extend to routine antenatal prophylaxis.

A number of studies have shown that administration of anti-D starting at 28 weeks' gestation will reduce the rate of alloimmunization to about 0.2% of women at risk.[63] The question, therefore, does not so much concern the effectiveness of antenatal prophylaxis, but whether the benefits justify the additional costs. One also needs to take into account which outcome measures are to be analysed. These might include cost per immunization prevented, or cost per case of HDFN prevented or cost per life saved. A number of studies have addressed this issue.[64] A full analysis requires accurate information on the current failure rate with postpartum prophylaxis, the anticipated reduction in alloimmunization, the anticipated prevention of loss of life and the cost of the additional anti-D. The costs of implementing an antenatal programme (which includes administration and organizational costs, as well as the anti-D immunoglobulin) are offset against the maternity and neonatal costs incurred as a result of alloimmunization. Analyses have shown that it is more cost-effective to treat primigravidae rather than all women – a consequence of primigravidae having a larger number of future pregnancies and greater savings in future healthcare costs. The most recent Scottish study suggests that antenatal prophylaxis for primigravidae would actually save money for the National Health Service (NHS).[65] It was estimated that this strategy to prevent immunization and its consequences, would result in net savings of £197 per alloimmunization prevented. Prophylaxis for all women would incur additional costs, at £2785 per alloimmunization prevented and £40 164 per fetal loss prevented. These costs are comparable to some existing healthcare services provided routinely. A key factor in planning implementation is the availability of sufficient supplies of anti-D immunoglobulin; these have now been secured for the UK. In the UK, a remaining problem with the implementation of antenatal prophylaxis is that the costs and the savings occur in different parts of the NHS budget, and cooperation is required between the obstetricians, midwives, general practitioners, hospital transfusion laboratories and the Blood Transfusion services for successful introduction.

6.7 Future developments

The use of monoclonal anti-D is an attractive alternative to the donor-derived polyclonal anti-D immunoglobulin since, in theory, this could ensure virtually unlimited supplies of standardized material produced by biotechnology. Various products have been under development over the past 15 years and a blend of IgG1 and IgG3 anti-Ds has been tested in phase I efficacy studies in volunteers, with considerable success in clearing D-positive red cells from the circulation and in suppressing the immune response (Section 5.6).[66] The major remaining difficulty is the implementation of comparative clinical trials, given that the current product is so effective and safe,[67] and in meeting regulatory concerns with material produced by cell lines in vitro.

6.8 References

1 Mollison PL, Engelfriet CP & Contreras M (1997). *Blood Transfusion in Clinical Medicine*, 10th edition. Oxford: Blackwell Scientific Publications, Chapter 12.

2 Woodrow JC (1970). Rh immunization and its prevention. *Series Haematologica*, **3**, No 3, 1–151.

3 Mourant AE, Kopec AC & Domaniewska-Sobczak K (1976). *The Distribution of Human Blood Groups and Other Polymorphisms*, 2nd edition. Oxford: Oxford University Press.

4 Pollack W, Ascari WQ, Kochesky RJ, O'Connor RR, Ho TY & Tripodi D (1971). Studies on Rh prophylaxis. 1. Relationship between doses of anti-Rh and size of antigenic stimulus. *Transfusion*, 11, 333–9.

5 Urbaniak SJ & Robertson AG (1981). A successful programme of immunizing Rh-negative male volunteers for anti-D production using thawed blood. *Transfusion*, **21**, 64–9.

6 Walker W, Murray S & Russell JK (1957). Stillbirth due to haemolytic disease of the newborn. *Journal of Obstetrics and Gynaecology of the British Empire*, 44, 573.

7 Hussey R & Clarke CA (1991). Deaths from Rh haemolytic disease of the fetus and newborn, 1977–87. *British Medical Journal*, **303**, 445–6.

8 Whitfield CR, Raafat A & Urbaniak SJ (1997). Underreporting from RhD haemolytic disease of the newborn and its implications: retrospective review. *British Medical Journal*, **315**, 1504–5.

9 Landsteiner K & Weiner AS (1940). An agglutinable factor in human blood recognized by immune sera for rhesus blood. *Proceedings of the Society for Experimental Biology and Medicine*, **43**, 223.

10 Chown B (1954). Anaemia from bleeding of the fetus into the mother's circulation. *Lancet*, 1, 1213–15.

11 Combined Study (1966). Prevention of Rh-haemolytic disease: results of the clinical trial. A combined study from centres in England and Baltimore. *British Medical Journal*, 2, 907–14.

12 Pollack W, Gorman JG, Freda VJ, Ascari WQ, Allen AE & Baker WJ (1968). Results of clinical trials of RhoGAM in women. *Transfusion*, 8, 151–3.

13 Medical Research Council (1974). Controlled trial of various anti-D dosages in suppression of Rh sensitization following pregnancy. Report of a working party on the use of anti-D immunoglobulin for the prevention of isoimmunization of Rh-negative women during pregnancy. *British Medical Journal*, ii, 75–80.

14 World Health Organisation (1971). Prevention of Rh sensitization. *Technical Report Series*, 468.

15 Consensus Conference on Anti-D Prophylaxis (1998). Proceedings of a Joint Meeting of the Royal College of Physicians of Edinburgh and the Royal College of Obstetricians and Gynaecologists, ed. SJ Urbaniak, *British Journal of Obstetrics and Gynaecology*, **105** (suppl 18).

16 Lee D, Contreras M, Robson SC Rodeck CH & Whittle MJ (1999). Joint Working Group of the British Blood Transfusion Society and the Royal College of Obstetricians and Gynaecologists. Recommendations for the use of anti-D immunoglobulin for Rh prophylaxis. *Transfusion Medicine*, **9**, 93–97.

17 Royal College of Obstetricians and Gynaecologists Guideline No 22 (1999). Use of anti-D immunoglobulin for Rh prophylaxis. http://www.rcog.org.uk/guidelines/antid.html.

18 Samson D & Mollison PL (1995). Effect on primary Rh immunization of delayed administration of anti-Rh. *Immunology*, **28**, 349–57.

19 McMaster Conference (1979). Conference on prevention of Rh immunization. *Vox Sanguinis*, **36**, 50–64.

20 Tovey LAD (1992). Haemolytic disease of the newborn and its prevention. In *ABC of Transfusion*, ed. M Contreras, pp. 22–5. London: BMJ Publishing Group,

21 National Blood Transfusion Service Immunoglobulin Working Party (1991). Recommendations for the use of anti-D immunoglobulin. *Prescriber's Journal*, **31**, 137–45.

22 Jakobowicz R, Williams L & Silberman F (1972). Immunization of Rh-negative volunteers by repeated injection of very small amounts of Rh-positive blood. *Vox Sanguinis*, **23**, 376–81.

23 Bowman JM (1978). The management of Rh-isoimmunization. *Journal of Obstetrics and Gynecology*, **52**, 1–16.

24 Crowther CA & Keirse MJNC (2000). Anti-D immunoglobulin administration in pregnancy for preventing Rhesus alloimmunization (Cochrane Review). In *The Cochrane Library*, Issue 1, http://www.update-software.com/clibhome/clib.htm.

25 Bowman JM & Pollock JM (1987). Failures of intravenous Rh immune globulin prophylaxis: an analysis of the reasons for such failures. *Transfusion Medicine Reviews*, **1**, 101–12.

26 Tovey LA, Townley A, Stevenson BJ & Taverner J (1983). The Yorkshire antenatal anti-D immunoglobulin trial in primigravidae. *Lancet*, **ii**, 244–6.

27 Huchet J, Defossez Y & Brossard Y (1988). Detection of transplacental haemorrhage during the last trimester. *Transfusion*, **28**, 506.

28 Bowman JM, Chown B, Lewis M & Pollock JM (1978). Rh isoimmunization during pregnancy: antenatal prophylaxis. *Canadian Medical Association Journal*, **118**, 623–7.

29 Lee D & Rawlinson VI (1995). Multicentre trial of antepartum low-dose anti-D immunoglobulin. *Transfusion Medicine*, **5**, 15–19.

30 Hughes-Jones NC, Ellis M, Ivona J & Walker W (1971). Anti-D concentration in mother and child in haemolytic disease of the newborn. *Vox Sanguinis*, **25**, 135.

31 Bowman JM & Pollock JM (1978). Antenatal prophylaxis of Rh isoimmunization: 28 week-gestation service program. *Canadian Medical Association Journal*, **118**, 627–30.

32 Herman M, Kjellman H & Ljunggren C (1984). Antenatal prophylaxis of Rh prophylaxis with 250 µg anti-D immunoglobulin. *Acta Obstetricia Gynecologica Scandinavica*, **124**, 1–15.

33 Trolle B (1989). Prenatal Rh-immune globulin prophylaxis with 300 micrograms immune globulin anti-D in the 28th week of pregnancy. *Acta Obstetricia Gynecologica Scandinavica*, **68**, 45–7.

34 Wagner FF, Gassner C, Muller TH, Schonitzer D, Schunter F & Flegel WA (1999). Molecular basis of weak D phenotypes. *Blood*, **93**, 385–93.

35 Avent ND & Reid ME (2000). The Rh group system: a review. *Blood*, **95**, 375–87.

36 Blanchette VS, Hume HA, Levy GJ, Luban NL & Strauss RG (1991). Guidelines for auditing pediatric blood transfusion practices. *American Journal of Diseases of Childhood*, **145**, 787–96.

37 Murphy MF & Lee D (1993). Dose of anti-D Ig for the prevention of Rh immunization after RhD incompatible platelet transfusions. *Vox Sanguinis*, **65**, 73.

38 British Committee for Standards in Haematology Guidelines (1999). The estimation of fetomaternal haemorrhage. *Transfusion Medicine*, 9, 87–92.

39 Duguid JKM & Bromilow IM (1999). Laboratory measurement of fetomaternal haemorrhage and its clinical relevance. *Transfusion Medicine Reviews*, 13, 43–8.

40 Johnson PRE, Tait RC, Austin EB, Shwe KH & Lee D (1995). The use of flow cytometry in the quantitation and management of large fetomaternal haemorrhage. *Journal of Clinical Pathology*, 48, 1005–8.

41 Nance SJ, Nelson JM, Arndt PA, Lam H-TC & Garratty G (1989). Quantitation of fetal-maternal hemorrhage by flow cytometry. A simple and accurate method. *American Journal of Clinical Pathology*, 91, 288–92.

42 Sebring ES & Polesky HF (1982). Detection of fetal hemorrhage in Rh immune globulin candidates. A rosetting technique using enzyme-treated Rh2Rh2 indicator erythrocytes. *Transfusion*, 22, 468–71.

43 Salama A, David M, Wittmann G, Stelzer A & Dudenhausen JW (1998). Use of the gel agglutination technique for determination of fetomaternal hemorrhage. *Transfusion*, 38, 177–80.

44 Bowman JM (1988). The prevention of Rh immunization. *Transfusion Medicine Reviews*, 2, 129–50.

45 Mathews CD & Mathews AE (1969). Transplacental haemorrhages in spontaneous and induced abortion. *Lancet*, i, 694–5.

46 Robson SC, Lee D & Urbaniak SJ (1998). Anti-D immunoglobulin in RhD prophylaxis. Commentaries. *British Journal of Obstetrics and Gynaecology*, 105, 129–34.

47 Everett C (1997). Incidence and outcome of bleeding before the 20th week of pregnancy: prospective study of general practice. *British Medical Journal*, 315, 32–4

48 Zipursky A & Israels LG (1967). The pathogenesis and prevention of Rh immunization. *Canadian Medical Association Journal*, 97, 1254–7.

49 Bowman JM, Pollock JM & Penston E (1986). Fetomaternal transplacental haemorrhage during pregnancy and after delivery. *Vox Sanguinis*, 51, 117–21.

50 Gilling-Smith C, Toozs-Hobson P, Potts DJ, Touquet R & Beard RW (1998). Failure to comply with anti-D prophylaxis recommendations in accident and emergency departments. *British Journal of Obstetrics and Gynaecology*, 105 (suppl 18), 24.

51 Bowman JM & Pollock JM (1985). Transplacental fetal hemorrhage after amniocentesis. *Obstetrics and Gynecology*, 66, 749–54.

52 Warren RC, Butler J, Morsman JM, McKenzie C & Rodeck CH (1985). Does chorionic villous sampling cause fetomaternal haemorrhage? *Lancet*, i, 691.

53 Rodeck CH, Sheldrake A, Beatie B & Whittle MJ (1993). Maternal serum alphafetoprotein after placental damage in chorionic villus sampling. *Lancet*, 341, 500.

54 Lau TK, Stock A & Rogers M (1995). Fetomaternal haemorrhage after external cephalic version at term. *Australia and New Zealand Journal of Obstetrics and Gynecology*, 35, 173–4.

55 Gunson HH, Stratton F & Phillips PK (1971). The use of modified cells to induce an anti-Rh response. *British Journal of Haematology*, 21, 683.

56 Gunson HH, Stratton F & Phillips PK (1976). The anti-Rh(D) responses of immunized volunteers following repeated antigenic stimuli. *British Journal of Haematology*, 32, 331–40.

57 Guidelines for the Blood Transfusion Services in the United Kingdom (1996), 3rd edn, Annexes 4, 4a.

58 Tabor E (1999). The epidemiology of virus transmission by plasma derivatives: clinical studies verifying lack of transmission of hepatitis B and C viruses and HIV type 1. *Transfusion*, **39**, 1160–8.

59 Watanabe KK, Busch MP, Schreiber GB & Zuck TF (2000). Evaluation of the safety of Rh immunoglobulin by monitoring viral markers among Rh-negative female blood donors. *Vox Sanguinis*, **78**, 1–16.

60 Power JP, Lawlor E, Davidson F, Holmes EC, Yap PL & Simmonds P (1995). Molecular epidemiology of an outbreak of infection with hepatitis C virus in recipients of anti-D immunoglobulin. *Lancet*, **346**, 372–3.

61 Turner ML & Ironside JW (1998). New-variant Creutzfeldt-Jacob disease: the risk of transmission by blood transfusion. *Blood Reviews*, **12**, 255–68.

62 Torrence GW & Zipursky A (1984). Cost-effectiveness of antepartum prevention of Rh immunization. *Clinical Perinatology*, **11**, 267–81.

63 Urbaniak SJ (1998). The scientific basis of antenatal prophylaxis. *British Journal of Obstetrics and Gynaecology*, **105** (suppl 18), 11–18.

64 Cairns JA (1998). Economics of antenatal prophylaxis. *British Journal of Obstetrics and Gynaecology*, **105** (suppl 18), 19–22.

65 Vick S, Cairns J, Urbaniak S, Whitfield C & Raafat A (1996). An economic evaluation of antenatal anti-D prophylaxis in Scotland. *Health Economics*, **5**, 319–28.

66 Kumpel BM, Goodrick MJ, Pamphilon DH et al. (1995). Human RhD monoclonal antibodies (BRAD-3 and BRAD-5) cause accelerated clearance of RhD+ red blood cells and suppression of RhD immunization in RhD− volunteers. *Blood*, **86**, 1701–9.

67 Robson SC (1998). Are obstetricians ready to prescribe monoclonal anti-D? *British Journal of Obstetrics and Gynaecology*, **105** (suppl 18), 30.

Fetal genotyping

Neil D Avent

University of the West of England, Bristol, UK

7.1 Introduction

Determination of the genetic status of a fetus has been a major area for the application of molecular biology in modern medicine. Indeed, the use of the polymerase chain reaction (PCR) to amplify DNA was first reported in a paper describing the prenatal diagnosis of sickle cell disease.[1] Four years later, this report was followed by the first description of an allele-specific PCR test, again for the prenatal diagnosis of sickle cell disease.[2] Without doubt, the PCR has revolutionized contemporary molecular biology because, within a few hours, an individual's DNA can be analysed for the presence or absence of an allele, providing the sequence of the gene of interest is known. This chapter describes the principles of PCR, it recounts the development of PCR-based methods for the analysis of fetal blood groups and it reviews PCR-based assays which are currently used for the management of alloimmunized pregnancies. Prospects and constraints for fetal genotyping from maternal blood will then be considered.

7.2 The polymerase chain reaction

7.2.1 Principle of the polymerase chain reaction

The PCR involves the amplification of a specific DNA target using synthetic oligonucleotides that have sequences complementary to regions flanking the target sequence. Heating DNA (normally to 94 °C) causes its denaturation into two single strands. On cooling the mixture, the oligonucleotides (so-called 'upstream' and 'downstream' primers) bind to their target sites. Once bound, a DNA polymerase uses the primers to start the synthesis of a new DNA molecule. This process requires deoxyribonucleotides, Mg^{2+} (an essential enzyme cofactor) and buffering to maintain an appropriate ionic strength and pH. The DNA polymerase is normally thermostable and will operate at a temperature optimum of 72–75 °C. Repeating the process of heating and cooling many times (20–30 cycles being the norm) results in an exponential increase in the target sequence in the PCR mix, with the molecular weight of the PCR product being dependent on the distance between the two primers when annealed to their target sequences. PCR products are normally visualized following gel electrophoresis and staining with ethidium bromide.

The PCR has many derivatives and adaptations introduced largely to enable the analysis of genomic polymorphisms. The most common adaptations are PCR restriction fragment length polymorphism (PCR-RFLP) analysis and the allele-specific primer amplification (ASPA). These are described in more detail below.

7.2.2 Polymerase chain reaction – restriction fragment length polymorphism analysis

PCR-RFLP analysis evolved from Southern blotting analysis. Southern blotting involves the digestion of genomic DNA with restriction endonucleases – enzymes which recognize and cleave DNA at specific sequences or restriction sites. DNA fragments are then separated using gel electrophoresis and visualized by transferring (blotting) the fragments onto a nylon or nitrocellulose membrane which is then incubated with a radioactively labelled DNA probe and autoradiographed. Fragments of digested genes are revealed as bands. Polymorphic genes often show differences in the sizes and numbers of distinct bands because of the existence of different numbers of restriction sites within the gene. This is because point mutations responsible for different alleles may disrupt (or create) restriction sites. The size differences of the DNA fragments after digestion give rise to the term 'restriction fragment length polymorphisms'. PCR-RFLP analysis is a development of this technique. An allelic region of the gene under investigation is first amplified by the PCR. Figure 7.1 illustrates the principle of PCR-RFLP. The resultant PCR product (amplicon) is then cleaved with an appropriate restriction enzyme and the fragments are separated electrophoretically. The presence (or absence) of different alleles may then be deduced from visual inspection of the bands representing the separated fragments.

7.2.3 Allele-specific primer amplification

ASPA has many different pseudonyms including allele-specific PCR (ASP), amplification refractory mutation system (ARMS) and analysis of single nucleotide polymorphism (SNP). This approach is commonly used for the detection of alleles caused by simple point mutations; these include many blood group polymorphisms such as K/k, Fy^a/Fy^b and RhE/e. The approach involves the use of PCR primers that match specifically one allele and, under the right conditions, will not bind and extend from the other allele(s). Normally, this involves the synthesis of a PCR primer with a perfect match to a known allele at its 3′ end. Thus, when this primer binds to its target allele, there is perfect base-pairing between the primer and the single-stranded template DNA, and extension from the 3′ end of the primer will proceed. When the primer binds to target DNA corresponding to a different allele, perfect base-pairing will not occur, and the thermostable DNA

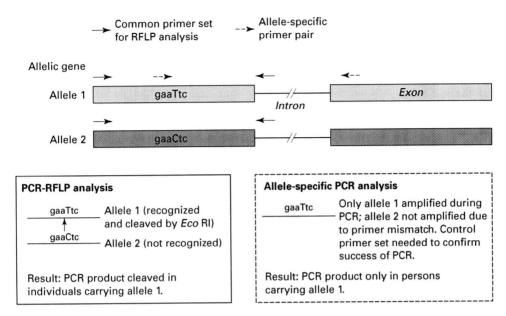

Figure 7.1   Adaptations of the PCR: PCR restriction fragment length polymorphism and allele-specific PCR.

An example of a single nucleotide polymorphism (thymine to cytosine) that causes the expression of two alleles. Using the PCR-restriction fragment-length polymorphism approach, one allele (thymine, T) is recognized by a restriction endonuclease (here *Eco*RI), while the other (cytosine, C) is not. By PCR amplification of the region of the gene surrounding the polymorphism, followed by cleavage of the PCR products by *Eco*RI, the identification of thymine-containing alleles can be performed by gel electrophoresis as they will be cleaved into two fragments. Using the allele-specific PCR approach, one of the primers used in the PCR reaction matches perfectly the thymine-containing allele (but not the cytosine-containing allele). As a perfect base-match is required by a DNA polymerase at the 3′ ends of PCR primers before DNA synthesis can proceed, only thymine-containing alleles will be amplified and detected by gel electrophoresis. Both techniques have internal control PCRs added in order to confirm the efficacy of restriction enzyme cleavage and PCR amplification.

polymerase will not extend from the 3′ end of the bound primer. Thus, the presence of a PCR product is indicative of the presence of a particular allele and the lack of a PCR product indicates the absence of an allele. Figure 7.1 illustrates the principle of allele-specific PCR.

It would be unwise to utilize a diagnostic test where a negative result is indicated by the absence of a PCR product without an internal control to show that the PCR was successful. Thus, ASP assays include a primer pair corresponding to a nonpolymorphic DNA target. This PCR product should be amplified from the DNA of all

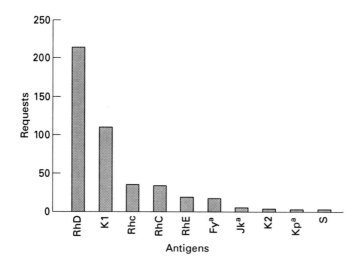

Figure 7.2   Genotyping requests referred to the International Blood Group Reference Laboratory (UK) from 1995 to 1999.
        Totals for each type of investigation are shown. Since RhC/c and RhD multiplex tests are used routinely for *RHD* investigations, they are not included in the totals for RhC and Rhc typing.

individuals. The absence of a band corresponding to the internal control would indicate that the PCR conditions were defective (poor template DNA, omission of a key reagent, inactive DNA polymerase etc.), rather than that the sample lacks the target allele. Thus, assay results are only reported when the presence of a positive control band(s) demonstrates the success of the PCR.

7.3 PCR-based typing for clinically significant blood groups

It may be useful to establish the blood group of a fetus following maternal allo-immunization to a clinically significant blood group antigen which the fetus has the potential to inherit from the father. In the majority of cases, this is the D antigen, but testing for other antigens such as K, Rhc, RhE and Fyᵃ may also be useful. Figure 7.2 shows the range of requests for genotyping referred to one major UK laboratory. Molecular genetic tests that define blood group status are based on the PCR amplification of fetal DNA (although serological tests are easier to perform when fetal red cells are available [Section 3.5.2]). Obviously, this is only possible when the molecular genetic basis of the blood group polymorphism under investigation has been defined. At present, the molecular genetic basis of almost all clinically significant blood group antigens has been elucidated. Most of these polymorphisms are caused by single base changes but others involve more complex genomic rear-

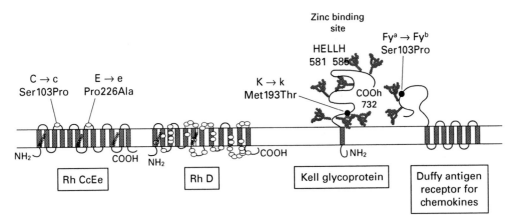

Figure 7.3   Polymorphic proteins of the red cell commonly implicated in HDFN.

This figure depicts the topography of erythrocyte membrane proteins that carry the blood group antigens commonly implicated in HDFN. The CcEe and D proteins are polytopic membrane proteins with 12 membrane spans. They express the C/c and E/e antigens and D antigen, respectively. D-negative individuals lack D proteins. There are 35 amino acid differences between the CcEe and D protein. These are shown as circles on the representation of the D protein. The Kell glycoprotein has a single membrane span, and a large extracellular C-terminal domain which expresses all the Kell system antigens. The K/k alleles involve a methionine 193 to threonine change. In K-positive individuals, this disrupts an N-glycosylation site (represented by branches of circles). The Fy^a and Fy^b blood group antigens are expressed on the large N-terminal domain of the Duffy glycoprotein which has a membrane domain comprising seven membrane-spanning segments.

rangements. The molecular bases of the antigens which may cause clinically signifi-cant maternal alloimmunization have been reviewed in detail previously[3,4] and are considered below only briefly, along with PCR-based tests for their identification.

7.3.1 The Rh system

7.3.1.1 Molecular biology of the Rh antigens

The Rh antigens are expressed on 30 kD nonglycosylated and palmitylated multi-spanning membrane proteins (termed the Rh proteins) that are tightly complexed with an ancestrally related glycosylated membrane protein called the Rh-associated glycoprotein.[5] There are two Rh protein species, D and CcEe, which have 30–35 amino acid differences between them. These variations define the differences that generate D and CcEe antigens. Amino acid changes within the second and fourth external loops of the RhCcEe proteins are responsible for the C/c (serine or proline at amino acid 103) and E/e (proline or alanine at amino acid 226) blood group polymorphisms (Figure 7.3). The RhD protein expresses at least six different epitope clusters as defined by site-directed mutagenesis studies.[6,7] Certain individuals with partial D phenotypes lack one or more of the D epitopes and, as a consequence, can become alloimmunized to those they lack. Thus, a partial D phenotype mother with a normal D-positive fetus may form anti-D, which may have the potential to affect subsequent pregnancies.

7.3.1.2 Molecular bases of the D-positive/D-negative polymorphism

Shortly after the first Rh cDNA was cloned,[8,9] Southern blotting studies revealed that there were two genes (named *RHCE* and *RHD*) at the *RH* locus. Both genes comprise 10 exons with intervening introns (Figure 7.4b). The molecular basis of the D-positive/D-negative polymorphism varies between different ethnic groups. Investigation of genomic DNA from Caucasians has indicated that the *RHD* gene is absent or deleted from D-negative individuals (Figure 7.4c).[10]

Most D-negative Africans have an *RHD* gene, called *RHD* pseudogene (*RHDψ*), which is grossly intact but contains multiple mutations and does not give rise to a transcript.[11,12] The mutations include a 37 base pair duplication at the intron 3/exon 4 boundary, missense mutations in exons 5 and 6, and a nonsense mutation in exon 6 (Figure 7.4a). The frequency of *RHDψ* in black D-negative phenotypes is high. *RHDψ* was found in 66% of South African D-negative blacks and 24% of D-negative African Americans.[12] Furthermore, 15% of South African D-negative blacks possessed a hybrid *RHD-RHCE-RHD* gene that is associated with the VS+V− blood group phenotype. The remaining 18% had the complete *RHD* gene deletion that accounts for the vast majority of D-negative phenotypes in Caucasians. So, in mixed-race populations, the occurrence of *RHDψ* will be frequent.

There are conflicting reports on the molecular genetic basis of the D-negative phenotype in Taiwanese and Japanese. One report indicates that a large proportion of D-negative Japanese possess *RHD* genes;[13] other reports describe complete *RHD* gene deletions.[14,15] Within Japanese and Chinese populations, there are individuals who appear to be D negative by normal serological methods, but anti-D can be adsorbed onto and eluted from the surface of their red cells. These so-called D-elute (D_{el}) phenotypes are characterized by the presence of an *RHD* gene, possibly indicating the presence of an altered RhD protein. In some individuals, the molecular basis of the D_{el} phenotype appears to involve a 1013 base pair deletion in the *RHD* gene, which includes exon 9.[16]

D-negative individuals with dCe(r′) and dcE (r″) haplotypes may also have intact or partially intact D genes.[17,18] This has been explained by the presence of hybrid *RH* genes comprising sequences derived from both the *RHCE* and *RHD* genes. In two instances, Caucasians expressing Cde (r′r′) phenotypes were found to have intact *RHD* genes with a nonsense mutation in exon 1 or a 4 base pair deletion in exon 4.[18,19]

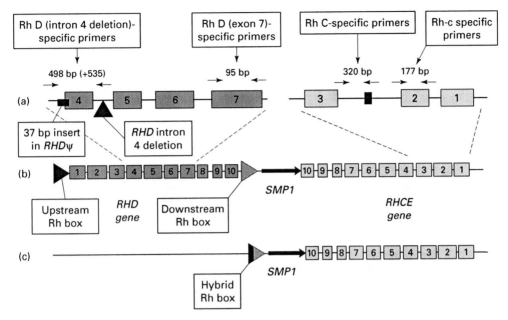

Figure 7.4　Schematic representation of RhDCc multiplex PCR.

(*a*) depicts the positions of the four amplimer pairs used in the multiplex PCR, with respect to their positions within the *RHCE* and *RHD* genes. The c-specific and C-specific primers anneal to targets within exon 2 and intron 2 of the *RHCE* gene, respectively. The *RHD* exon 7 set anneal to target sequences within that exon, while the reverse primer of the intron 4 set anneal to the site of the D-specific deletion. The forward primer is located 5′ of the site of the internal 37 base pair duplication found at the intron 3/exon 4 boundary of *RHD*ψ.

(*b*) shows the gene organization of the *RH* locus in D-positive persons. The gene order *RHD-SMP1-RHCE* is depicted, but, interestingly, *RHD* and *RHCE* are in tail to tail configuration and are separated by a gene of unknown function, *SMP1*. The positions of the two RH boxes (approximately 9000 base pairs) are shown.

(*c*) shows the gene organization of the *RH* locus in D-negative individuals. The entire *RHD* gene is deleted, leaving a hybrid RH box structure, the 5′ end of which has upstream RH box sequences, the 3′ end has downstream RH box sequences. RH boxes are thought to be repeat sequences related to L1 transposable elements. (Adapted from Wagner and Flegel[35]).

7.3.1.3 RhD genotyping tests

Prenatal testing for *RHD* status using PCR was first described by Bennett et al.[20] This assay detected the presence or absence of the D gene using primers specific for exon 10 of the *RHD* gene. Arce et al.[21] identified a small genomic deletion within intron 4 of the *RHD* gene and described a PCR assay capable of amplifying both *RHCE* and *RHD* introns. Two products of 1200 and 600 base pairs are obtained, the

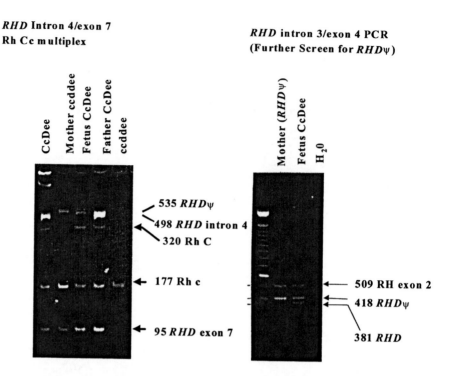

RHD Intron 4/exon 7
Rh Cc multiplex

RHD intron 3/exon 4 PCR
(Further Screen for RHDψ)

CcDee
Mother ccddee
Fetus CcDee
Father CcDee
ccddee

Mother (RHDψ)
Fetus CcDee
H₂0

535 RHDψ
498 RHD intron 4
320 Rh C

177 Rh c

95 RHD exon 7

509 RH exon 2
418 RHDψ
381 RHD

Figure 7.5   Multiplex assays for RhD, Rhc and RhC typing.
The left-hand panel shows a photograph of a polyacrylamide gel of a genotyping
experiment to demonstrate the presence of RHDψ in a fetus. The primers used are shown
in Figure 7.4a. Sizes of the intron 3/exon 4/intron 4 PCR products differ by 37 base pairs
according to the presence of RHDψ (which has a 37 base pair insert at the intron 3/exon
4 boundary). Amplification of the fetal DNA has resulted in two bands of 498 and 535
base pairs consistent with the presence of both RHDψ and RHD (i.e. the fetus is
heterozygous and RhD positive). The RhC-specific band of 320 base pairs in the fetus
confirms that a Cde gene complex has been inherited from the father.
The right-hand panel shows the result of a specific screening test for RHDψ in this
pregnancy where intron 3/exon 4 is amplified yielding products of 381 base pairs (wild-
type RHD) and 418 base pairs (RHDψ).

smaller product arising from, and so indicating, the presence of the *RHD* intron.
Other workers have exploited sequence differences in exon 7 where the *RHD* gene
shows the widest divergence from the *RHCE* gene.[22]

Assays which detect the presence or absence of a single region of the RHD gene
remain in widespread use, although many workers have reported false-positive
results in Caucasian as well as nonCaucasian individuals.[18,23,24] The limitations of
these assays have become more obvious as the molecular bases underlying the
different partial D phenotypes have emerged.[5,25,26] Since the majority of partial D

phenotypes involve hybrid *RH* genes where exchange of DNA has occurred between the *RHCE* and *RHD* genes, *RHD* genotyping, if directed to these regions of exchange, would incorrectly type some partial D phenotypes as D negative.

To overcome the limitations inherent in the detection of just one region of the *RHD* gene, the early assays were further developed and incorporated into second generation multiplex tests. These assays simultaneously detect the presence of at least two regions of the *RHD* gene.[13,18,24,27–29] Although these multiplex assays more accurately predict the presence of partial D phenotypes, they continue falsely to type most D-negative individuals of African descent as D positive.

The discovery of *RHDψ* heralded the development of improved PCR-based tests to detect the D-negative phenotype in individuals of African descent. The 37 base pair duplication has been exploited in a new multiplex test which is able to discriminate the major Caucasian and Black D-negative alleles, while simultaneously defining RhC/c status. This multiplex test is depicted in Figure 7.4a and the PCR products after electrophoretic separation are shown in Figure 7.5.

Many requests for *RHD* typing are to support the clinical management of pregnant women with anti-C+D. In such cases, it is probably good practice to type the fetus for *RHC* as well as *RHD*. Hadley et al.[30] reported a case of a D-negative fetus with severe HDFN delivered by a mother with apparent anti-C+D. On further investigation, the mother's antibody was shown to be anti-G (which recognizes D-positive or C-positive cells).

7.3.1.4 RhC/c and RhE/e genotyping

Transcript and genomic sequencing of exon 5 of the *RHCE* gene reveal that a single amino acid change (proline 226 to alanine) accounts for the E/e polymorphism. The situation regarding the C/c polymorphism is more complex. Initially, it was thought that six nucleotide substitutions dispersed throughout *RHCE* exons 1 and 2 causing four amino acid changes (cysteine 16 to tryptophan; methionine 60 to isoleucine; serine 68 to asparagine; serine 103 to proline) were responsible for expression of the C and c antigens, respectively. However, analyses of Rhc transcripts isolated from black individuals indicated that there is variation within five of the nucleotide substitutions and that only the cytosine 309 to thymine substitution (encoding the change serine 103 to proline) is critical for C/c polymorphic variation.

Rhc and RhE genotyping tests were first introduced following the description of the regions of the *RHCE* gene responsible for the polymorphisms (exon 2 C/c and exon 5 E/e). Le van Kim et al.[31] described an allele-specific PCR test to define c and E status, and Faas et al.[32] refined the test to differentiate E/e status. RhC typing is not straightforward because the *RHD* gene shares with the *RhC* allele of *RHCE* the nucleotide at position 306 critical for RhC expression. Initial C/c genotyping tests were aimed at the exon 1 localized nucleotide polymorphism that predicts the cysteine 16 to tryptophan change in the CcEe protein (C→c). However, the cysteine 16 allele associates poorly with C status in Blacks, and is a poor choice for C/c genotyping. A report describing a 109 base pair insert into the *RhC* allele of *RHCE* allowed definitive RhC genotyping.[33] Although intronic, this polymorphism showed perfect correlation with RhC phenotype. Recent work using multiplexing of primers specific for *RHD* and the *RhC* and *Rhc* alleles of *RHCE* allows the simultaneous definition of RhC/c and RhD blood group status.[12] This multiplex test is depicted in Figure 7.4a and the PCR products after electrophoretic separation are shown in Figure 7.5.

7.3.1.5 Rh zygositity testing

It is normal practice when considering amniocentesis for fetal genotyping to determine the Rh phenotype of the father. If the father is homozygous (RhD/RhD), amniocentesis for genotyping should not be necessary; the fetus would be D positive. However, Rh phenotypes cannot accurately predict genotype. For example, a father of Rh phenotype CDe (R_1) may be of genotype CDe/CDe (R_1R_1), CDe/Cde (R_1r') or even CDe/-D-. Unless PCR tests are available to identify specific haplotypes, then accurate Rh genotyping is not possible. No tests are presently published to identify r' or r'' haplotypes. However, a recent report has described a method to define R_o (cDe) haplotypes. This PCR-based test exploits the discovery of a sequence-length polymorphism in intron 2 of the *Rhc* allele of *RHCE*. In all cde and cDE phenotype individuals tested, a repeat of six guanine/cytosine/adenine/cytosine nucleotides was found, but in all cDe phenotype individuals these repeat sequences were absent.[34] This observation may form the basis for a test to differentiate between cDe/cDe and cDe/cde fathers, the most common request for zygosity testing.

Recent work on the genomic organization of the *RHD* and *RHCE* genes provides the basis for a method to screen for the Caucasian cde haplotype.[35] In D-positive genomes, the *RHD* gene is flanked by two highly homologous DNA segments (named '*RHD* boxes') that are about 9000 base pairs in size (Figure 7.4b). The two *RHD* boxes (upstream and downstream) are highly (98.6%) homologous. In the deletion-type (cde) D-negative genome, the *RHD* deletion occurs within the upstream and downstream *RHD* boxes, and a residual hybrid (5'-upstream–3'-downstream) *RHD* box is left. A PCR-based test for this hybrid box is now available to detect the cde haplotype. This test approach is useful for zygosity testing.

7.3.2 Kell system

7.3.2.1 Molecular basis of Kell antigen expression

Antigens of the Kell system are expressed by the Kell glycoprotein, a membrane-bound enzyme that has significant homology to zinc-dependent neutral metalloendopeptidases that are known to process peptide hormones (Figure 7.3).[36] The Kell glycoprotein has recently been shown to cleave proteolytically big endothelin-3 to produce ET-3, a potent bioreactive peptide with multiple functional roles.[37] There are currently 22 Kell system antigens, of which K/k, Js[a] and Kp[a] have been implicated in HDFN. Following the cloning of the first Kell cDNA in 1991,[38] the major clinically significant K/k (KEL1/KEL2) polymorphism was defined as a single point mutation in exon 6 of the *KEL* gene, altering amino acid 193 from methionine (K) to threonine (k). The presence of methionine in K-positive individuals disrupts an N-glycosylation signal motif, asparagine-X-threonine, and this may explain why the K antigen is so immunogenic in K-negative individuals.

7.3.2.2 KEL genotyping

The description of the molecular basis of the K/k (K1/K2) blood group polymorphism permitted the application of PCR-RFLP and PCR-ASPA assays for the prenatal definition of K status.[39] The PCR-RFLP test is based on the amplification of exons 6 and 7 of the KEL gene (resulting in a 740 base pair product) followed by digestion with *Bsm* I; K-positive DNA is cleaved with *Bsm* I, while K-negative DNA is not. Thus, two fragments of 540 and 200 base pairs are observed in K-positive individuals, but the *Bsm* I-resistant PCR product of 740 base pairs is observed in K-negative individuals. During 1996, four further reports described improved K and K/k assays which included internal controls either to confirm that amplification had occurred (in ASPA assays)[40–42] or to confirm restriction endonuclease cleavage (in RFLP tests).[43]

Fetal anaemia, caused by other Kell system antigens, is comparatively rare. Anti-Kp[a] (KEL3) and anti-Js[a] (KEL6) can cause fetal anaemia. PCR-based diagnostic tests specific for the detection of these alleles have been described elsewhere.[44,45]

7.3.3 Duffy system

7.3.3.1 Molecular basis of Duffy antigen expression

The Duffy antigens are expressed on the red cell promiscuous chemokine receptor known as Duffy antigen receptor for chemokines (DARC) which has seven membrane-spanning domains with a large extracellular N-terminus where the Fy[a], Fy[b] and Fy6 antigens are located (Figure 7.3). The *Fy[a]/Fy[b]* polymorphism is associated with a single acid change, glycine 42 to aspartic acid, although this was originally reported to be at amino acid 44.[46–49] Further work revealed the molecular basis of the erythroid-silent Fy(a−b−) phenotype in Blacks. A single base change in the promoter region of the *FY* gene (thymine to cystosine) disrupts a GATA (nucleotide sequence: guanine/adenine/thymine/adenine) motif, which functions as a binding site for the erythroid-specific transcription factor GATA-1. This mutation causes the complete lack of Fy glycoprotein on red cells, but, interestingly, Fy is

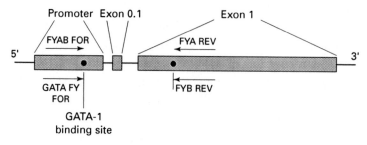

Figure 7.6   Structure of the *FY* gene locus and location of PCR primers for *FY* genotyping.
The two exon structure of the *FY* gene is shown. The positions of the PCR primers are also illustrated, and include a promoter region primer for *Fyª* and *Fyᵇ* genotyping, and also a GATA-FY primer for the mutated GATA-1 binding site found in Fy(a−b−) individuals (adapted from Olsson et al.[50]).

expressed normally in nonerythroid tissues such as endothelial cells of postcapillary venules.

7.3.3.2 Fy genotyping

Initially, PCR-RFLP tests were described for the determination of the *FY*A and *FY*B alleles based on the cleavage of PCR products with the restriction endonuclease *Ban* I. The GATA (thymine to cytosine) promoter expression was identified by a PCR-RFLP using the restriction endonuclease *Sty* I.[49] Allele-specific tests that could differentiate these alleles were subsequently described.[50,51] The tests exploit *Fyª* or *Fyᵇ* allele-specific reverse primers paired with forward primers specific for either the normal or mutated GATA-1 sequences in the promoter region of the gene (Figure 7.6).

7.3.4 Kidd system

Kidd system antigens may elicit antibodies which can cause severe HDFN, albeit rarely. The Kidd blood group antigens are expressed on the red cell membrane urea transporter and are caused by a single nucleotide polymorphism that causes an amino acid change, aspartic acid 280 to asparagine (Jkª→Jkᵇ).[52,53] A PCR test suitable for the prenatal diagnosis of Jkª/Jkᵇ status has been published,[54] although it gives incorrect genotypic assignment to the extremely rare Jk (a−b−) phenotype, which types as Jk(a−b+). The molecular basis of the Jk(a−b−) phenotype has been defined in Polynesians and Finns and is caused by splice site mutations and the disruption of a concensus N-glycan addition site.[55,56] In all Jk(a−b−) phenotypes tested, silent *Jkᵇ* alleles are present.

7.3.5 ABO system

Several techniques for ABO genotyping have been described.[57,58] ABO genotyping is complicated by the large number of different group O alleles and the many hybrid

ABO genes that express variant A and B subgroups. A discussion of the complexities of ABO genetics is outside the scope of this chapter. Although ABO genotyping is technically feasible, it is performed only rarely because fetal anaemia due to anti-A or anti-B tends to be mild in Caucasians, although it may be more severe in some other populations (Section 2.6.1).

7.4 Noninvasive testing

The fetal genotyping tests described in the previous Sections utilize genomic DNA isolated from cells contained in amniotic fluid or chorionic villi. These cells or tissues are obtained using invasive procedures. Thus, the benefit of knowing the fetal genotype must be measured against the small risk of performing amniocentesis or chorionic villous sampling. Noninvasive testing by the analysis of fetal DNA or RNA in maternal blood would circumvent these risks and might herald the more widespread use of prenatal genetic testing.[59] As a result of the ease with which maternal and fetal D status can be determined serologically, *RHD* genotyping has been used as a test bed to explore the use of noninvasive methods.

7.4.1 Detection of fetal RHD targets in genomic DNA extracted from fetal leukocytes in maternal blood

Using a sensitive 'nested' PCR approach, Lo et al. showed that D-specific PCR products could be amplified from DNA derived from leukocytes isolated from the blood of D-negative women with D-positive fetuses.[60] The nature of the fetal cells in the maternal circulation was not identified but subsequent studies showed that they presumably included erythroid and lymphoid cells as well as fetal trophoblasts.[59] A significant disadvantage of this approach was the inability to demonstrate positively the D-negative genotype (i.e. the absence of the *RHD* gene). Negative test results might indicate the presence of a D-negative fetus or the absence of fetal DNA in the test sample. Thus, it is unlikely that this methodology will be used in clinical practice.

7.4.2 The detection of fetal RhD cDNA derived from RNA extracted from maternal blood

The detection of fetal RhD mRNA via synthesis of cDNA was first described by Hamlington et al.[61] The method was found to have an overall accuracy of 75% on analysis of 96 D-negative women, but was less reliable early in pregnancy.[62] Using a similar approach, Al-Mufti et al.[63] correctly identified 28 of 35 RhD-positive fetuses using a CD71-sorted fraction of cells from maternal peripheral blood, followed by RNA extraction and cDNA synthesis. They concluded that the mRNA detection procedure is more sensitive than the detection of fetal genomic DNA in maternal peripheral blood. Clearly, this methodology has some merit, but it is unclear if it can be successfully applied to clinical diagnosis because RNA samples tend to be extremely unstable and are rapidly degraded. Furthermore, in common with techniques based on the analysis of fetal DNA, the high error rate associated with this technique highlights the fundamental requirement for an internal control to demonstrate the presence of fetal cells. Finning et al.[64] attempted to develop a suitable control for this method based on the detection of epsilon (i.e. fetal) globin mRNA, but, unfortunately, significant amounts of epsilon globin mRNA were also present in some adults.

7.4.3 Detection of fetal RHD targets in genomic DNA extracted from maternal plasma

Lo et al.,[65] using DNA extracted from maternal plasma, were first able to demonstrate the presence of fetal Y chromosomes in maternal blood. These studies were later extended to include the analysis of *RHD* blood group genes.[66,67] The methods that were exploited to detect fetal DNA included real-time PCR (Taq-man™ chemistry) and normal liquid-phase PCR. The advantages of this technique include the fact that fetal DNA is rapidly degraded *postpartum*. This reduces the risk of falsely typing a D-negative fetus as D positive due to the presence of D-positive DNA from a previous pregnancy. In one study, it was found that the mean half-life for fetal DNA in material blood was 16.3 minutes, and that most women had undetectable levels of Y chromosome DNA 2 hours after delivery.[68] The origin of fetal DNA in maternal plasma is unclear, but it may be derived from the breakdown of fetal trophoblasts. The level of fetal DNA in maternal plasma has been reported to range between 0.39% and 11.9% of total DNA.[69]

Further work is required to develop appropriate controls for procedures such as those described above before the tests may reliably be used for fetal genotyping.

7.5 Future perspectives

The first few years of the third millennium are seeing the completion of the human genome project. The billionth base pair was deposited in October 1999, the complete sequence of chromosome 22 was published in December 1999 and a first draft of the complete human sequence was completed shortly thereafter. The completion of this project is precipitating the widespread development of rapid throughput tests for the diagnosis of genetic disposition to certain diseases. The technology that is being used for these types of analyses is developing at an astounding pace. Perhaps the most significant of these developments is DNA microarraying where tens of thousands of individual spots of DNA probes can be placed on microscope slides. These DNA probes (either oligonucleotides or cDNAs) are spatially addressed, and, when probed with genomic DNA or cDNA, can identify the presence of certain alleles or the expression of specific mRNAs. This technology can be readily adapted to such areas as fetal genotyping and will enable the detection of rare partial and weak D alleles.

7.6 References

1 Saiki RK, Scharf, S, Faloona, FA et al. (1985). Enzymatic amplification of β-globin genomic sequences and restriction site analysis for diagnosis of sickle cell anaemia. *Science*, **230**, 1350–4.

2 Wu DY, Ugozzoli L, Pal BK & Wallace RB (1989). Allele-specific enzymatic amplification of β-globin genomic DNA for diagnosis of sickle cell anaemia. *Proceedings of the National Academy of Sciences USA*, **86**, 2757–60.

3 Avent, ND (1997). Human blood group antigen expression: its molecular bases. *British Journal of Biomedical Science*, **54**, 16–37.

4 Reid ME & Yazdanbakhsh K (1998). Molecular insights into blood groups and implications for blood transfusion. *Current Opinions in Hematology*, **5**, 93–102.

5 Avent ND & Reid ME (2000). The Rh blood group system: a review. *Blood*, **95**, 375–87.

6 Liu W, Smythe JS, Scott ML, Jones JW, Voak D & Avent ND (1999). Site-directed mutagenesis of the human Rh D antigen: definition of D epitopes on the sixth external domain of the D protein expressed on K562 cells. *Transfusion*, **39**, 17–25.

7 Liu W, Avent ND, Jones JW, Scott ML & Voak D (1999). Molecular configuration of Rh D epitopes as defined by site-directed mutagenesis and expression of mutant Rh constructs in K562 erythroleukemia cells. *Blood*, **94**, 3986–96.

8 Cherif-Zahar B, Bloy C, Le van Kim et al.(1990). Molecular cloning and protein structure of a human blood group Rh polypeptide. *Proceedings of the National Academy of Sciences USA*, **87**, 6243–7.

9 Avent ND, Ridgwell K, Tanner MJA & Anstee DJ (1990). cDNA cloning of a 30 kDa erythrocyte membrane protein associated with Rh (Rhesus)-blood-group-antigen expression. *Biochemical Journal*, **271**, 821–5.

10 Colin Y, Cherif-Zahar B, Le van Kim C, Raynal V, van Huffel V & Cartron J-P (1991). Genetic basis of the RhD-positive and RhD-negative blood group polymorphism as determined by Southern analysis. *Blood*, **78**, 2747–52.

11 Daniels GL, Green C & Smart E (1997). Differences between RhD-negative Africans and RhD-negative Europeans. *Lancet*, **350**, 862–3.

12 Singleton BK, Green CA, Avent ND et al. (2000). An RHD pseudogene containing a 37 bp duplication and a nonsense mutation is present in most Africans with the Rh D-negative blood group phenotype. *Blood*, **95**, 12–18.

13 Okuda H, Kawano M, Iwamoto S et al. (1997). The *RHD* gene is highly detectable in Rh D− negative Japanese donors. *Journal of Clinical Investigation*, **100**, 373–9.

14 Fukumori Y, Hori Y, Ohnoki S et al. (1997). Further analysis of Del (D-elute) using polymerase chain reaction (PCR) with RHD gene-specific primers. *Transfusion Medicine*, **7**, 227–31.

15 Sun CF, Chou CS, Lai NC & Wang WT (1998). RHD gene polymorphisms among RhD-negative Chinese in Taiwan. *Vox Sanguinis*, **75**, 52–7.

16 Chang JG, Wang JC, Yang TY et al. (1998). Human RhDel is caused by a deletion of 1,013 bp between introns 8 and 9 including exon 9 of RHD gene. *Blood*, **92**, 2602–4.

17 Hyland CA, Wolter LC & Saul A (1994). Three unrelated Rh D gene polymorphisms identified among blood donors with Rhesus CCee (r′r′) phenotypes. *Blood*, **84**, 321–4.

18 Avent ND, Martin PG, Armstrong-Fisher SS et al. (1997). Evidence of genetic diversity underlying Rh D−, weak D (Du) and partial D phenotypes as determined by multiplex polymerase chain reaction analysis of the RHD gene. *Blood*, **89**, 2568–77.

19 Andrews KT, Wolter LC, Saul A & Hyland CA (1998). The RhD-trait in a white patient with the RhCCee phenotype attributed to a four-nucleotide deletion in the *RHD* gene. *Blood*, **92**, 1839–40 (letter).

20 Bennett PR, Le van Kim C, Colin Y et al. (1993). Prenatal determination of fetal Rh D type by DNA amplification. *New England Journal of Medicine*, **329**, 607–10.

21 Arce MA, Thompson ES, Wagner S, Coyne KE, Ferdman BA & Lublin DM (1993). Molecular cloning of RhD cDNA derived from a gene present in RhD-positive, but not RhD negative individuals. *Blood*, **82**, 651–5.

22 Wolter LC, Hyland CA & Saul A (1993). Rhesus D genotyping using polymerase chain reaction. *Blood*, **82**, 1682–3.

23 Simsek S, Bleeker PM & von dem Borne AE (1994). Prenatal determination of fetal RhD type. *New England Journal of Medicine*, **330**, 795–6.

24 Pope J, Navarette C, Warwick R & Contreras M (1995). Multiplex PCR analysis of the Rh D gene. *Lancet*, **346**, 375–6.

25 Flegel WA, Wagner FF, Muller TH & Gassner C (1998). Rh phenotype prediction by DNA typing and its application to practice. *Transfusion Medicine*, **8**, 281–302.

26 Avent ND (1999). The Rh blood group system: insights from recent advances in molecular biology. *Transfusion Medicine Reviews*, **13**, 245–66.

27 Aubin JT, Le van Kim C, Mouro I et al. (1997). Specificity and sensitivity of RHD genotyping methods by PCR-based DNA amplification. *British Journal of Haematology*, **98**, 356–64.

28 Gassner C, Schmarda A, Kilga-Nogler S et al. (1997). RHD/CE typing by polymerase chain reaction using sequence-specific primers. *Transfusion*, **37**, 1020–6.

29 van Wijk M-PA, Faas BHW, de Ruijter JAM et al. (1998). Genotyping of *RHD* by multiplex polymerase chain reaction analysis of all *RHD* specific exons. *Transfusion*, **38**, 1015–21.

30 Hadley AG, Poole GD, Anderson NA & Robson M (1996). Haemolytic disease of the newborn due to anti-G. *Vox Sanguinis*, **71**, 108–12.

31 Le van Kim C, Mouro I, Brossard Y, Chavinie J, Cartron JP & Colin Y (1994). PCR-based determination of Rhc and RhE status of fetuses at risk of Rhc and RhE haemolytic disease. *British Journal of Haematology*, **88**, 193–5.

32 Faas BH, Simsek S, Bleeker PM et al. (1995). Rh E/e genotyping by allele-specific primer amplification. *Blood*, **85**, 829–32.

33 Poulter M, Kemp TJ & Carritt B (1996). DNA-based rhesus typing: simultaneous determination of RHC and RHD status using the polymerase chain reaction. *Vox Sanguinis*, **70**, 164–8.

34 Kemp TJ, Poulter M & Carritt B (1999). Microsatellite variation within the human RHCE gene. *Vox Sanguinis*, **77**, 159–63.

35 Wagner FF & Flegel WA (2000). The RHD gene deletion occurred in the Rhesus box. *Blood*, **15**, 3662–8.

36 Lee S (1997). Molecular basis of Kell blood group phenotypes. *Vox Sanguinis*, **73**, 1–11.

37 Lee S, Lin M, Mele A et al. (1999). Proteolytic processing of big endothelin-3 by the Kell blood group protein. *Blood*, **94**, 1440–50.

38 Lee S, Zambas ED, Marsh WL & Redman CM (1991). Molecular cloning and primary structure of Kell blood group protein. *Proceedings of the National Academy of Sciences USA*, **88**, 6353–7.

39 Lee S, Wu X, Reid ME, Zelinski T & Redman CM (1995). Molecular basis of the Kell (K1) phenotype. *Blood*, **85**, 912–16.

40 Avent ND & Martin PG (1996). Kell typing by allele specific PCR (ASP). *British Journal of Haematology*, **93**, 728–30.

41 Lee S, Bennett PR, Overton T, Warwick R, Wu X & Redman CM (1996). Prenatal diagnosis of Kell blood group genotypes: KEL1 and KEL2. *American Journal of Obstetrics and Gynecology*, **175**, 455–9.

42 Hessner MJ, McFarland JG & Endean DJ (1996). Genotyping of KEL1 and KEL2 of the human Kell blood group system by the polymerase chain reaction with sequence-specific primers. *Transfusion*, **36**, 495–9.

43 Murphy MT, Fraser RH & Goddard JP (1996). Development of a PCR-based diagnostic assay for the determination of KEL genotype in blood donor samples. *Transfusion Medicine*, **6**, 133–7.

44 Lee S, Wu X, Reid M & Redman C (1995). Molecular basis of the K:6,-7 [Js(a+b−)] phenotype in the Kell blood group system. *Transfusion*, **35**, 822–5.

45 Lee S, Wu X, Son S et al. (1996). Point mutations characterize KEL10, the KEL 3, KEL4 and KEL21 alleles, and the KEL17 and KEL11 alleles. *Transfusion*, **36**, 490–4.

46 Chaudhuri A, Zbrzezna V, Polyakova J & Pogo AO (1995). The coding sequence of Duffy blood group gene in humans and simians: restriction fragment length polymorphism, antibody and malarial parasite specificities, and expression in nonerythroid tissues in Duffy negative individuals. *Blood*, **85**, 615–21.

47 Iwamoto S, Omi T, Kajii E & Ikemoto S (1995). Genomic organization of the glycoprotein D gene: Duffy blood group Fy^a/Fy^b alloantigen system is associated with a polymorphism at the 44-amino acid residue. *Blood*, **85**, 622–6.

48 Mallinson G, Soo KS, Schall TJ, Pisacka M & Anstee DJ (1995). Mutations in the erythrocyte chemokine receptor (Duffy) gene: the molecular basis of the Fy^a/Fy^b antigens and identification of a deletion in the Duffy gene of an apparently healthy individual with the Fy(a−b−) phenotype. *British Journal of Haematology*, **90**, 823–9.

49 Tournamille C, Le Van Kim C, Gane P, Cartron J-P & Colin Y (1995). Molecular basis and PCR-DNA typing of the Fy^a/Fy^b blood group polymorphism. *Human Genetics*, **95**, 407–10.

50 Olsson ML, Hansson C, Avent ND, Akesson IE, Green CA & Daniels GL (1998). A clinically applicable method for determining the three major alleles at the Duffy (FY) blood group locus using polymerase chain reaction with allele-specific primers. *Transfusion*, **38**, 168–73.

51 Mullighan CG, Marshall SE, Fanning GC, Briggs DC & Welsh KI (1998). Rapid haplotyping of mutations in the Duffy gene using the polymerase chain reaction and sequence-specific primers. *Tissue Antigens*, **51**, 195–9.

52 Olives B, Mattei MG, Huet M et al. (1995). Kidd blood group and urea transport function of human erythrocytes are carried by the same protein. *Journal of Biological Chemistry*, **270**, 15607–10.

53 Olives B, Merriman M, Bailly P et al. (1997). The molecular basis of the Kidd blood group polymorphism and its lack of association with type 1 diabetes susceptibility. *Human Molecular Genetics*, **6**, 1017–20.

54 Irshaid NM, Thuresson B & Olsson ML (1998). Genomic typing of the Kidd blood group locus by a single-tube allele-specific primer PCR technique. *British Journal of Haematology*, **102**, l010–14.

55 Lucien N, Sidoux-Walter F, Olives B et al. (1998). Characterization of the gene encoding the human Kidd blood group/urea transporter protein. Evidence for splice site mutations in Jk null individuals. *Journal of Biological Chemistry*, **273**, 12973–80.

56 Irshaid NM, Henry SM & Olsson ML (2000). Genomic characterization of the Kidd blood group gene: different molecular basis of the Jk(a−b−) phenotype in Polynesians and Finns. *Transfusion*, **40**, 69–74.

57 Olsson ML & Chester MA (1995). A rapid and simple ABO genotype screening method using a novel B/O2 versus A/O2 discriminating nucleotide substitution at the ABO locus. *Vox Sanguinis*, **69**, 242–7.

58 Gassner C, Schmarda A, Nussbaumer W & Schonitzer D (1996). ABO glycosyltransferase genotyping by polymerase chain reaction using sequence-specific primers. *Blood*, **88**, 1852–6.

59 Bianchi DW (1999). Fetal cells in the maternal circulation: feasibility for prenatal diagnosis. *British Journal of Haematology*, **105**, 574–83.

60 Lo Y-MD, Bowell PJ, Selinger M et al. (1993). Prenatal determination of fetal RhD status by analysis of peripheral blood of rhesus negative mothers. *Lancet*, **341**, 1147–8.

61 Hamlington J, Cunningham J, Mason G, Mueller R & Miller D (1997). Prenatal detection of rhesus D genotype. *Lancet*, **349**, 540.

62 Cunningham J, Yates Z, Hamlington J, Mason G, Mueller R & Miller D (1999). Non-invasive RNA-based determination of fetal Rhesus D type: a prospective study based on 96 pregnancies. *British Journal of Obstetrics and Gynaecology*, **106**, 1023–8.

63 Al-Mufti R, Howard C, Overton T et al. (1998). Detection of fetal messenger ribonucleic acid in maternal blood to determine fetal RhD status as a strategy for noninvasive prenatal diagnosis. *American Journal of Obstetrics and Gynecology*, **179**, 210–14.

64. Finning KM, Martin PG, Soothill P & Avent ND (1999). Noninvasive prenatal diagnosis of fetal blood group status. *Transfusion Medicine*, **9** (suppl 1), 32.

65 Lo YMD, Corbetta N, Chamberlain PF, Rai V, Sargent IL & Redman CWG (1997). Presence of fetal DNA in maternal plasma and serum. *Lancet*, **350**, 485–7.

66 Lo YMD, Hjelm NM, Fidler C et al.(1998). Prenatal diagnosis of fetal RhD status by molecular analysis of maternal plasma. *New England Journal of Medicine*, **339**, 1734–8.

67 Faas BH, Beuling EA, Christiaens GC, von dem Borne AE & van der Schoot CE (1998). Detection of fetal RHD-specific sequences in maternal plasma. *Lancet*, **352**, 1196.

68 Lo YM, Zhang J, Leung TN, Lau TK, Chang AM & Hjelm NM (1999). Rapid clearance of fetal DNA from maternal plasma. *American Journal of Human Genetics*, **64**, 218–24.

69 Lo YM, Tein MS, Lau TK et al. (1998). Quantitative analysis of fetal DNA in maternal plasma and serum: implications for noninvasive prenatal diagnosis. *American Journal of Human Genetics*, **62**, 768–75.

Laboratory assays to determine the severity of haemolytic disease of the fetus and newborn

Andrew G Hadley

International Blood Group Reference Laboratory, Bristol, UK

8.1 Introduction

The clinical management of alloimmunized pregnancies relies on the use of laboratory assays first to screen for the presence of blood group antibodies and then, once detected, to forecast their potential clinical significance. Screening is discussed in Chapter 3. This chapter considers laboratory tests that measure or characterize blood group antibodies in an attempt to forecast the severity of fetal haemolysis and to identify those cases where amniocentesis or percutaneous fetal umbilical cord blood sampling may be warranted in order to determine more directly the extent of fetal haemolysis. These invasive procedures carry risks, such as transplacental haemorrhage leading to exacerbation of maternal alloimmunization and the worsening of fetal anaemia (Chapter 10). It is important, therefore, that laboratory assays should reliably predict disease severity because failure to do so will expose some pregnancies to these risks unnecessarily.

Numerous techniques have been developed to predict the severity of HDFN. These assays may be serological, quantitative or cellular in nature. In all cases, the aim is to establish thresholds of antibody activity or trends in activity which are predictive of fetal haemolysis. This chapter discusses the advantages and limitations of these approaches, emphasizing the need for a structured and sequential application of assays of increasing complexity in order to generate clinically useful information in a cost-effective manner.

8.2 Serological assays

The majority of antibodies which cause HDFN do not agglutinate red cells suspended in saline. Red cells suspended in saline tend to repel one another and the maximum distance between the lipid bilayers of red cell membranes is approximately 30 nM. The maximum distance between the two antigen-binding

Table 8.1 Summary of studies into the relationship between anti-D titres and the severity of HDFN

	Fetal outcome		Samples tested	Reference
Unaffected	Affected			
Titres* ≦8 in 154 of 161 cases	Titres *>8 in 27 of 34 cases		Samples taken during week 32; first immunized pregnancy	12
Titres*<64 in 78 of 106 cases	Titres*>64 in nine of nine cases		Samples taken during week 32; immunized during a previous pregnancy	12
Titres<32 in five of seven cases	Titres≧32 in 19 of 22 cases		Data refer to highest titre from each case	13
Titres<32 in 10 of 10 cases	Titres≧32 in nine of 10 cases requiring exchange transfusion, and 19 of 19 cases requiring IUT		Not stated	14
Not stated	Titres greater than the normal range in 12 of 25 'severely affected' cases		Samples taken during 32nd week of gestation	15
Not stated	Titres greater than the normal range in 13 of 24 'severely affected' cases		Samples taken at end of gestation	15
Titres<64 in 106 of 146 cases	Titres≧64 in 33 of 33 cases requiring exchange transfusion		Samples taken within 2 weeks of delivery	16
Titres<16 in 17 of 83 cases	Titres≧16 in 128 of 133 cases requiring exchange transfusion		Data refer to highest titre from each case.	10
Titres<32 in nine of 19 cases	Titres>32 in 20 of 23 cases requiring exchange transfusion or IUT		Samples taken <54 days (mean 7 days) before delivery	17

Notes:

IUT = intrauterine transfusion.

* = titre by agglutination in albumin.

sites on IgG is 14 nM and, so, IgG antibodies to antigens close to the lipid bilayer (anti-D, for example) cannot crosslink between red cells and cause haemagglutination.[1]

Suspension of red cells in saline containing a colloidal medium such as bovine serum albumin or treatment of red cells with enzymes such as papain, trypsin or bromelian reduces their negative charge and renders them susceptible to haemagglutination by IgG anti-D.[2,3] However, methods based on the use of colloidal media or enzymes also detect IgM antibodies and are not ideally suited to the characterization of the level of IgG antibodies which are the causative agent in HDFN. Assays using enzyme-modified red cells are relatively sensitive and antibodies reactive solely in these assays do not cause HDFN.[4,5] However, some workers consider these assays to have a role in the early detection of antibodies which may then be followed during pregnancy in case they subsequently become detectable in the indirect antiglobulin test.[6]

The indirect antiglobulin test uses an anti-IgG reagent to agglutinate IgG-sensitized red cells. The titration of antisera in the indirect antiglobulin test may, therefore, be used to indicate the level of IgG blood group antibodies; antisera are generally titrated by doubling dilution. Dilutions of antisera and red cells are usually incubated at 37 °C, and the titre of the antibody taken as the reciprocal of the highest dilution which gives haemagglutination after the addition of antiglobulin reagent. Suitable methods for this purpose have been described in detail elsewhere.[7] Titration studies to monitor antibody levels should begin during the first trimester or as soon as the antibody is detected in order to establish baseline values for comparison with titres obtained later in the pregnancy. Titrations should be performed every 2–4 weeks to reveal trends in antibody levels which help to predict the severity of fetal haemolysis. Recommendations for the use of serological testing during pregnancy have been prepared by several expert committees, including the American Association of Blood Banks[8] and the British Committee for Standards in Haematology.[9]

Although antibody titration is an inherently imprecise procedure, the technique does provide an indication of risk when performed under standardized conditions by experienced personnel. HDFN is uncommon in babies from women with anti-D titres of less than 16. In the USA, a 'critical titre' of 16 is generally accepted as an indicator of the need for direct fetal monitoring.[8] Others have questioned the safety of basing clinical management on the use of a critical titre of 16; van Dijk et al. found that 20% of anti-D antibodies with titres of less than 16 were associated with cases requiring exchange transfusion.[10] Critical titres for antibodies other than anti-D have not been established; anti-K, for example, may cause fetal anaemia at low titres.[11] Table 8.1 summarizes the data from several studies which have evaluated the accuracy with which anti-D titres forecast fetal outcome.

8.3 Quantitative assays

Given the imprecision of estimating antibody concentration by titration, several quantitative assays have been developed to measure more accurately the level of red cell-binding IgG anti-D in maternal serum. Assays based on the use of flow cytometry,[15] ELISA,[18,19] and radioimmunoassay[14] have all been reported to correlate with clinical severity better than antibody titration by indirect antiglobulin test. However, these assays are not used routinely.

In the UK, levels of anti-D (and sometimes anti-c) are generally quantified by AutoAnalyzer.[20] This apparatus mixes red cells, an enzyme such as bromelain and an agent to potentiate haemagglutination such as methyl cellulose and serum. The mixture is passed through incubation coils and then settling coils which allow agglutinated red cells to be separated from nonagglutinated cells. The nonagglutinated cells are then lysed and passed through a colourimeter which measures the released haemoglobin.

It is generally accepted that AutoAnalyzer results have a greater predictive value than titration results. However, there are few published comparisons of the two techniques and the greater predictive value of the AutoAnalyzer may be marginal.[21] Nevertheless, the AutoAnalyzer has several advantages over manual titration. It offers the ability to process a larger number of samples with greater reproducibility than is possible using manual titration.[20] Severe HDFN is very rare in women with anti-D levels of less than 4 IU/ml (or 0.8 μg/ml).[22] However, the converse does not hold, and several studies have found that antibody levels above 6 IU/ml are commonly found in cases where the infant is unaffected.[22,23] Importantly, the reproducibility of the AutoAnalyzer allows small increases in antibody concentration to be identified and this commonly indicates a worsening of fetal anaemia. Nicolaides and Rodeck found that fetal anaemia developed within 2–3 weeks when maternal anti-D concentrations increased by 15 IU/ml.[24]

8.4 Cellular assays

The failure of quantitative assays to predict reliably disease severity presumably reflects the various factors, in addition to antibody concentration, which influence disease severity (Section 1.3.2). Important among these factors may be differences in the functional or biological activity of antibodies from different individuals. The functional activity of antibodies is amenable to evaluation by the use of cellular assays which measure the ability of maternal antibodies to promote interactions between red cells and either monocytes or K lymphocytes. The basis of these assays is shown diagrammatically in Figure 8.1.

The adherence and phagocytosis of red cells by monocytes is measured in the

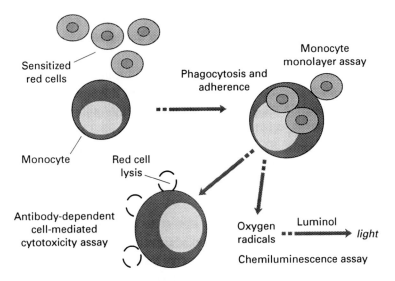

Figure 8.1   Diagram illustrating four cellular assays.

monocyte monolayer assay (MMA),[25] the metabolic response of monocytes to sensitized red cells may be measured in the chemiluminescence test (CLT)[19] and the lysis of red cells by monocytes or K lymphocytes is measured in antibody-dependent cell-mediated cytotoxicity assays, with monocytes (M-ADCC) or K lymphocytes (K-ADCC) as effector cells.[15,26]

Monocytes and K lymphocytes differ in the way they interact with IgG-sensitized red cells; monocyte-based assays reflect the interaction of IgG anti-D-sensitized red cells with Fcγ receptor I while K lymphocyte-based assays reflect interactions with Fcγ receptor III.[27] Monocyte-based assays preferentially detect IgG3 antibodies while the K-ADCC assay is sensitive to poorly characterized functional differences between antibodies which are not revealed in monocyte-based assays.[18,23,28] Although K lymphocytes are unlikely to participate significantly in red cell destruction in utero, the functional heterogeneity of different human monoclonal IgG1 anti-Ds in the K-ADCC assay correlates with their ability to promote the binding of red cells to macrophages via Fcγ receptor III in cryostat sections of human spleen.[29]

8.4.1 The K lymphocyte-mediated ADCC assay

The K-ADCC assay was the first cellular test to be evaluated for the potential to predict the severity of HDFN.[26,30] The assay involves the treatment of red cells with a proteolytic enzyme such as bromelain or papain. The red cells are then labelled with 51-sodium chromate (^{51}Cr) and added to peripheral blood mononuclear cells (depleted of monocytes by adherence) and serum. The mixture of red cells, serum and lymphocytes is incubated for 4–16 hours at 37°C and then the ^{51}Cr released from lysed red cells into the supernatant is determined using a gamma counter. Lysis is usually expressed as a percentage of maximum lysis in the presence of a detergent such as Triton X100.

Urbaniak et al. investigated a relatively small sample of 10 women with high levels of anti-D and showed that results from the K lymphocyte-mediated ADCC assay discriminated those women whose babies had mild HDN from those with severe HDN.[26] The K-ADCC assay has also been used to predict the severity of HDFN due to anti-c.[31] In contrast to these reports, Hadley et al. did not find a correlation between results from the K-ADCC assay and the severity of HDFN.[19]

8.4.2 The monocyte-mediated ADCC assay

The M-ADCC assay is somewhat similar to the K lymphocyte-mediated assay except that peripheral blood mononuclear cells are used as effector cells and red cells are washed after sensitization because fluid-phase serum IgG inhibits interactions between red cell-bound IgG and Fcγ receptor I.[15] The release of ^{51}Cr from damaged red cells may be increased by the addition of hypotonic saline.

The M-ADCC assay has been evaluated in a number of retrospective and prospective studies.[32] In a prospective study of 482 women with anti-D and D-positive fetuses, results from the M-ADCC assay correlated with disease severity better than titration results by indirect antiglobulin test or flow cytometric quantitation of red cell-bound IgG.[32] Moreover, in no cases in which M-ADCC assay results remained below a critical level until delivery did the infants suffer from severe HDFN. Based on these data, the M-ADCC assay has been used routinely in the Netherlands to assess cases of maternal alloimmunization to D.[33]

8.4.3 The monocyte monolayer assay

The monocyte monolayer assay involves the microscopic evaluation of red cell adherence and phagocytosis by adherent monolayers of monocytes.[34] In brief, mononuclear cells are separated from blood by density gradient centrifugation and monocyte monolayers are prepared by incubating mononuclear cells in Chamber Slides; nonadherent lymphocytes are then removed by aspiration. Sensitized red cells are then added to the monolayer and incubated for 1 hour at 37°C. The slides are then rinsed to remove nonadherent red cells and the cells stained with Wright/Giemsa. Monocytes are examined microscopically and the frequency of cells with adherent or phagocytosed red cells is estimated.

The superiority of the monocyte monolayer assay over manual titration with respect to predicting the severity of HDFN has been reported.[25] Assays with over 20% active monocytes predicted the requirement for treatment in 95% of cases; results less than 20% predicted a lack of requirement for treatment in 83% of cases.

Monocyte monolayer assay results were also reported to be a better predictor of disease severity than analysis of amniotic fluid.[34] However, other studies have not corroborated these findings.[35,36] Moreover, monocyte monolayer assay results appear to be very dependent on antibody subclass and false-positive results tend to be associated with sera containing mostly IgG3 anti-D.[28]

8.4.4 The chemiluminescence test

The CLT involves the incubation of sensitized red cells and monocytes in the presence of luminol which converts the metabolic biproducts of phagocytosis into light (chemiluminescence). The light is then measured in a luminometer.

Several retrospective and prospective studies have shown that results from the CLT correlate with fetal outcome better than results from the AutoAnalyzer.[37,38] Results from some of these studies are summarized in Table 8.2. However, it does not necessarily follow that results from the CLT can or should affect clinical management. In a 5-year prospective study involving 132 women with D-positive fetuses and over 5 IU/ml anti-D, the CLT correctly predicted outcomes more often than the AutoAnalyzer (84.9% of cases compared with 71.2% of cases, $P<0.01$).[39] Of 56 women managed at a single fetal medicine centre, 30 women had between one and five amniocenteses. Seven women received a total of 15 amniocenteses which were deemed 'negative' because the babies were unaffected by HDFN and absorbance OD_{450} results corresponded to Liley zones 1 or low 2. In retrospect, it would have been preferable had these procedures been avoided. When used to analyse maternal blood taken within 7 days of these amniocenteses, CLT results were consistently negative (less than 30%) while AutoAnalyzer results were less than 15 IU/ml in only six instances. Twenty-one women whose babies were severely affected by HDFN received a total of 43 amniocenteses, giving results consistent with fetal haemolysis (Liley zones 2M–3). CLT results were above 30% in 36 instances, but falsely predicted a lack of haemolysis in seven instances. Results from the AutoAnalyzer were similar, correctly predicting haemolysis in 35 instances, but falsely predicting a lack of haemolysis in eight cases. Overall, the CLT results were a better predictor of the appropriateness of amniocentesis ($P<0.01$).

In conclusion, it seems reasonable to use CLT results over 30% to prompt amniocenteses even when anti-D levels by AutoAnalyzer are less than 15 IU/ml; such results were invariably associated with haemolysis. This conclusion is subject to the caveat that the CLT would be expected to prompt 'inappropriate' amniocenteses in rare cases with blocking antibodies or defective placental transfer of IgG (Section 1.3.2.8). However, it is probably less safe to use negative CLT results as the basis for not performing amniocenteses.

Table 8.2 Summary of studies comparing the ability of the AutoAnalyzer and the chemiluminescence test to predict the severity of HDFN

Severity of HDFN	% sera with positive results*			Reference
	Unaffected or mild[1]	Moderate[2]	Severe[3]	
Study 1[4]	(*n* = 23)	(*n* = 8)	(*n* = 1)	19
AutoAnalyzer	48	100	100	
CLT	0	75	100	
Study 2[5]	(*n* = 8)	(*n* = 7)	(*n* = 4)	40
AutoAnalyzer	100[5]	100	100	
CLT	0	100	100	
Study 3[6]	(*n* = 8)	(*n* = 9)	(*n* = 10)	27
AutoAnalyzer	75	89	100	
CLT	12	78	100	
Study 4[7]	(*n* = 47)	(*n* = 24)	(*n* = 61)	39
AutoAnalyzer	28	54	85	
CLT	8	79	97	

Notes:

* A positive result is over 5 IU/ml (studies 1, 2 and 3) or over 15 IU/ml (Study 4) anti-D by AutoAnalyzer or a chemiluminescence test (CL) response of over 20% of the response to a positive control. All data shown are from women with D-positive fetuses.

[1] Hb > 12.5 g/dl at delivery, no exchange transfusions.

[2] Hb = 10.0–12.5 g/dl at delivery, ± exchange transfusions.

[3] Hb < 10.0 g/dl at delivery or intrauterine transfusions and/or intrauterine death.

[4] Sera containing IgG anti-D were collected during the last 8 weeks of pregnancy.

[5] Sera containing over 5 IU/ml anti-D were selected; all samples were taken during the last 8 weeks of pregnancy.

[6] Sera containing over 1 IU/ml anti-D were collected from 27 women.

[7] Sera containing over 5 IU/ml anti-D were collected from 132 women and tested prospectively over a 5-year period. Data shown relate to the highest AutoAnalyzer result or CLT result obtained for each pregnancy.

8.5 A strategy for antenatal testing

A primary aim of laboratories involved in antenatal testing is to provide obstetricians with clinically useful information in the most cost-effective manner. Information may be regarded as 'clinically useful' when it improves the appropriateness and timeliness of the invasive monitoring procedures – which remain the only way of establishing actual fetal haemolysis. Laboratory testing is performed against a background where most antibodies detected antenatally do not cause HDFN. Thus, cost-effectiveness derives in part from a structured approach to testing so that the more technically demanding assays are selectively provided for 'at-risk' pregnancies.

Serological screening is appropriate for all pregnant women in order to detect the presence of red cell antibodies (reviewed in Chapter 3). Antibody titration by the indirect antiglobulin test may be appropriate when the specificity of an antibody indicates the potential to be clinically significant. Quantitation of anti-D by AutoAnalyzer is preferred in the UK; quantitation is best suited to regional centres with a proven record of reproducibility. Functional or cellular assays should be used only for those relatively rare women with anti-D levels over 5 IU/ml whose fetuses are at risk of moderate or severe disease and who have probably been referred to a fetal medicine centre specializing in the management of HDFN. In these rare cases, cellular assays may provide additional information. Significant CLT or M-ADCC assay results might prompt direct fetal monitoring when anti-D concentrations are in the 'grey area' between 5 and 30 IU/ml. Negative M-ADCC results might be used to prevent or postpone amniocenteses. Cellular assays are specialized tests which need to be performed regularly and validated carefully. Given the rarity of cases requiring these tests, quality and cost-effectiveness are best achieved by providing these assays from specialist reference laboratories.

8.6 References

1 van Oss CJ & Absolom DR (1983). Zeta potentials, van der Waals forces and haemagglutination. *Vox Sanguinis*, **44**, 183–90.

2 Lewis M & Chown B (1957). A short albumin method for the determination of isohemagglutinins, particularly incomplete Rh antibodies. *Journal of Laboratory and Clinical Medicine*, **50**, 494–7.

3 Goldsmith K (1955). Papain-treated red cells in the detection of incomplete antibodies. *Lancet*, **i**, 76

4 Issit PD (1991). Lack of clinical significance of 'enzyme-only' red cell antibodies. *Transfusion*, **31** (suppl), 39.

5 Clark D, Greiss MA & Urbaniak SJ (1999). A prospective study of routine antenatal enzyme antibody screening demonstrates lack of clinical value in predicting haemolytic disease of the newborn. *British Journal of Haematology*, **106**, 824–6.

6 Garner SF, Devenish A, Barbar H, Contreras M (1991). The importance of monitoring 'enzyme-only' red cell antibodies during pregnancy. *Vox Sanguinis*, **61**, 219–20.

7 Walker RH, Hoppe PA, Judd WJ et al. (1990). *American Association of Blood Banks Technical Manual*. Arlington, VA: AABB.

8 Judd WJ, Luban NLC, Ness PM, Silberstein LE, Stroup M & Widmann FK (1990). Prenatal and perinatal immunohematology: recommendations for serologic management of the fetus, newborn infant, and obstetric patient. *Transfusion*, **30**, 175–83.

9 Voak D, Mitchell R, Bowell P, Letsky E, De Silva M & Whittle M (1996). Guidelines for blood grouping and red cell antibody testing during pregnancy. *Transfusion Medicine*, 6, 71–4.

10 van Dijk BA, Dooren MC & Overbeeke MAM (1995). Red cell antibodies in pregnancy: there is no 'critical titre'. *Transfusion Medicine*, 4, 199–202.

11 Vaughan JL, Warwick R, Letsky E, Nicoloni U, Rodeck CH & Fisk NM (1994). Erythropoietic suppression in fetal anemia because of Kell alloimmunization. *American Journal of Obstetrics and Gynecology*, 171, 247–52.

12 Bowman JM & Pollock JM (1965). Amniotic fluid spectrophotometry and early delivery in the management of erythroblastosis fetalis. *Pediatrics*, 35, 815–35.

13 Gall SA & Miller JM (1981). Rh isoimmunization: a 24 year experience at Duke University Medical Center. *American Journal of Obstetrics and Gynecology*, 140, 902–6.

14 Zupanska B, Brojer E, Richards Y, Lenkiewicz B, Seyfried H & Howell P (1989) Serological and immunological characteristics of maternal anti-Rh(D) antibodies in predicting the severity of haemolytic disease of the newborn. *Vox Sanguinis*, 56, 247–53.

15 Engelfriet CP & Ouwehand WH (1990). ADCC and other cellular bioassays for predicting the clinical significance of red cell alloantibodies. *Bailliere's Clinical Haematology*, 3, 321–37.

16 Gottvall T, Hilden J-O & Selbing A (1994). Evaluation of standard parameters to predict exchange transfusions in the erythroblastotic newborn. *Acta Obstetricia et Gynecologica Scandinavica*, 73, 300–6.

17 Filbey D, Garner SF, Hadley AG & Shepard SL (1996). Quantitative and functional assessment of anti-RhD: a comparative study of non-invasive methods in antenatal prediction of Rh hemolytic disease. *Acta Obstetricia et Gynecologica Scandinavica*, 75, 102–7.

18 Kumpel BM & Hadley AG (1990). Functional interactions of red cells sensitized by IgG1 and IgG3 human monoclonal anti-D with enzyme-modified monocytes and FcR-bearing cell lines. *Molecular Immunology*, 27, 247–56.

19 Hadley AG, Kumpel BM, Leader KA, Poole GD & Fraser ID (1991). Correlation of serological, quantitative and cell-mediated functional assays of maternal alloantibodies with the severity of haemolytic disease of the newborn. *British Journal of Haematology*, 77, 221–28.

20 Gunson HH, Phillips PK & Stratton F (1972). Manipulative and inherent errors in anti-D quantitation using the AutoAnalyzer. *Journal of Clinical Pathology*, 25, 198–205.

21 Morley G, Gibson M & Eltringham D (1977). Use of discriminant analysis in relating maternal anti-D levels to the severity of haemolytic disease of the newborn. *Vox Sanguinis*, 32, 90–8.

22 Bowell P, Wainscoat JS, Peto TEA & Gunson HH (1982). Maternal anti-D concentrations and outcome in rhesus haemolytic disease of the newborn. *British Medical Journal*, 285, 327–9.

23 Hadley AG & Kumpel BM (1993). The role of Rh antibodies in haemolytic disease of the newborn. *Bailliere's Clinical Haematology*, 6, 423–44.

24 Nicolaides KH & Rodeck CH (1992). Maternal serum anti-D antibody concentration and assessment of rhesus isoimmunization. *British Medical Journal*, 304, 1155–6.

25 Nance S, Nelson J, O'Neill P & Garratty G (1984). Correlation of monocyte monolayer assay, maternal antibody titres, and clinical course in hemolytic disease of the newborn (HDN). *Transfusion*, 24, 415.

26 Urbaniak SJ, Greiss MA, Crawford RJ & Fergusson MJC (1984). Prediction of the outcome of

rhesus haemolytic disease of the newborn: additional information using an ADCC assay. *Vox Sanguinis*, **46**, 323–9.

27 Hadley AG, Garner SF & Taverner JM (1993). AutoAnalyzer quantification, monocyte-mediated cytotoxicity and chemiluminescence assays for predicting the severity of haemolytic disease of the newborn. *Transfusion Medicine*, **3**, 195–200.

28 Garner SF, Gorick BD, Lai WYY et al. (1995). Prediction of the severity of HDN: quantitative IgG anti-D subclass determinations explain the correlation with functional assay results. *Vox Sanguinis*, **68**, 169–76.

29 Kumpel BM & Davenport RD (1996). Comparison of two FcγRIII-mediated assays of anti-D functional activity, using spleen and K cells. *Transfusion Medicine*, **6**, 20S.

30 Urbaniak SJ, Greiss MA, Crawford RJ & Fergusson MCJ (1981). Prediction of the severity of rhesus haemolytic disease of the newborn by an ADCC assay. *Lancet*, **ii**, 142–3.

31 Greiss MAM & Urbaniak SJ (1984). Abstracts of the *18th Congress of the International Society of Blood Transfusion*, Munich, Germany, p. 225.

32 Engelfriet CP, Overbeeke MAM, Dooren MC, Ouwehand WH & von dem Borne AEG Kr (1994). Bioassays to determine the clinical significance of red cell alloantibodies based on Fc receptor-induced destruction of red cells sensitized by IgG. *Transfusion*, **34**, 617–26.

33 Engelfriet CP, Reesink HW, Bowman JM et al. (1995). International Forum. Laboratory procedures for the prediction of the severity of haemolytic disease of the newborn. *Vox Sanguinis*, **69**, 61–9.

34 Nance SJ, Nelson JM, Horenstein J, Arndt PA, Platt LD & Garratty G (1989). Monocyte monolayer assay: an efficient non-invasive technique for predicting the severity of hemolytic disease of the newborn. *American Journal of Clinical Pathology*, **92**, 89–92.

35 Lucas GF, Hadley AG, Nance SJ & Garratty G (1993). Predicting hemolytic disease of the newborn: a comparison of the monocyte monolayer assay and the chemiluminescence test. *Transfusion*, **33**, 484–7.

36 Sacks DA, Nance SJ, Garratty G, Petrucha RA, Horenstein J & Fotheringham N (1993). Monocyte monolayer assay as a predictor of severity of hemolytic disease of the fetus and newborn. *American Journal of Perinatology*, **10**, 428–31.

37 Buggins AG, Thilaganathan B, Hambley H & Nicolaides KH (1994). Predicting the severity of rhesus alloimmunization: monocyte-mediated chemiluminescence versus maternal anti-D antibody estimation. *British Journal of Haematology*, **88**, 199–200.

38 Hadley AG (1995). In vitro assays to predict the severity of hemolytic disease of the newborn. *Transfusion Medicine Reviews*, **9**, 302–10.

39 Hadley AG, Wilkes A, Goodrick J, Penman D, Soothill P & Lucas G (1998). The ability of the chemiluminescence test to predict clinical outcome and the necessity for amniocenteses in pregnancies at risk of haemolytic disease of the newborn. *British Journal of Obstetrics and Gynaecology*, **105**, 231–4.

40 Hadley AG, Poole GD & Fraser ID (1992). Predicting the severity of haemolytic disease of the newborn: prospective evaluation of the chemiluminescence test. *Vox Sanguinis*, **63**, 291–2.

Assessing the severity of haemolytic disease of the fetus and newborn: clinical aspects

Sherif Abdel-Fattah and Peter Soothill

St. Michael's Hospital, Bristol, UK

9.1 Introduction

With the established use of postnatal anti-D prophylaxis for D-negative women, together with its increasing use for routine antenatal prophylaxis, the incidence of sensitization to D has markedly fallen. This is reflected by the reduction in the overall number of cases of HDFN (Section 5.3.2).[1] However, women with low antibody levels or in their first sensitized pregnancies continue to be referred to tertiary fetal medicine units for specialized management. Considerable effort is, therefore, spent by fetal medicine specialists in monitoring the disease course, predicting its progression and deciding on the need and timing of intrauterine transfusions.

The most accurate test to assess the degree of fetal anaemia, and thus the need for transfusion, is direct fetal haemoglobin measurement by fetal blood sampling. However, cordocentesis can cause an increase in the antibody concentration[2,3] and is associated with about a 1% fetal loss rate[4] and so is not an appropriate first-line investigation. Fetal blood sampling is best reserved for cases where severe fetal anaemia is already suspected and so intrauterine transfusion is likely to follow. At amniocentesis, the needle is rarely passed transplacentally and, therefore, the risk of boosting the antibody level is less than with cordocentesis, although the procedure still has small but significant risks of causing miscarriage or preterm labour. In recent years, several noninvasive methods for the prediction of fetal anaemia have been assessed and these are now allowing the use of invasive testing to be deferred, usually until transfusion is necessary.

In this chapter, the methods used to predict fetal anaemia, both invasive and noninvasive, will be discussed.

9.2 Noninvasive assessment

9.2.1 Previous obstetric history

In a woman's first sensitized pregnancy, the risk of significant fetal anaemia is low and fetal hydrops is a rare occurrence. The disease tends to become more severe with each subsequent pregnancy, with fetal anaemia occurring at a progressively earlier gestational age. This is likely to be due to the antibody-boosting effect of small fetomaternal haemorrhages during pregnancy and at delivery. Also, if hydrops has occurred in one pregnancy, it is very likely to occur again and it has been estimated that, once hydrops or a stillbirth has occurred from HDFN due to anti-D, there is a 90% chance that the next D-positive fetus, if untreated, will die in utero.[5] It has also been estimated that, after one previous stillbirth at term, subsequent stillbirths in utero will usually (>50%) occur before 35 weeks' gestation, but, after more than one stillbirth, before 32 weeks.[6]

A long-standing 'rule of thumb' for the management of patients with a previous affected pregnancy is to aim to time the first intervention approximately 10 weeks before the earliest previous intrauterine transfusion, fetal or neonatal death, or birth of a severely affected baby.[7] The reason for this policy is that, at this time interval, the fetus will often be anaemic but hydrops is unlikely to have developed. It is important to note that fetal death or hydrops due to red cell alloimmunization before 18 weeks' gestation is exceptionally rare. Therefore, in the absence of hydrops, cordocentesis should not be attempted before this gestational age, particularly because the fetal loss rate is significantly higher when the procedure is undertaken before 20 weeks.[8]

9.2.2 Antibody levels

All pregnant women should have their blood group status determined and have an antibody screen at their first antenatal visit. For D-negative women with no evidence of sensitization at booking, it is common practice in the UK to repeat the antibody screen at 28 and 34 weeks. Details of the various screening tests and laboratory aspects of measuring and characterizing red cell antibodies are described elsewhere (Section 3.3 and Chapter 8). In this chapter, the clinical use of the serological information generated in the management of red cell-alloimmunized pregnancies will be considered.

9.2.2.1 Anti-D

The maternal serum antibody titre is a guide to the severity of the disease, but this test is most useful in either first sensitized pregnancies or in those with only mildly affected previous pregnancies.[9] Although there are variations between laboratories, each should report the titre below which severe fetal haemolytic disease is considered unlikely (usually 1:32) and above which further investigations and monitoring are indicated. When the titre is below the threshold, it should be repeated initially every 2–4 weeks and with increasing frequency towards the end of the pregnancy. If the threshold is crossed, the antibody titre becomes an inadequate measure to rely on for management, although a rapid rise should always be taken as an indication of severe disease. Automated methods (Section 8.3) for measuring anti-D levels have been developed. Results from these methods are more precise than titres; levels of anti-D are reported in terms of μg/ml or IU/ml (1 IU = 5 μg). An anti-D titre of 1:32 is approximately 4 IU/ml. It has been suggested that amniocentesis is only indicated if the levels exceed 4 IU/ml[10] and, in more than 1200 sensitized pregnancies, the fetus was likely to be only minimally affected at levels less than 4 IU/ml (less than 5% of neonates required exchange transfusion for hyperbilirubinaemia).[11] The risks of more serious fetal disease increased with the antibody level and, at more than 10 IU/ml, the chances of the pregnancy being seriously affected increased greatly and either invasive testing or delivery if the pregnancy had exceeded 36 weeks were indicated.

More recently, a cross-sectional study of 237 pregnancies between 17 and 38 weeks' gestation determined the association between maternal anti-D levels and fetal haemoglobin. With maternal anti-D levels of less than 15 IU/ml, the fetus was, at most, mildly anaemic with a haemoglobin deficit of less than 3 g/dl, while, when the levels were over 15 IU/ml, the risk of severe fetal anaemia was high.[12] It was also reported that, with an anti-D concentration of less than 5 IU/ml, the possibility of fetal anaemia is only 3%, but, with levels of 30 IU/ml or higher, there was at least a 59% chance of fetal anaemia and at least a 36% chance that the degree of anaemia was severe.[6] It is, therefore, reasonable to reserve invasive testing for pregnancies with a maternal anti-D concentration of over 15 IU/ml. However, a steep rise in an antibody level between tests should be regarded as a strong indicator of increasing severity of the disease and a warning that intervention may be required soon. Also, antibody levels should be interpreted with all the other information and not used as a management cut-off alone.

Recently, there have been concerns about the considerable overlap between the ranges of anti-D levels in women whose fetuses were subsequently found to be severely affected, and in those with nonaffected fetuses.[12] One reason for this overlap might be the presence of differences in biological activity of the antibodies in different women. The chemiluminescence test (CLT) is a cellular assay which can provide a measure of the biological activity of antibodies and, therefore, potentially their ability to promote the lysis of the fetal D-positive red cells (Section 8.4.4). Recent studies have shown that CLT results were able to predict the fetal outcome and haemoglobin deficit with greater precision than the anti-D levels measured by AutoAnalyzer. The clinical application of this test, particularly its potential role in avoiding invasive testing, requires further work.[13,14]

9.2.2.2 Other red cell antibodies

There are at least 100 known red blood cell surface antigens other than the D antigen and some of them can cause HDFN.[2] With the recent marked decline in the incidence of alloimmunization to D due to the use of anti-D prophylaxis, a relative increase in the proportion of cases of alloimmunization due to other antigens has been noted. However, it is important to note that anti-D is still the most common and important cause of haemolytic disease of the fetus.[5] Antibodies to some of the nonD antigens, especially anti-K, anti-c and anti-E, can cause severe fetal haemolytic disease and death and so require intrauterine transfusion and timed delivery, as with anti-D. Other antibodies like anti-e, anti-C, anti-Fy[a] and anti-Jk[a] can cause significant, but usually less severe, haemolytic disease.[15-18] Severe haemolytic disease due to other antibodies has only been described in sporadic case reports (Section 2.7).

There are no routine methods at present to measure the levels of nonD antibodies (except anti-c) and so assessment relies only on antibody titration. However, the titres are not reliable predictors of the severity of the disease and no intervention threshold titres have been identified so far, probably because of the relatively small numbers of cases of severe disease with each antibody.[19] The current approach for managing these cases is by serial monitoring of the maternal titres during the pregnancy, with further investigations considered if there are steep rises of the titres. Cases with high-titre[5] (over 64) antibodies of unknown disease potential should be investigated and monitored. The value of determining bilirubin levels in amniotic fluid by absorbance measurement at a wavelength of 450 nm when antibodies other than anti-D are present is unknown. However, they are certainly unreliable in women with anti-K (Section 9.6.1), and earlier resort to fetal blood sampling should be considered in these cases.

9.2.3 Ultrasound findings

9.2.3.1 Fetal hydrops

The sequence of events leading to the development of hydrops in severely anaemic fetuses is not fully understood and several theories have been proposed. Severe anaemia causes tissue hypoxia[20] which further results in hypoxic endothelial damage and increased capillary permeability. This may lead to protein loss into the interstitial space, hypoproteinaemia and, consequently, ascites.[21] Generalized oedema follows and is associated with worsening hypoproteinaemia. In response to red cell haemolysis and fetal anaemia, extramedullary haematopoiesis occurs and erythopoietic islets may cause distortion of the hepatic parenchyma, so increasing portal and umbilical venous pressures. This would impair hepatic function and protein synthesis, resulting in severe hypoproteinaemia and decreased colloid osmotic pressure which would further worsen the hydropic process.[22,23]

The presence of fetal hydrops in a red cell-alloimmunized case is a definite indication of severe fetal anaemia. The ultrasonographic features of hydrops include ascites, pleural effusions, pericardial effusions, scalp oedema, subcutaneous oedema and polyhydramnious. For hydrops to develop, the haemoglobin deficit must be more than about 6 standard deviations below the normal mean for gestational age.[24] Therefore, urgent intrauterine fetal transfusion is necessary once hydrops is detected. In alloimmunized pregnancies without fetal hydrops, weekly ultrasound scans can be used to detect early hydropic changes. The earliest sign on ultrasound scanning of anaemic hydrops (as opposed to other causes of hydrops, e.g. chromosomal abnormalities, cardiac anomalies, arrythmias or structural thoracic abnormalities) is fetal ascites which appears as free fluid within the peritoneal cavity.

9.2.3.2 Prehydropic changes

There have been many attempts to identify sonographic features of fetal anaemia which occur before the development of fetal hydrops and, for example, visualization of both sides of the fetal bowel wall[25] or polyhydramnious[26] have been suggested. The mechanism for the development of polyhydramnious in anaemia is not clear, although it might be due to the hyperdynamic circulation resulting from the fetal anaemia, leading to increased glomerular perfusion and, so, fetal polyuria. One study has suggested that the earliest sonographic feature of haemolytic disease is enlargement of the heart, and especially the right atrium, as the fetal circulation adjusts to the decreased haemoglobin concentration.[27] Another study proposed that enlargement of the fetal liver would compress the hepatic vessels, leading to decreased venous drainage of the umbilical vein and, therefore, umbilical vein dilatation.[28] However, the correlation between several of these suggested parameters and the degree of fetal anaemia as assessed by fetal blood sampling was examined and all parameters were found to be unreliable in predicting fetal anaemia in the absence of hydrops.[29]

9.2.3.3 Fetal liver and spleen size

Measurements of the liver and spleen have also been suggested as potentially reliable predictors of worsening fetal anaemia. The rationale behind this is that the liver is the major erythropoietic organ in the fetus from 8 weeks' gestation onwards, with the bone marrow gradually taking over this role in the third trimester. The spleen is also an important additional erythropoietic site in the fetus, producing up to one-third of the red blood cells from about 18 weeks until term.[30] Hepatosplenomegaly develops as extramedullary haematopoiesis increases in response to red cell haemolysis and is a well-known manifestation of haemolytic disease in newborns. In addition to its role in extramedullary erythropoiesis, splenomegaly may also be related to the rapid destruction of the antibody-coated red blood cells, which predominantly occurs in the spleen.

Two studies have described the measurement of the fetal liver length in a parasagittal plane and reported its usefulness as a predictor of fetal anaemia.[31,32] Other studies measured the fetal splenic perimeter in a transverse plane of the abdomen and noted that splenomegaly in nonhydropic fetuses predicted a haemoglobin deficit of over 5 standard deviations from the normal for gestational age with a sensitivity of 94%. Splenomegaly was found to be an excellent predictor of severe fetal anaemia in cases with no previous transfusion, but the measurements did not correlate when there was a previous transfusion or with milder degrees of anaemia. There was also a trend towards a better correlation between splenomegaly and anaemia with advancing gestational age, suggesting that splenic measurements may be a more useful tool after 30 weeks' gestation.[30,33]

Although some of these results were encouraging, it appears that when high-quality Doppler measurements are available (Section 9.5) these morphometric measurements add little useful independent information for the prediction of anaemia. So, in conclusion, our current practice is to look very carefully for the earliest features of ascites rather than any other structural measurement or appearance.

9.2.4 Fetal heart rate monitoring

9.2.4.1 Abnormal cardiotocography patterns

Some of the most pathological fetal heart rate patterns on antepartum cardiotocography (CTG) have been associated with fetal anaemia. Good correlations between abnormal CTG patterns a few days before delivery and the level of umbilical cord haemoglobin, presence of hydrops and perinatal fetal loss have been noted, with a sinusoidal pattern and late decelerations being strongly associated with severe anaemia. However, these patterns are only evident in severe disease and are often preterminal.[34,35]

The role of antepartum CTGs in detecting mild to moderate anaemia or anaemia at earlier gestational ages is less encouraging. An association has been noted between fetal anaemia in the second trimester (20–26 weeks' gestation) and abnormal fetal heart rate patterns which include fetal tachycardia, reduced baseline variability and the presence of prolonged decelerations. However, the sensitivity of these pathological fetal heart rate patterns for predicting fetal anaemia was only 33%.[36] Antepartum CTGs in third trimester pregnancies have been analysed according to 25 different classifications and the positive predictive values of abnormal fetal heart rate patterns to predict fetal anaemia ranged widely, according to the classification used, but the negative predictive value was always low.[37] Although a common association between sinusoidal fetal heart rate pattern and severe fetal anaemia is consistently found, most moderately anaemic fetuses were noted to have normal reactive CTGs.[38]

9.2.4.2 Computerized analysis

One potential problem with CTG interpretation is that it is subjective and prone to inter- and intraobserver variation. The usefulness of computerized analysis of short- and long-term fetal heart rate variability to predict mild to moderate fetal anaemia has been assessed to avoid the possible effects of subjective interpretation. A strong correlation between fetal heart rate variability and fetal haematocrit have been found even after adjusting for the effects of gestational age. When short-term variation was less than 5 ms or the long-term variation was less than 30 ms, the positive predictive values for fetal haematocrit of less than 30 were 85% and 90%, and the negative predictive values were 56% and 57%, respectively. The extent of the reduction in fetal heart rate variation was also positively correlated with the degree of fetal anaemia. However, there were false-negative cases and it was concluded that anaemia cannot be excluded by normal fetal heart rate variation.[39]

In our view, antepartum CTGs are of very limited use in the monitoring of fetuses at risk of developing anaemia. In addition, abnormal fetal heart rate patterns, including reduced variability, are also associated with various other fetal pathological conditions like intrauterine growth restriction and pre-eclampsia, and these conditions should be carefully excluded before assuming that the abnormal patterns are due to fetal anaemia.

9.2.5 Fetal Doppler ultrasonography

Doppler ultrasonography is a noninvasive method of studying fetal haemodynamics. While studies of the uterine and umbilical arteries give information on the perfusion of the placental circulations, results from the vessels supplying fetal organs can detect the haemodynamic changes that occur in response to pathological conditions. In normal pregnancy, the mean blood velocity in the descending thoracic aorta, common carotid artery and middle cerebral arteries increases with gestational age, possibly reflecting a progressive increase in cardiac output to fulfil the demands of the growing fetus.[40] The ideal measurement to describe both the physiological fetal haemodynamics and their changes in response to pathological conditions such as anaemia would be the absolute volume flow in a particular vessel. Volume flow (Q) is calculated from the product of the time-averaged mean velocity and the cross-sectional area of the vessel lumen. However, a large degree of error was found to occur with these measurements, particularly in relation to the vessel diameter, which is further compounded when the measurement is cubed in the equation to derive the flow. Therefore, these have been largely replaced by the time-averaged mean velocity (TAV) (the area under the spectral curve), the time-averaged maximum velocity (the average of the velocities making the spectral curve) and the peak systolic velocity (the maximum Doppler shift at the peak of the spectral curve).[41–43]

In theory, the concept of Doppler blood velocity evaluation being useful in the identification of anaemic fetuses is mainly based on the assumption of decreased blood viscosity with a decrease in fetal red blood cell count. Direct measurement of blood viscosity is technically difficult,[44,45] but decreased viscosity should result in an increase of peak blood velocity measurable by Doppler. It is likely that this effect will be more pronounced in the central part of the cardiovascular system such as the cardiac outflow tracts and the descending aorta.[46] Early studies were difficult to assess because of a mixture of methodologies used. Kirkinen et al.[47] reported a close correlation between umbilical venous blood flow and postpartum haematocrit in cases of immunization to D. Griffin et al.[48] noted a weak relationship of uncertain clinical significance between the time-averaged maximal velocity in the descending aorta and the haematocrit. Rightmire et al.[49] found a significant negative correlation between the fetal haematocrit and the time-averaged mean velocity in the fetal aorta. In contrast, Copel et al.[50] reported that peak aortic velocity indices appeared to be of limited usefulness in the prediction of the need for transfusion.

9.2.5.1 Fetal aorta

The statistically significant negative correlation between fetal haemoglobin concentration and the Doppler blood flow velocities in the descending fetal aorta was further confirmed in later studies. The finding of a time-averaged mean velocity in the aorta above the normal range suggests that the fetus is probably anaemic, whereas, if the velocity is at or below the normal mean for gestation, anaemia is unlikely. Since the cross-sectional area of fetal vessels, including the aorta, does not change in the presence of anaemia, it was suggested that the increased velocity must reflect greater blood flow from increased cardiac output. The correlation between fetal anaemia and cardiac output is probably mediated, as it is in postnatal life, by an increase in stroke volume. This can be caused by several mechanisms including decreased viscosity, hypoxic peripheral vasodilatation and, therefore, decreased peripheral resistance, or hypoxic stimulation of chemoreceptors leading to more myometrial contractility.[51]

The effectiveness of several ultrasonographic and Doppler parameters in the prediction of anaemia severity has been compared.[52,53] Increased flow velocities in the descending thoracic aorta were consistently shown to be significantly associated with the degree of anaemia. However, one study of gestational age-dependent 95% confidence limits of peak aortic velocities found that the prediction of fetal anaemia was possible with a sensitivity of 64%, specificity of 74%, positive predictive value of 73% and negative predictive value of 66%.[46] The authors of this paper considered that these figures were too low to be clinically useful.

9.2.5.2 Middle cerebral artery

In 1990, Vyas et al.[54] found an increase in the middle cerebral artery time-averaged mean blood velocity in cases of fetal anaemia. They suggested that this increase was the consequence of decreased blood viscosity and not due to peripheral vasodilatation as a compensatory mechanism for anaemic tissue hypoxia. In a larger study,[55] an inverse relationship between the middle cerebral artery peak velocity and the haematocrit was found, with all anaemic fetuses having peak velocities above the normal mean for gestational age. The authors reported that, by relying on the middle cerebral artery peak velocity, up to one-half of cordocenteses they would have performed on previous policies could be avoided. The increase in fetal haematocrit following intrauterine transfusion also results in a rapid statistically significant reduction in the middle cerebral artery peak velocity.[56]

A recent large multicentre study[57] involving 110 pregnancies at risk of developing fetal anaemia due to red cell alloimmunization reported that moderate and severe fetal anaemia can be detected by an increased peak velocity in the middle cerebral artery, with a sensitivity of 100% and with a false-positive rate of 12%. They found that the optimal threshold values for the peak velocity were 1.29 times the median of gestational age for mild anaemia, 1.50 times the median for moderate anaemia and 1.55 times the median for severe anaemia. The authors also suggested that the agreement of results from different centres involved in the study indicated the reproducibility of this measurement. The middle cerebral artery was selected because cerebral arteries respond quickly to hypoxaemia, due to the strong dependence of brain tissue on oxygen and, so, fetal anaemia is expected to produce rapid haemodynamic changes in this vessel.[57] This is recent confirmation that Doppler studies have an important place in the clinical management of these patients.

9.2.5.3 Splenic artery

Splenic artery Doppler has also been studied for the prediction of fetal anaemia. The spleen is a major site for the final destruction of fetal erythrocytes that have been damaged by circulating antibodies and also contributes to erythropoiesis in severe anaemia. One study described the measurement of an angle which reflects the average rate of deceleration during diastole (a straight line from the peak systole to the end of diastole) in the splenic artery Doppler waveform.[58] The authors reported a statistically significant correlation between the extent of the reduction of this angle and the degree of fetal anaemia. However, the numbers were small (41 measurements in 22 pregnancies) and the false-negative rate was not reported. Larger numbers, as well as data on the reproducibility of this measurement, are essential before we can assume any clinical benefits.

9.2.5.4 Venous Dopplers

The role of fetal venous Doppler studies to detect anaemia has also been assessed. Hecher et al.[52] studied the effect of fetal anaemia on the velocities in the ductus venosus, the right hepatic vein and the inferior vena cava, as well as the middle cerebral artery, the descending thoracic aorta and the atrioventricular valves, in 38 alloimmunized pregnancies. There was a trend for increased velocities in all venous and arterial vessels and increased diastolic peak velocities across the mitral and tricuspid valves. However, a statistically significant increase was found only for the velocities in the ductus venosus, thoracic aorta and middle cerebral artery. For these vessels, a regression analysis was performed and only the time-averaged mean velocity in the thoracic aorta was significantly associated with the degree of anaemia. The authors concluded that Doppler studies of the venous blood flow did not provide further information over and above the arterial measurements to allow the severity of fetal anaemia to be predicted. Another study[59] found that ductus venosus time-averaged blood velocities were significantly higher in anaemic than normal fetuses and the velocities returned to normal values the day after a transfusion. Increased ductus venosus velocity was thought to indicate increased volume flow through the foramen ovale to the fetal brain as a compensatory mechanism to the decreased oxygen content caused by fetal anaemia. The return of the time-averaged blood velocity to normal the day after the transfusion reflected the corrected fetal haematocrit and increased blood viscosity, and, possibly, the return of normal cardiac contractility.[59]

9.2.5.5 Overview of the use of Doppler

Multivariate regression analyses have been used to determine the best possible combination of various ultrasonographic and Doppler measurements to allow the prediction of the severity of fetal haemolytic anaemia. These included measurements of the fetal liver, spleen, umbilical vein diameter, placental thickness and Doppler measurements of umbilical venous maximum flow velocity and fetal aorta time-averaged mean velocities, together with anti-D antibody concentrations. Umbilical venous maximum velocity was found to be the most important single diagnostic parameter. While the information from the fetal aorta blood velocity measurements resulted in an improvement of the prediction equation, the morphological measurements were of no benefit.[53,60] Careful attention to the previous obstetric history and serial antibody quantification is equally important.[60]

9.3 Invasive testing

9.3.1 Amniocentesis

9.3.1.1 Amniotic fluid optical density

Bevis[61] in 1952 demonstrated that the severity of fetal haemolytic disease can be predicted by serial amniocentesis. Bilirubin is an end product of fetal red cell destruction and, therefore, the fetus with haemolytic anaemia tends to have elevated serum bilirubin levels. Although most of the fetal bilirubin is removed via the placenta, a significant amount is excreted into the fetal urine and appears in the amniotic fluid. Bevis showed that an increase in the bilirubin levels in the amniotic fluid correlates with the degree of fetal anaemia.

In 1961, Liley[62] suggested a management protocol for pregnancies complicated by anti-D by using the finding that the amniotic fluid bilirubin concentration can be quantified spectrophotometrically by the deviation in absorption at a wavelength of 450 nm (ΔOD_{450}). He described three prognostic zones according to the outcome of pregnancy and the severity of the disease as assessed by the haemoglobin at delivery. Liley's chart became the principal tool for the management of pregnancies complicated by alloimmunization to D for many years. Amniocentesis was performed when the maternal antibody level was more than 4 IU/ml, or 10 weeks before the gestation at which the patient had had a previous fetal death or delivery of a severely affected baby. In the third trimester of pregnancy, the accuracy of predicting the severity of the disease by the Liley chart was high.

The major disadvantage of Liley's chart is that it was devised for managing alloimmunized pregnancies in the third trimester. With the marked improvement in neonatal care and improved prognosis for very preterm babies over the last decade, management of these pregnancies gradually became more directed towards the second trimester. Attempts to extrapolate Liley's curves backward, to be used in the second trimester, met with limited success.[63–65] One study correlated fetal haemoglobin obtained by fetal blood sampling with ΔOD_{450} in pregnancies between 16 and 25 weeks' gestation and found that 68% of fetuses who were severely anaemic and required intrauterine transfusions, including 10 hydropic fetuses, would have been misdiagnosed as only mildly to moderately affected (mid zone) by the extrapolated Liley chart. It was therefore concluded that the ΔOD_{450} measurement before 27 weeks' gestation was not useful.[66] What later became clear is that the relationship between ΔOD_{450} and gestational age in normal pregnancies is not linear and so the extrapolation was incorrect. Queenan and coworkers[67] in 1993 produced normal ΔOD_{450} values between 14 and 40 weeks' gestation and suggested a new chart with four zones for the management of anti-D alloimmunized pregnancies. The reliability of the Queenan chart has been studied, with conflicting reports resulting.[68,69]

As described above, it is vital that the correct gestational age chart is used to interpret the results, but other technical problems can also occur. Contamination of the amniotic fluid with blood or meconium can cause marked differences in the reading – with serious implications, as these substances also absorb light at the same wavelength as bilirubin. In addition, bilirubin can undergo degradation by light and the specimen should, therefore, be transported to the laboratory in a light-resistant container.[9] Also, this technique provides only an indirect assessment of the degree of fetal anaemia. Even without technical difficulties, disease severity varies at any given ΔOD_{450}.[70] Another issue is that the development of the use of ΔOD_{450} was only based on cases with anti-D alloimmunization. Alloimmunization to K results in a different pathophysiology and produces fetal anaemia more as a result of erythroid precursor suppression at the progenitor cell level, rather than haemolysis (Section 2.5.3).[71] Therefore, fetuses of women with anti-K may have low serum and amniotic fluid bilirubin levels; if ΔOD_{450} is used in these cases, false reassurance is likely to be given.[72,73]

9.3.1.2 Fetal blood group genotyping

Perhaps the most important advance in the assessment of alloimmunized pregnancies in recent years is the ability to genotype the fetus by using the polymerase chain reaction (PCR) to analyse DNA derived from fetal amniocytes (Chapter 7).[74] This technique is of great benefit when alloimmunized women have heterozygous partners – so that the fetus has a 50% chance of being antigen negative and therefore unaffected. Previously, the main approach to determining the fetal blood group status involved obtaining fetal blood through cordocentesis, with its associated risks. Amniocentesis to obtain fetal amniocytes avoids these risks and can be done at an earlier gestational age than cordocentesis, so a negative result can provide early reassurance that the fetus will be unaffected and unnecessary invasive procedures avoided.[75] Alternatively, a positive result allows early antenatal management planning. Fetal blood sampling can then be scheduled with a view to a therapeutic procedure timed when the fetus is expected to be anaemic rather than as a diagnostic procedure for the presence or absence of anaemia. The option of termination of pregnancy at an early stage can also be a possibility for women with severe disease and a history of pregnancy losses as a result of alloimmunization.[75]

Reports of the accuracy of the PCR technique in determining the fetal blood group status have been very encouraging. Although false-positive and false-negative rates were very low ranging between 0 and 1.5 %,[76–78] false results could have very serious clinical implications. Misdiagnosis of a fetus as D positive might be followed by further invasive testing, usually by cordocentesis, subjecting a D-negative fetus to unnecessary risks. Conversely, a diagnosis which falsely identifies a D-positive fetus as D negative might lead to either omission or delay of the appropriate management with possible unfavourable outcome.[79] Therefore, at present, the results of this technique should still be interpreted with a knowledge of the possibility of an incorrect result.

9.3.2 Fetal blood sampling

Fetal blood sampling was first undertaken with fetoscopic guidance, but cordocentesis under ultrasound guidance then became the standard technique and played a major role in the management of fetal haemolytic disease. The technique has obvious advantages when assessing a fetus at risk of developing anaemia. Direct measurement of the fetal haemoglobin and haematocrit gives definitive information on the severity of anaemia. In addition, tests indicating red cell antibody binding (Section 3.3.1), haemolysis and fetal erythropoietic response as well as blood grouping can be undertaken.

The indications for fetal blood sampling are similar to those used to decide when to perform the first amniocentesis for ΔOD_{450}. These include a rapid rise in the maternal antibody level or its increase above the threshold for the local laboratory, a severe past obstetric history or signs suggestive of fetal anaemia on ultrasound scan or Doppler flow velocimetry. Cordocentesis can be performed as early as 18–20 weeks' gestation.[80] When sampling for this indication, equipment should be available on-site for rapid determination of the fetal haemoglobin and haematocrit within 1–2 minutes while the needle is still in the umbilical vein. If the fetus is found to be anaemic, intravascular fetal blood transfusion can then start immediately, which necessitates having blood ready for transfusion when cordocentesis is performed in these cases, thereby avoiding an extra invasive procedure.

9.3.2.1 Fetal haemoglobin and haematocrit

In normal pregnancies, the mean fetal haemoglobin increases linearly from 17 to 40 weeks' gestation.[24] The severity of red cell alloimmunization should be assessed and treated according to the deviation of the fetal haemoglobin from the normal mean for gestation. If the fetal haemoglobin is within 2 g/dl (2 standard deviations) of the normal and the direct antiglobulin test is positive, the fetus is only mildly affected and careful monitoring for increased severity is required rather than intrauterine transfusion or early delivery. Fetuses with haemoglobin deficit between 2 and 7 g/dl are moderately anaemic and require intrauterine blood transfusion. In fetuses with severe anaemia and ultrasonographic evidence of hydrops, the haemoglobin deficit is almost always over 7 g/dl and urgent intrauterine transfusion is required.[24] These measurements are rightly regarded as the 'gold-standard' in the assessment of severity in red cell-alloimmunized cases.

9.3.2.2 Fetal blood reticulocyte, erythropoietin and erythroblast counts

Indicators of the fetal compensation to haemolysis can provide information about the disease severity, in addition to the haemoglobin concentration. Reference ranges of the fetal reticulocyte count and its changes in alloimmunized pregnancies have been reported by various authors.[81–83] When fetuses are subjected to varying degrees of anaemia, they compensate by both cardiovascular adjustments and increased erythropoiesis. The erythroblast count is an indirect measure of extramedullary haematopoiesis, while reticulocytes are the products of both medullary and extramedullary erythropoiesis. The reticulocyte count increases linearly with fetal anaemia and has been found to have exceeded the 97.5th centile for gestational age when the fetal haemoglobin deficit was >2 g/dl. In contrast, when the erythroblast count exceeded the 97.5th centile for gestational age, the haemoglobin deficit was >7 g/dl.[84] It appears that the fetus responds to mild or moderate degrees of anaemia by stimulating medullary haematopoiesis. As in postnatal life, this is associated with an increase in the proportion of immature erythrocytes (reticulocytes) released into the circulation. Extramedullary haematopoiesis in the fetal liver starts with severe anaemia which results in erythroblastosis.[84] Indeed, fetal serum erythropoietin concentration was only found to be increased in cases of severe anaemia when the haemoglobin deficit was >7 g/dl, which indicates that tissue oxygenation is maintained in mild anaemia, probably through placental clearance of lactate and increased cardiac output and peripheral perfusion.[20,85] However, fetal plasma erythropoietin does not seem to increase in response to even severe anaemia before 24 weeks' gestation.[86] Most importantly, the risk of developing anaemia in the following few weeks is increased when the reticulocyte count and direct antiglobulin test titre are elevated.[82]

9.3.2.3 Fetal bilirubin levels

As already discussed, elevated serum bilirubin levels are expected in fetuses with active haemolysis. In normal pregnancies, umbilical venous total bilirubin increases progressively with advancing gestational age. Umbilical venous total bilirubin levels in antigen-positive fetuses were found to be inversely related to haemoglobin concentration and rose with gestational age at a rate significantly greater than expected.[87] Bilirubin levels often exceeded the 97.5th centile before the development of fetal anaemia, although this may be slightly misleading because anaemia in this study[87] was defined as a haematocrit <30 rather than a gestational age-adjusted centile. Although fetal bilirubin levels may be an indication of the risk of developing severe fetal haemolytic anaemia, this is unlikely to be clinically useful.

9.4 Conclusions

Noninvasive tests to predict fetal anaemia are of value not only in avoiding unnecessary invasive procedures but also in deciding on the appropriate timing of intervention in fetuses with severe disease. However, none of the tests described can alone provide a 100% accurate prediction, so the assessment of patients with this condition should be comprehensive and include all possible relevant information. The obstetric history and antibody levels should be taken into consideration together with the results of ultrasonographic and Doppler blood velocity examinations. In the absence of fetal hydrops, other ultrasonographic parameters and antepartum CTGs, when normal, are of very limited value in predicting the severity of fetal anaemia and, therefore, no management decisions should be undertaken on the basis of these tests alone. Doppler blood velocity studies appear to be the most valuable single noninvasive test.

Amniotic fluid ΔOD_{450} still has a role in providing information on the extent of fetal anaemia in the third trimester when noninvasive tests are not conclusive, particularly in a patient with a previous history of affected pregnancies and antibody levels suggestive of a progressive disease. Fetal blood group genotyping by amniocentesis should be a part of the routine management of pregnancies in sensitized women with heterozygous partners. Fetal blood sampling by cordocentesis allows direct assessment of the degree of fetal anaemia. Normal reference ranges are available for the relevant fetal blood indices, endproducts of red cell haemolysis (bilirubin) and indicators of erythropoiesis (erythropoietin and reticulocytes), and can, therefore, provide information on the extent of the disease and the fetal compensatory responses. Cordocentesis is most useful during the second trimester or when intrauterine transfusion is likely to be required.

9.5 References

1 Hughes RG, Craig JIO, Murphy WG & Greer IA (1994). Causes and clinical consequences of rhesus (D) haemolytic disease of the newborn: a study of a Scottish population, 1985–90. *British Journal of Obstetrics and Gynaecology*, **101**, 297–300.

2 Bowell PJ, Selinger M, Furgeson J, Giles G & Mackenzie IZ (1988). Antenatal fetal blood sampling for the management of alloimmunized pregnancies: effect upon maternal anti-D potency levels. *British Journal of Obstetrics and Gynaecology*, **95**, 759–64.

3 Nicolini U, Kochenour NK, Greco P et al. (1988). Consequences of fetomaternal haemorrhage after intrauterine transfusion. *British Medical Journal*, **297**, 1379–81.

4 Soothill PW (1999). Fetal blood sampling before labor. In *High Risk Pregnancy, Management Options*, eds. DK James, PJ Steer, CP Weiner & B. Gonik, pp. 225–23. London: WB Saunders.

5 Bowman JM (1994). Intrauterine and neonatal transfusion. In *Scientific Basis of Transfusion*

Medicine. Implications for Clinical Practice, eds. KC Anderson & NM Ness. London: WB Saunders, pp. 403–20.

6 Nicolaides KH (1993). Management of red blood cell isoimmunized pregnancies. In *Ultrasound in Obstetrics and Gynecology*, eds. FA Chervenak, GC Isaacson & S Campbell. London: Little, Brown & Co, pp. 1543–55

7 Whitfield CR (1970). A three-year assessment of an action-line method of timing intervention in Rhesus isoimmunization. *American Journal of Obstetrics and Gynecology*, **108**, 1239–44.

8 Orlandi F, Damiani G, Jahil C, Lairicella S, Bertolini O & Maggie A (1990). The risks of early cordocentesis (12–21 weeks): analysis of 500 cases. *Prenatal Diagnosis*, **10**, 425–8.

9 Rodeck CH & Deans A (1999). Red cell alloimmunization. In *Fetal Medicine: Basic Science and Clinical Practice*, eds. CH Rodeck & MJ Whittle. London: Churchill Livingston, pp. 785–804.

10 Bowell PJ, Wainscoat JS, Peto TEA & Gunson HH (1982). Maternal anti-D concentrations and outcome in rhesus haemolytic disease of the newborn. *British Medical Journal*, **285**, 327–9.

11 MacKenzie IZ, Selinger M & Bowell PJ (1993). Management of red cell isoimmunization in the 1990s. In *Progress in Obstetrics and Gynaecology*, Vol 9, ed. J. Studd. Edinburgh: Churchill Livingston, pp. 31–53.

12 Nicolaides KH & Rodeck CH (1992). Maternal serum anti-D antibody concentration and assessment of rhesus isoimmunization. *British Medical Journal*, **304**, 1155–6.

13 Hadley AG, Garner SF & Taverner JM (1993). AutoAnalyzer quantification, monocyte-mediated cytotoxicity and chemiluminescence assays for predicting the severity of haemolytic disease of the newborn. *Transfusion Medicine*, **3**, 195–200.

14 Hadley AG, Wilkes A, Goodrick J, Penman D, Soothill P & Lucas G (1998). The ability of the chemiluminescence test to predict clinical outcome and the necessity for amniocenteses in pregnancies at risk of haemolytic disease of the newborn. *British Journal of Obstetrics and Gynaecology*, **105**, 231–4.

15 Bowman JM (1990). Treatment options for the fetus with alloimmune hemolytic disease. *Transfusion Medicine Reviews*, **4**, 191–207.

16 Filbey D, Hanson U & Wesstrom G (1995). The prevalence of red cell antibodies in pregnancy correlated to the outcome of the newborn: a 12 year study in central Sweden. *Acta Obstetricia et Gynecologica Scandinavica*, **74**, 686–92.

17 Geifman-Holtzman O, Wojtowycz M, Kosmas E & Artal R (1997). Female alloimmunization with antibodies known to cause hemolytic disease. *Obstetrics and Gynecology*, **89**, 272–5.

18 Goodrick MJ, Hadley AG & Poole G (1997). Haemolytic disease of the fetus and newborn due to anti-Fy^a and the potential clinical value of Duffy genotyping in pregnancies at risk. *Transfusion Medicine*, **7**, 301–4.

19 Van Dijk BA, Dorren MC & Overbeeke MA (1995). Red cell antibodies in pregnancy: there is no 'critical titre'. *Transfusion Medicine*, **5**, 199–202.

20 Soothill PW, Nicolaides KH, Rodeck CH, Clewell WH & Lindridge J (1987). Relationship of fetal hemoglobin and oxygen content to lactate concentration in Rh isoimmunized pregnancies. *Obstetrics and Gynecology*, **69**, 268–71.

21 Nicolaides KH, Warenski JC & Rodeck CH (1985). The relationship of fetal plasma protein concentration and hemoglobin level to the development of hydrops in rhesus isoimmunization. *American Journal of Obstetrics and Gynecology*, 152, 341–4.

22 Bowman JM (1978). The management of Rh isoimmunization. *Obstetrics and Gynecology*, 52, 1–16.

23 Socol ML, MacGregor SN, Pielet BW, Tamura RK & Sabbagha RE (1987). Percutaneous umbilical transfusion in severe rhesus isoimmunization: resolution of fetal hydrops. *American Journal of Obstetrics and Gynecology*, 157, 1369–75.

24 Nicolaides KH, Soothill PW, Clewell WH, Rodeck CH, Mibashan RS & Campbell S (1988). Fetal haemoglobin measurement in the assessment of red cell isoimmunization. *Lancet*, 1, 1073–5.

25 Benacerraf BR & Frigoletto FD (1985). Sonographic sign for the detection of early fetal ascites in the management of severe isoimmune disease without intrauterine transfusion. *American Journal of Obstetrics and Gynecology*, 152, 1039–41.

26 Chitkara U, Wilkins I, Lynch L, Mehalek K & Berkowitz RL (1988). The role of sonography in assessing severity of fetal anemia in Rh- and Kell-isoimmunized pregnancies. *Obstetrics and Gynecology*, 71, 393–8.

27 Queenan JT (1982). Current management of the Rh-sensitized patient. *Clinical Obstetrics and Gynecology*, 25, 293–301.

28 De Vore GR, Mayden K, Tortora M, Berkowitz RL & Hobbins JC (1981). Dilation of the fetal umbilical vein in rhesus hemolytic anemia: a predictor of severe disease. *American Journal of Obstetrics and Gynecology*, 141, 464–6.

29 Nicolaides KH, Fontanarosa M, Gabbe SG & Rodeck CH (1988). Failure of ultrasonographic parameters to predict the severity of fetal anemia in rhesus isoimmunization. *American Journal of Obstetrics and Gynecology*, 158, 920–6.

30 Oepkes D, Meerman RH, Vandenbussche FP, Van Kamp IL, Kok FG & Kanhai HHH (1993). Ultrasonographic fetal spleen measurements in red blood cell-alloimmunized pregnancies. *American Journal of Obstetrics and Gynecology*, 169, 121–8.

31 Vintzileos AM, Campbell WA, Storlazzi E, Mirochnik MH, Escoto DT & Nochimson DJ (1986). Fetal liver ultrasound measurements in isoimmunized pregnancies. *Obstetrics and Gynecology*, 68, 162–7.

32 Roberts AB, Mitchell JM & Pattison NS (1989). Fetal liver length in normal and isoimmunized pregnancies. *American Journal of Obstetrics and Gynecology*, 161, 42–6.

33 Bahado-Singh R, Oz U, Mari G, Jones D, Paidas M & Onderoglu L (1998). Fetal splenic size in anemia due to Rh-alloimmunization. *Obstetrics and Gynecology*, 92, 828–32.

34 Rochard F, Schifrin BS, Legrand H, Blottiere J & Sureau C (1976). Nonstressed fetal heart rate monitoring in the antepartum period. *American Journal of Obstetrics and Gynecology*, 126, 699–706.

35 Visser GHA (1982). Antepartum sinusoidal and decelerative heart rate patterns in Rh disease. *American Journal of Obstetrics and Gynecology*, 143, 538–44.

36 Nicolaides KH, Sadovsky G & Visser GHA (1989). Heart rate patterns in normoxemic, hypoxemic, and anemic second-trimester fetuses. *American Journal of Obstetrics and Gynecology*, 160, 1034–40.

37 Nicolaides KH, Sadovsky G & Cetin E (1989). Fetal heart rate patterns in red blood cell alloimmunized pregnancies. *American Journal of Obstetrics and Gynecology*, 161, 351–6.

38 Sadovsky G, Visser GHA & Nicolaides KH (1988). Heart rate patterns in fetal anemia. *Fetal Therapy*, 3, 216–23.

39 Economides DL, Selinger M, Ferguson J, Bowell PJ, Dawes GS & Mackenzie IZ (1992). Computerized measurement of heart rate variation in fetal anemia caused by rhesus allo-immunization. *American Journal of Obstetrics and Gynecology*, 167, 689–93.

40 Bilardo CM, Campbell S & Nicolaides KH (1988). Mean blood velocities and flow impedance in the fetal descending thoracic aorta and common carotid artery in normal pregnancy. *Early Human Development*, 18, 213–21.

41 Eik-Nes SH, Brubakk AO & Ulstein MK (1980). Measurement of human blood flow. *British Medical Journal*, 280, 283–4.

42 Gill RW (1985). Measurement of blood flow by ultrasound. Accuracy and sources of error. *Ultrasound and Medical Biology*, 11, 625–31.

43 Campbell S, Harrington K & Hecher K (1995). The fetal arterial circulation. In *A Colour Atlas of Doppler Ultrasonography in Obstetrics*, eds. K Harrington & S Campbell, pp. 59–69. London: Edward Arnold.

44 Giles WB & Trudinger BJ (1986). Umbilical cord whole blood viscosity and the umbilical artery flow velocity time waveforms: a correlation. *British Journal of Obstetrics and Gynaecology*, 93, 466–70.

45 Welch R, Rampling MW, Anwar A, Talbert DG & Rodeck CH (1994). Changes in hemo-rheology with fetal intravascular transfusion. *American Journal of Obstetrics and Gynecology*, 170, 726–32.

46 Steiner H, Schaffer H, Spitzer D, Batka M, Graf AH & Staudach A (1995). The relationship between peak velocity in the fetal descending aorta and hematocrit in rhesus isoimmuniza-tion. *Obstetrics and Gynecology*, 85, 659–62.

47 Kirkinen P, Jouppila P & Eik-Nes S (1983). Umbilical vein blood flow in rhesus isoimmuniza-tion. *British Journal of Obstetrics and Gynaecology*, 90, 640–3.

48 Griffin D, Cohen-Overbeek T & Campbell S (1983). Fetal and utero-placental blood flow. *Clinics in Obstetrics and Gynecology*, 10, 565–602.

49 Rightmire DA, Nicolaides KH, Rodeck CH & Campbell S (1986). Midtrimester fetal blood flow velocities in rhesus isoimmunization: relationship to gestational age and to fetal hema-tocrit in the untransfused patient. *Obstetrics and Gynecology*, 68, 233–6.

50 Copel JA, Grannum PA, Green JJ, Belanger K & Hobbins JC (1989). Pulsed Doppler flow-velocity waveforms in the prediction of fetal hematocrit of the severely isoimmunized preg-nancy. *American Journal of Obstetrics and Gynecology*, 161, 341–4.

51 Nicolaides KH, Bilardo CM & Campbell S (1990). Prediction of fetal anemia by measurement of the mean blood velocity in the fetal aorta. *American Journal of Obstetrics and Gynecology*, 162, 209–12.

52 Hecher K, Snijders R, Campbell S & Nicolaides K (1995). Fetal venous, arterial, and intracar-diac blood flows in red blood cell isoimmunization. *Obstetrics and Gynecology*, 85, 122–8.

53 Oepkes D, Brand R, Vandenbussche FP, Meerman RH & Kanhai HHH (1994). The use of ultrasonography and Doppler in the prediction of fetal haemolytic anaemia: a multivariate analysis. *British Journal of Obstetrics and Gynaecology*, 101, 680–4.

54 Vyas S, Nicolaides KH & Campbell S (1990). Doppler examination of the middle cerebral artery in anemic fetuses. *American Journal of Obstetrics and Gynecology*, **162**, 1066–8.

55 Mari G, Adrignolo A, Abuhamad AZ et al. (1995). Diagnosis of fetal anemia with Doppler ultrasound in the pregnancy complicated by maternal blood group immunization. *Ultrasound Obstetrics and Gynecology*, **5**, 400–5.

56 Mari G, Rahman F, Olofsson P, Ozcan T & Copel JA (1997). Increase of fetal hematocrit decreases the middle cerebral artery peak systolic velocity in pregnancies complicated by rhesus alloimmunization. *Journal of Maternal and Fetal Medicine*, **6**, 206–8.

57 Mari G, for the Collaborative Group for Doppler Assessment of the Blood Velocity in Anaemic Fetuses (2000). Noninvasive diagnosis by Doppler ultrasonography of fetal anaemia due to maternal red-cell alloimmunization. *New England Journal of Medicine*, **342**, 9–14.

58 Bahado-Singh R, Oz U, Deren O et al. (1999). A new splenic artery Doppler velocimetry index for prediction of severe fetal anemia associated with Rh alloimmunization. *American Journal of Obstetrics and Gynecology*, **180**, 49–54.

59 Oepkes D, Vandenbussche FP, Van Bel F & Kanhai HHH (1993). Fetal ductus venosus blood flow velocities before and after transfusion in red cell-alloimmunized pregnancies. *Obstetrics and Gynecology*, **82**, 237–41.

60 Iskaros J, Kingdom J, Morrison JJ & Rodeck C (1998). Prospective non-invasive monitoring of pregnancies complicated by red cell alloimmunization. *Ultrasound Obstetrics and Gynecology*, **11**, 432–7.

61 Bevis DCA (1952). The antenatal prediction of haemolytic disease of the newborn. *Lancet*, **ii**, 395–8.

62 Liley AW (1961). Liquor amnii analysis in management of pregnancy complicated by rhesus sensitization. *American Journal of Obstetrics and Gynecology*, **82**, 1359–70.

63 Harman CR, Manning FA, Bowman JM & Lange IR (1983). Severe Rh disease; poor outcome is not inevitable. *American Journal of Obstetrics and Gynecology*, **145**, 823–9.

64 Scott JR, Kochenour NK, Larkin RM & Scott MJ (1984). Changes in the management of severely Rh immunized patients. *American Journal of Obstetrics and Gynecology*, **149**, 336–41.

65 Ananth U & Queenan JT (1989). Does midtrimester ΔOD_{450} of amniotic fluid reflect severity of Rh disease? *American Journal of Obstetrics and Gynecology*, **161**, 47–9.

66 Nicolaides KH, Rodeck CH, Mibashan RS & Kemp JR (1986). Have Liley charts outlived their usefulness? *American Journal of Obstetrics and Gynecology*, **155**, 90–4.

67 Queenan JT, Tomai TP, Ural SH & King JC (1993). Deviation in amniotic fluid optical density at a wavelength of 450 nm in Rh-immunized pregnancies from 14 to 40 weeks' gestation: a proposal for clinical management. *American Journal of Obstetrics and Gynecology*, **168**, 1370–6.

68 Scott F & Chan FY (1998). Assessment of the clinical usefulness of the Queenan chart versus the Liley chart in predicting severity of rhesus iso-immunization. *Prenatal Diagnosis*, **18**, 1143–8.

69 Spinnato JA, Clark AL, Ralston KK, Greenwell ER & Goldsmith LJ (1998). Hemolytic disease of the fetus: a comparison of the Queenan and extended Liley methods. *Obstetrics and Gynecology*, **92**, 441–5.

70 Liley AW (1963). Errors in the assessment of hemolytic disease from amniotic fluid. *American Journal of Obstetrics and Gynecology*, **86**, 485–94.

71 Vaughan JI, Warwick R, Letsky E, Nicolini U, Rodeck CH & Fisk NM (1994). Erythropoietic

suppression in fetal anemia because of Kell alloimmunization. *American Journal of Obstetrics and Gynecology*, **171**, 247–52.

72 Berkowitz RL, Beyth Y & Sadovsky E (1982). Death in utero due to Kell sensitization without excessive elevation of the delta OD450 value in amniotic fluid. *Obstetrics and Gynecology*, **60**, 746–9.

73 Weiner CP & Widness JA (1996). Decreased fetal erythropoiesis and hemolysis in Kell hemolytic anemia. *American Journal of Obstetrics and Gynecology*, **174**, 547–51.

74 Bennett PR, Le Van Kim C, Colin Y et al. (1993). Prenatal determination of fetal Rh D type by DNA amplification. *New England Journal of Medicine*, **329**, 607–10.

75 Fisk NM, Bennett P, Warwick RM et al. (1994). Clinical utility of fetal Rh D typing in alloimmunized pregnancies by means of polymerase chain reaction on amniocytes or chorionic villi. *American Journal of Obstetrics and Gynecology*, **171**, 50–4.

76 Simsek S, Bleeker PM & von dem Borne AEG Kr (1994). Prenatal determination of fetal Rh D type. *New England Journal of Medicine*, **330**, 795–6.

77 Lighten A, Overton T, Sepulveda W, Warwick RM, Fisk NM & Bennett PR (1995). Accuracy of prenatal determination of Rh D type status by polymerase chain reaction using amniotic cells in Rh D-negative women. *American Journal of Obstetrics and Gynecology*, **173**, 1182–5.

78 Van den Veyver IB & Moise KJ Jr (1996). Fetal Rh D typing by polymerase chain reaction in pregnancies complicated by rhesus alloimmunization. *Obstetrics and Gynecology*, **88**, 1061–7.

79 Moise KJ Jr & Schumacher B (1997). Anaemia. In *Fetal Therapy, Invasive and Transplacental*, eds. NM Fisk & KJ Moise Jr, pp. 141–63. Cambridge: Cambridge University Press.

80 Daffos F, Capella-Pavlovsky M & Forestier F (1985). Fetal blood sampling during pregnancy with use of a needle guided by ultrasound: a study of 606 consecutive cases. *American Journal of Obstetrics and Gynecology*, **153**, 655–60.

81 Nicolaides KH, Thilaganathan B & Mibashan RS (1989). Cordocentesis in the investigation of fetal erythropoiesis. *American Journal of Obstetrics and Gynecology*, **161**, 1197–200.

82 Weiner CP, Williamson RA, Wenstrom KD, Sipes SL, Grant SS & Widness JA (1991). Management of fetal hemolytic disease by cordocentesis. I. Prediction of fetal anemia. *American Journal of Obstetrics and Gynecology*, **165**, 546–53.

83 Boulot P, Cattaneo A, Taib J et al. (1993). Hematologic values of fetal blood obtained by means of cordocentesis. *Fetal Diagnosis and Therapy*, **8**, 309–16.

84 Nicolaides KH, Thilaganathan B, Rodeck CH & Mibashan RS (1988). Erythroblastosis and reticulocytosis in anemic fetuses. *American Journal of Obstetrics and Gynecology*, **159**, 1063–5.

85 Thilaganathan B, Salvesen DR, Abbas A, Ireland RM & Nicolaides KH (1992). Fetal plasma erythropoietin concentration in red blood cell-isoimmunized pregnancies. *American Journal of Obstetrics and Gynecology*, **167**, 1292–7.

86 Moya FR, Grannum PA, Widness JA, Clemons GK, Copel JA & Hobbins JC (1993). Erythropoietin in human fetuses with immune hemolytic anemia and hydrops fetalis. *Obstetrics and Gynecology*, **82**, 353–8.

87 Weiner CP (1992). Human fetal bilirubin levels and fetal hemolytic disease. *American Journal of Obstetrics and Gynecology*, **166**, 1449–54.

Antenatal therapy for haemolytic disease of the fetus and newborn

Kenneth J Moise Jr and Paul W Whitecar
University of North Carolina School of Medicine, Chapel Hill, North Carolina, USA

10.1 Introduction

Intrauterine blood transfusion of anaemic fetuses represents one of the great successes of fetal therapy. The therapeutic success of other potential therapies for HDFN, such as plasmapheresis, intravenous immune globulin, immunoabsorption, oral tolerance and chemotherapeutic agents, has been met with more mixed views.

10.2 Plasmapheresis and intravenous immune globulin

10.2.1 Plasmapheresis

An interest in plasmapheresis for the in utero treatment of HDFN preceded the improved perinatal survival realized in the late 1980s with modern intrauterine transfusion techniques. Most of the literature has reported single cases or relatively small case series (Table 10.1). Many of the studies used the historical control of the outcome of the patient's previous affected pregnancy to assess a therapeutic effect. In addition, plasmapheresis has often been combined with intrauterine transfusion or intravenous immune globulin (IVIG) making assessment of its effect more difficult. Despite these limitations, a review of the published cases reveals a perinatal survival of 69%. This would appear to warrant further scientific investigation into the use of plasmapheresis as an adjunct in the management of the severely alloimmunized patient. A randomized clinical trial was attempted by the Canadian Apheresis Study Group, but, unfortunately, insufficient enrolment necessitated premature termination of the study.

Reported protocols vary considerably but all involve repeated procedures due to a rebound increase in antibody titre. In animal studies, Bystryn and coworkers[20] experimentally lowered antibody levels by exchange transfusion. Antibody levels were noted to rebound to over 200% of the initial levels with increases of up to 50–80% being seen even in the first 48 hours. Using weekly plasmaphereses,

Table 10.1 Reports of plasmaphereses for severe alloimmunization to D

Author	Reference	Number of patients	IVIG	Intrauterine transfusion	Number of fetal deaths	Number of neonatal deaths
Besalduch et al., 1991	1	1	Yes	Yes	0	0
Odendaal et al., 1991	2	9	No	No	1	0
Al-Omari, 1989	3	50	No	No	10	3
Berlin et al., 1985	4	1	Yes	Yes	0	0
Eklund, 1985	5	1	No	Yes	0	0
Van't Veer-Korthof et al., 1981	6	22	No	No	6	0
Hauth et al., 1981	7	2	No	Yes	0	1
Robinson & Tovey, 1980	8	14	0	Yes	3	2
James et al., 1979	9	1	No	No	0	0
Gunston et al., 1979	10	1	No	No	0	0
Graham-Pole et al., 1977	11	8	No	Yes	3	2
Tilz et al., 1977	12	12	No	No	0	0
Fraser et al., 1976	13	106	No	Yes	29	20
Pole et al., 1974	14	2	No	Yes	0	0
Fias et al., 1973	15	1	No	No	0	0
Kovacs et al., 1973	16	1	No	No	0	0
Clarke et al., 1970	17	8	No	Yes	1	1
Bowman et al., 1968	18	1	No	Yes	0	0
Powell, 1968	19	8	No	Yes	2	2

Note: Overall perinatal survival: 64%.

Robinson and Tovey[8] noted three different patterns of antibody titre equally distributed among their patients. Some patients were noted to have an initial suppression of their anti-D titre which then remained low throughout the gestation; a second group remained suppressed until 32 weeks' gestation when a marked rise occurred. The titres in the third group remained high despite repeated procedures with a rapid rebound to pre-pheresis levels at short intervals. Interestingly, all cases exhibited a dramatic rise in titre after delivery ranging from 66% to 1566% of baseline.

Most reports suggest starting plasmapheresis after 12 weeks' gestation. This approach seems reasonable in view of the documented transplacental passage of up to 60% of maternal levels of IgG1 and 30% of IgG3 antibodies by this gestation.[21] Some authors advocate the removal of 2–3 l of plasma two to five times weekly,[11] while others[3] feel that smaller volumes (500 ml–1 l) removed once weekly produce less rebound in antibody titre. The plasma that has been removed requires replacement; saline, plasma protein fraction, D-negative plasma and albumin have all been used as replacement. If plasmapheresis is to be used today, with modern concerns regarding viral transmission through blood products, albumin would seem to be the preferred fluid. Automated cell separators have been routinely used for the procedure. Citrate is employed in the machine's extracorporeal circuit to prevent coagulation. Robinson and Tovey[8] reported a 15% incidence of complications in 261 procedures in pregnant women. These included delayed vertigo, headache, allergic reaction to plasma, peripheral oedema and syncope; 10 cases involved mild citrate toxicity. The latter is usually heralded by circumoral paresthesia and can be treated with oral calcium. In some cases, intravenous calcium gluconate is required at the conclusion of the procedure.

The role for plasmapheresis today is probably limited to patients with a previous history of early perinatal loss and when technical limitations preclude successful intrauterine transfusion. In these cases, plasmapheresis may serve as a method to prolong the interval until an initial intrauterine transfusion can be undertaken.

10.2.2 Intravenous immunoglobulin

IVIG has been used effectively in the antenatal treatment of HDFN. In the largest series reported to date, Margulies and coworkers[22] described the exclusive use of IVIG in 24 patients with severe HDFN. Over one-half of the patients had experienced a previous pregnancy with a fetal or neonatal death, with 12% of the previous pregnancies involving two or more perinatal losses. All patients in the series carried a D-positive fetus, three having undergone cordocentesis in the case of a heterozygous paternal genotype. Patients received a total dose of 2 g/kg of IVIG administered over 5 consecutive days (400 mg/kg/day); the dose was repeated at 2–3-week intervals throughout the pregnancy. The patients were divided into three groups based on gestational age at the initiation of IVIG therapy: less than 20 weeks' gestation (group 1), 20–28 weeks' gestation (group 2) and over 28 weeks' gestation (group 3). There was a total of three fetal losses in groups 1 and 2. All three fetuses were noted to be hydropic at the start of therapy. There were no neonatal deaths, yielding a perinatal survival rate for the series of 88%. One-half of the neonates in group 1, one third in group 2 and 88% of group 3 required exchange transfusions leading the authors to conclude that IVIG is not effective if initiated after 28 weeks' gestation. Interestingly, the maternal anti-D titres fell in all three groups, although this difference was not statistically significant in group 2.

In a follow-up case-controlled study of 69 patients, this same group of investigators compared the outcome of pregnancies that received IVIG prior to 20 weeks' gestation in conjunction with subsequent intrauterine transfusion with the use of intrauterine transfusions only after 20 weeks.[23] Again, the study group represented cases of severe HDFN in that 73% of the IVIG group and 56% of the intrauterine transfusion group had experienced previous perinatal losses. Significant differences were noted between the groups. Hydrops at the first intrauterine transfusion occurred in 25% of the IVIG group as compared with 75% of the transfusion alone group (RR = 0.36). The first transfusion was performed a median of 1.5 weeks later in the patients who had received IVIG. Fetal death was 2.5-fold more likely in the transfusion-only group (51% versus 20%; RR = 0.39). Neonatal death occurred in 8% of the IVIG group as compared with 21% in the transfusion-only group, although this difference did not achieve statistical significance.

The mechanism of action of IVIG in cases of severe haemolytic disease is not well understood. At least three different explanations for its effect have been postulated: decreased production of maternal anti-red cell antibodies, decreased placental transport of antibodies and fetal reticuloendothelial blockade. Dooren and coworkers[24] randomized 20 patients to receive either intravascular intrauterine transfusion alone or intrauterine transfusion in conjunction with the direct fetal infusion of IVIG. No significant differences in transfusion requirement or clinical outcome could be demonstrated between the two groups. However, the average fetal IVIG dose of 85 mg/kg was fairly low compared with the 500 mg/kg dose usually employed to treat neonatal HDFN.[25] In a case report, Alonso and coworkers[26] used a dose of IVIG of between 406 and 481 mg/kg and administered this directly to the fetus on four occasions at the time of cordocentesis. Fetal haematocrit was noted to increase and absorbance $\Delta OD_{(450)}$ values decreased with advancing gestation. To further elucidate the protective mechanism of IVIG, one investigation compared six pregnancies treated with maternal IVIG with seven control sensitized women who were only followed with serial cordocenteses.[27] No obvious inhibitory effect on the transplacental passage of anti-D or the maternal anti-D production was noted. Finally, Besalduch and coworkers[1] reported a case in which IVIG was used in a patient with early hydrops fetalis secondary to anti-E alloimmunization. These authors used a pepsin-treated product resulting in a purified IgG preparation lacking Fc domains. Fetal hydrops and hepatosplenomegaly were noted to resolve with repeated administration. The authors postulated that effectiveness in their case was related to the suppression of maternal antibody levels since their product could not have crossed the placenta. Yu and Lennon[28] have recently proposed a mechanism to explain the potential ability of IVIG to cause the accelerated catabolism of circulating anti-red cell antibodies. An intracellular Fc receptor abundant in endothelial cells normally binds the IgG that has entered the cell through pinocytosis and presents it back to the surface of the cell for release back into the microcirculation. In cases of excess circulating IgG secondary to IVIG, the protective intracellular Fc receptors become saturated allowing for the accelerated catabolism of free IgG molecules that enter the endothelial cells. These data would lead one to conclude that, given in sufficient doses, IVIG may exert its

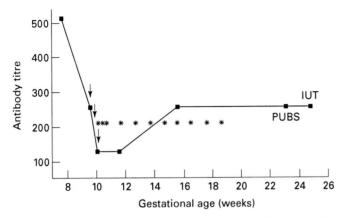

Figure 10.1   Case of alloimmunization to D managed with plasmapheresis × 3 (vertical arrows) followed by 1 g/kg infusions (*) of intravenous immune globulin (IVIG). PUBS is percutaneous umbilical blood sampling; IUT is intrauterine transfusion; fetal haematocrit was 29%.

predominant therapeutic role by blocking the fetal reticuloendothelial system; a secondary role would be the suppression of the level of maternal antibody.

Currently, the authors' centre offers a combination of plasmapheresis and IVIG to those patients with a previous fetal loss prior to 20 weeks' gestation. This approach is based on a randomized trial of 383 adult patients with Guillain–Barré syndrome.[29] In this trial, patients received one of three therapies: five plasmaphereses, 2 g/kg IVIG, or five plasmaphereses followed by a 2 g/kg course of IVIG. Patients in the latter group showed a trend towards more favourable outcome. In a case report, Berlin et al.[4] used a combined plasmaphereses/IVIG approach when problems with continued venous access precluded continued plasmaphereses in the patient's second pregnancy. A total of 10 l of plasma was exchanged over 4 days at 25 weeks' gestation. This was followed by an IVIG dose of 0.4 g/kg/day over 5 consecutive days. The patient's anti-D concentration became markedly reduced and did not return to pretreatment levels for 6–7 weeks. The infant was delivered at 35 weeks and was noted to have a cord haemoglobin of 12.5 g/dl.

The authors' protocol in a patient with severe red cell alloimmunization involves a single volume plasmapheresis every other day for three procedures in the 10th week of gestation. Albumin is used for volume replacement. After the third procedure, the patient is administered a 1 g/kg loading dose of IVIG diluted in normal saline after 25 mg of intravenous diphenhydramine HCl. The infusion is started at a rate of 60 cm³/hour and increased by 30 cm³/hour every 30 minutes to a maximum rate of 240 cm³/hour. A second dose of 1 g/kg is given the following day. The patient is then treated with a weekly dose of 1 g/kg until 20 weeks' gestation (Figure 10.1).

This dosing regimen gives plasma levels of IgG equivalent to the regimen of 0.4 g/kg daily for 5 days that has been previously used and is generally well tolerated. In the case of a heterozygous paternal genotype, an amniocentesis is undertaken at 15 weeks' gestation and DNA-based techniques used to determine the fetal red cell antigen status (Section 7.3). Chorion villus biopsy is not used in these cases due to the risk of a secondary amnestic response to fetomaternal haemorrhage.[30] Typical side-effects encountered during IVIG administration include urticaria and severe headache. We have found that premedication with 1000 mg of oral acetaminophen several hours prior to the scheduled infusion can prevent this latter complication. In some situations, a change to a different manufacturer will produce fewer reactions in some patients. On occasion, patients will complain of a desquamation of the palmar surface of the hands; the aetiology of this phenomenon is unknown. Standard noninvasive and invasive fetal testing is then used to determine the timing of the first intrauterine transfusion.

In the UK, plasmapheresis and IVIG are almost never used for the treatment of HDFN because of the high success rates of transfusion therapy. However, there is a consensus that plasmapheresis and IVIG are most likely to be of value in those patients with the most severe HDFN since they may lead to a delay in the requirement for very early transfusion and avoidance of the associated risks.

10.3 Intrauterine transfusion

10.3.1 History

The first successful treatment for haemolytic disease of the fetus was described by Liley in 1963 when he introduced the technique of intraperitoneal transfusion.[31] No further modifications in technique occurred until 1981. In that year, Rodeck and coworkers[32] described the intravascular transfusion of the fetus by directing a needle into chorionic plate vessels under visualization through a fetoscope. The following year, a group in Denmark reported the intravascular transfusion of a fetus by umbilical venous puncture under ultrasound guidance.[33] By 1986, two schools of thought had emerged regarding the optimal method for intravascular transfusion. A group of investigators at Yale proposed an exchange intravascular technique similar to that used to treat HDFN in the neonate.[34] A second group at the Mount Sinai Medical Center in New York championed the direct intravascular transfusion approach.[35] As more experience was gained with the two techniques, the direct intravascular transfusion became more widely adopted by many centres in the USA because it was associated with a shorter procedure time. Exchange transfusion was never taken up in Europe, mostly because the aim of exchange transfusion in the neonate is to reduce severe hyperbilirubinaemia and this is not relevant in the fetus because of the removal of bilirubin across the placenta. Interest in intravascular transfusion led to a virtual abandonment of the intraperitoneal transfusion by most centres treating red cell alloimmunization.

10.3.2 Access site

Initial attempts to gain access to the fetal circulation utilized the umbilical cord insertion at the placental interface. The cord insertion proximate to the fetal umbilicus should be avoided as vagal innervation is thought to be present in this portion, increasing the likelihood of fetal bradycardia. Weiner and coworkers[36] also noted that puncture of the midsegment of the umbilical cord was associated with a 2.5-fold higher incidence of fetal bradycardia as compared with puncture at the placental insertion. The vessel of interrogation should be the umbilical vein instead of one of the umbilical arteries. In one series of 750 diagnostic or therapeutic cordocenteses, the incidence of fetal bradycardia was 21% with puncture of the umbilical artery as compared with 3% with umbilical venous puncture.[36] Several authors have conjectured that this may be due to spasm of the muscularis of the umbilical artery. In 1982, Bang and coworkers[33] first described the use of the intrahepatic portion of the fetal umbilical vein as the site for intrauterine transfusion. In a subsequent series of 214 procedures, Nicolini and coworkers[37] reported a 2.3% incidence of fetal bradycardia utilizing this approach. In an effort to detect hepatic damage, liver enzymes were measured in 13 fetuses transfused using the intrahepatic vein and compared with 13 control fetuses who underwent transfusion using the placental cord insertion. No differences were noted at the time of subsequent intrauterine transfusion. These authors proposed that the absence of the umbilical artery at the anatomical level of the intrahepatic vein explained their low incidence of fetal bradycardia. An additional advantage proposed by the authors was that blood loss from the cord puncture site would be minimized by absorption from the peritoneal cavity. Despite these theoretical advantages, intrauterine transfusion using the intrahepatic vein has been reported to be associated with an increase in the fetal stress hormones of noradrenaline, cortisol and beta-endorphin.[38,39] Similar changes were not detected in these levels when the cord placental insertion was used as the site of transfusion. Puncture of the intrahepatic vein is technically more challenging than using the placental insertion, predominantly due to fetal movement. In addition, the fetus must present with its spine towards the maternal back to allow access. However, in cases of poor visualization of a cord insertion into a posterior placenta, the use of the intrahepatic vein is a viable option.

Direct cardiac puncture has been reported as a method of access for intrauterine transfusion, although it has been associated with a high rate of fetal death.[40] In one series of 158 cases of diagnostic cardiocentesis for the prenatal diagnosis of haemoglobinopathies, the corrected fetal loss rate was 5.6%, significantly higher than the 1% loss rate generally quoted for cordocentesis.[41]

10.3.3 Method of transfusion

Prior to the advent of intravenous transfusion, it was generally accepted that the hydropic fetus appeared unable to absorb red cells effectively from its peritoneal cavity after intraperitoneal transfusion.[42] Harman and coworkers[43] compared the experience at one referral centre between two time periods when either intravenous or intraperitoneal techniques were exclusively used. Patients were matched for severity of disease, placental location and gestational age at the start of transfusions. Several important outcome differences were noted. When the fetuses were divided into nonhydropic and hydropic groups at the time of the first transfusion, survival was only slightly improved in nonhydropic fetuses using intravenous transfusion (96%) as compared with intraperitoneal transfusion (83%). In the hydropic fetuses however, survival was markedly improved with intravenous transfusion (86% versus 48%). Intravenous transfusion resulted in the need for fewer neonatal exchange transfusions as compared with intraperitoneal transfusion (mean of 0.8 versus 1.8) as well as a shorter stay in the intensive care nursery (mean of 6.1 versus 8.2 days). It therefore appears that direct intravenous transfusion represents the preferred method of transfusion of the anaemic fetus. The intraperitoneal transfusion, however, remains a practical method for delivering red cells to the nonhydropic fetus when there is difficulty with access to the umbilical cord or intrahepatic umbilical vein. Bowman[44] has proposed a formula for the maximum intraperitoneal transfusion volume (ml) that has withstood the test of time. The volume of red cells to be infused is calculated by subtracting 20 from the gestational age in weeks and multiplying this by a factor of 10. Blood in the peritoneal reservoir can be expected to be absorbed over a 7–10-day period.

Serial haematocrits from fetuses transfused intravenously reveal a marked decline between procedures of approximately 1% per day.[35] In order to avoid this problem, the authors evaluated whether a combined intraperitoneal/intravenous technique would result in a more stable fetal haematocrit between intrauterine transfusions.[45] The technique involved administering enough packed red cells (haematocrit of 75–85%) by intravenous transfusion to achieve a final fetal haematocrit of 35–40%. A standard intraperitoneal transfusion was then undertaken. The hypothesis was that the intraperitoneal infusion would serve as a reservoir, allowing for the slow absorption of red cells between procedures. Four transfusion techniques in 19 fetuses were compared. A combined direct intraperitoneal/intravenous technique achieved a more stable fetal haematocrit compared with direct intravenous transfusion alone, resulting in a decline in haematocrit of 0.01% per day between transfusions compared with a decline of 1.14% per day. Nicolini and coworkers[46] compared 17 intravenous transfusions with 32 combined intraperitoneal/intravenous procedures. A final fetal haematocrit of 40% was targeted for the intravenous portion of the procedure. The volume of blood (ml) used for the intraperitoneal transfusion was calculated from the formula:

$$Hct_{post\ IVT/IPT} = \frac{[Vol_{IPT,\ ml}\ (hct_{post\ IPT} - hct_{initial})\ ] + hct_{post\ IPT}}{Vol_{IVT,\ ml}}$$

where:

IVT = intravenous transfusion
IPT = intraperitoneal transfusion
Hct = haematocrit.

Assuming complete absorption of the blood infused into the peritoneal cavity, a theoretical final haematocrit of 50–60% was used by these investigators to determine the volume for the intraperitoneal transfusion. Although the decline in haematocrit per day was identical for intravenous transfusion and combined intravenous/intraperitoneal transfusion, the combined procedure achieved a significantly longer interval between transfusions and also maintained a higher initial fetal haematocrit at subsequent transfusion. These data have led several centres to use a combined intravenous/intraperitoneal approach to intrauterine transfusion.

Reports of intrauterine transfusions in twin gestations have been limited to case reports. In one series of nine pregnancies complicated by alloimmunization to D, five of the cases required intrauterine transfusion.[47] Four of the five cases were noted to be dichorionic and diamniotic by first trimester ultrasound using the lambda sign. In one case, only one of the fetal pair was D positive illustrating the need to sample each fetus for antigen testing in such cases. In the authors' one case of monochorionic gestation, the intrauterine transfusion of one fetus was quickly followed by the movement of donor red cells through intraplacental anastomoses, as illustrated by a Kleihauer–Betke stain (Section 6.3.1) at the time of sampling, in the second twin. In the subsequent intrauterine transfusions, the transfusion of only one member of the twin pair resulted in adequate levels of haemoglobin in both twins. This case illustrates the complexity of intrauterine transfusions in twin gestations. Caution against overtransfusion should be undertaken in the monozygotic gestation. In addition, the use of the intrahepatic portion of the umbilical vein may be the preferred target for vascular access when transfusing a twin gestation and when the corresponding placental cord insertions are difficult to identify.

10.3.4 Amount to transfuse

The endpoint for the completion of an intrauterine transfusion varies considerably. Most centres use a target haematocrit to decide when a transfusion is completed. Advocates of direct intravenous transfusions will usually transfuse to a final value

Table 10.2 Transfusion coefficient for calculating transfusion volume

Target increase in fetal haematocrit	Transfusion coefficient
10%	0.02
15%	0.03
20%	0.04
25%	0.05
30%	0.06

of 50–65%. This will allow for a reasonable interval between procedures based on a projected decline in haematocrit of 1% per day. However, one should be cautious in transfusing the fetus to nonphysiological values of haematocrit. Welch and coworkers[48] demonstrated that a marked rise in whole blood viscosity is associated with fetal haematocrits above 50%. Centres that use a combined technique will usually use a final target haematocrit of 35–40% for the intravascular portion of the procedure.

Several authors have proposed formulae to calculate the volume of red blood cells to be transfused. The method of Mandelbrot and coworkers[49] requires the calculation of the fetoplacental volume (ml) from the ultrasound estimate of the fetal weight as the initial step (1.046 + fetal weight in grams × 0.14). The volume (ml) to be transfused is then calculated using the following formula:

$$V_{transfused} = \frac{V_{fetoplacental} \times (hct_{final} - hct_{initial})}{Hct_{transfused\ blood}}$$

Giannina and coworkers[50] proposed a simpler method of calculating the volume of packed red cells needed for intrauterine transfusion. Assuming a haematocrit of approximately 75% for the donor unit, they calculated a series of transfusion coefficients for raising the initial fetal haematocrit to a desired final value (Table 10.2). The operator simply multiplies the coefficient by the ultrasound-estimated fetal weight to achieve the final desired fetal haematocrit. Both the equation by Mandelbrot and the technique of Giannina yield similar results when tested prospectively; however, both overestimated the final fetal haematocrit by a value of 8%.

After the first intrauterine transfusion, subsequent procedures are scheduled at 14–21-day intervals until suppression of fetal erythropoiesis is noted on Kleihauer–Betke stains (Section 6.3.1). This usually occurs by the third intrauterine transfusion. Thereafter, the interval for repeat procedures can be determined based on the decline in haematocrit for the individual fetus – usually a 3–4-week interval.

10.3.5 The severely anaemic fetus

The severely anaemic fetus at 18–24 weeks' gestation is less able to adapt to acute correction of its anaemia. Monitoring of the umbilical venous pressure during intravenous transfusion has been found useful in such cases.[51] An increase of more than 10 mm Hg predicted fetal death within 24 hours after transfusion with a sensitivity of 80%. Radunovic and coworkers[52] noted a 37% mortality within 72 hours of intravenous transfusion in fetuses presenting with severe anaemia and hydrops. These authors recommended that, in the severely anaemic fetus, the final posttransfusion haematocrit after intravenous transfusion should not exceed a value of 25% or a 4-fold increase from the pretransfusion value. At the authors' centre, the umbilical venous pressure has been chosen to determine when to conclude an intravenous transfusion in a very anaemic fetus in the early second trimester. Periodic evaluation of the pressure is undertaken and the procedure concluded when the change in pressure approaches 10 mm Hg. A second intravenous transfusion is performed within 48 hours to correct the fetal haematocrit into the normal range; the third procedure is scheduled in 7–10 days. Thereafter, repeat transfusions are undertaken based on fetal haematocrits and Kleihauer–Betke stains. Others choose to evaluate progress of the transfusion by ultrasound assessment of blood flow and fetal heart rate and proceed directly to the full transfusion (even with hydrops) in a single procedure, with the second transfusion at about 2 weeks.

10.3.6 Adjunctive measures

Another important development in the field of fetal transfusion has been the use of fetal paralysis during the procedure. Prior to this modification, fetal movement often resulted in injury to fetal viscera during intraperitoneal transfusion or umbilical cord damage during intravenous transfusion. Fetal paralysis was first introduced by de Crespigny and coworkers[53] in Australia. Initial use in the United States involved the intramuscular injection of (d)-tubocurarine into the fetal thigh under ultrasound guidance.[54] Later, pancuronium bromide was used intravascularly.[55] More recently, short-acting agents such as atracurium besylate and vecuronium bromide have been utilized.[56,57] These latter agents do not appear to cause the fetal tachycardia and loss of short-term heart rate variability associated with pancuronium.[58] A vecuronium dose of 0.1 mg/kg ultrasound-estimated fetal weight produces immediate cessation of fetal movement after intravascular injection at the start of the intrauterine transfusion. Fetal paralysis can be expected for 1–2 hours. We have observed no untoward effects in neonates treated in this manner. However, the use of fetal paralysis is not indicated when the placenta is anteriorly placed and the needle is not passed through the amniotic fluid.

Prophylactic antibiotics have not been studied in association with intrauterine transfusion, and various centres have developed their own preferences. If they are to be used, a broad spectrum cephalosporin with coverage that includes gram-positive skin flora would appear to be appropriate.

10.3.7 Outcome

Overall survival after intrauterine transfusion varies with centre, experience and the presence of hydrops fetalis. No randomized or multicentred trials have been undertaken, therefore, to assess whether one type of procedure is superior to another in relation to fetal survival. An overview of the reported literature is presented in Table 10.3. Overall survival was noted to be 84%; up to one-quarter fewer hydropic fetuses survive with intrauterine transfusion (70%) as compared with fetuses who undergo their first intrauterine transfusion when they are not hydropic (survival of 92%).

Immediate follow-up studies of infants treated with intravenous transfusions in utero have revealed a need for 'top-up' transfusions in the early months of life. Typically, these infants are born with a virtual absence of reticulocytes, with a red cell population consisting mainly of transfused red cells containing adult haemoglobin. Exchange transfusions for hyperbilirubinaemia are rarely necessary. However, at 1 month of age, these infants often require a simple transfusion due to symptoms associated with anaemia. In one series of 36 infants who had undergone intrauterine transfusions, 50% required top-up transfusions at a mean age of 38 days, with a range of 20–68 days.[81] Studies of these infants indicate erythroid hypoplasia of the bone marrow accompanied by low levels of circulating erythropoietin and reticulocytes.[82] This led Ovali and coworkers[83] to study the use of exogenous erythropoietin in neonates after intrauterine transfusions. Twenty infants were randomized to receive 200 IU/kg of recombinant human erythropoietin or saline placebo subcutaneously three times a week between the second and eighth week of life. Infants in the treatment group required a mean of 1.8 red cell transfusions as compared with a mean of 4.2 transfusions in the placebo group. Absolute reticulocyte counts rose earlier and achieved higher levels in the treatment group as compared with controls.

As a result of this phenomenon, weekly haematocrit and reticulocyte determinations are recommended for the first 1–2 months of life in infants who have undergone intrauterine transfusions.[84] Proposed criteria for the transfusion of infants vary in the literature and are usually related to infants born prematurely. A more conservative approach is advocated by Maier and coworkers.[85] A threshold for haematocrit used by these authors is 32% if the infant is asymptomatic and 28% with symptoms. Citing the blunting of the normal erythropoietic effect by transfusion, Shannon and coworkers[86] proposed a threshold value for haematocrit of 30% or 20% in conjunction with symptoms. If erythropoietin is to be used, initiation in the first week of life in the infant with a persistently low circulating reticulocyte count may prove beneficial. Supplemental iron therapy is unnecessary due to the high levels of circulating iron in these infants secondary to ongoing haemolysis in utero.[87] Supplemental folate therapy (0.5 mg/day) should be considered.

Investigations regarding long-term neurological sequelae in infants who have been treated with intrauterine transfusions are limited. Hardyment and coworkers[88] reported a series of fetuses treated with intraperitoneal transfusion between 1966 and 1975; survival was only 48%. Twenty-one of the 27 infants underwent evaluation and evidence of cerebral palsy was found in two (10%). Advancements in the treatment of HDFN are resulting in the survival of increasing numbers of moribund and severely anaemic fetuses. It is therefore important to review the recent data on the follow-up of infants treated by intravenous transfusion (Table 10.4).

Doyle and coworkers[89] evaluated 38 surviving infants at 2 years of age. The authors noted one case of cerebral palsy, one case of mild disability with a mental developmental index of 72, and one case of severe developmental delay associated with seizures. Comparison with a group of 51 randomly selected infants of normal birth weight who underwent a similar assessment at 2 years of age yielded no significant differences in the incidence of sensorineural outcomes. Mean developmental index was found to be higher in the transfused group. Janssens and coworkers[61] studied 69 infants between 6 months and 6 years of age. Seven per cent of the children exhibited some evidence of neurological handicap; three infants (4%) were diagnosed with cerebral palsy. Sixteen per cent of the children were noted to have developmental delay; six cases showed mild delay while five additional cases exhibited severe delay. The overall rate of 10% disability in their group was found to be comparable to a cohort of normal Dutch children (6% disabled) and a cohort of high-risk children (12% disabled). We followed 40 surviving infants for up to 62 months of age.[90] One case of spastic hemiplegia was detected. Gesell and McCarthy developmental scores were similar to norms for the general population. Grab and coworkers[59] followed 30 infants and noted mild sensorineural disabilities in two. One infant exhibited delayed speech development at 24 months; the second had mild psychomotor developmental delay at 1 year of age that had resolved by 6 years of life.

Hearing loss in the neonate has been reported in association with high bilirubin levels.[91] Since red cell destruction can lead to higher than normal levels of bilirubin in utero, as well as elevated levels in neonatal life, it would appear that HDFN could be associated with sensorineural hearing loss. Janssens and coworkers[61] found a 14% rate in 58 children screened at 9 months. However, five of the cases were thought to be conductive in nature due to the association with middle ear or respiratory infection and the transient nature of the findings. Hudon and coworkers[90]

Table 10.3 Literature reports of intravascular transfusion

Authors	Reference	Technique	Number of patients	Number of survivors (total)	Number of survivors (hydrops)	Number of survivors (no hydrops)
Lepercq et al., 1999	47	IVT	9	9	NM	NM
Grab et al., 1999	59	IVT	43	35	7/11	28/32
Babinszki et al., 1998	60	IVT	41	36	NM	NM
Janssens et al., 1997	61	IVT	92	73	24/37	49/55
Inglis et al., 1996	62	IVT	19	19	3/3	16/16
Merchant et al., 1994	63	IVT	7	7	2/2	5/5
Plockinger et al., 1994	64	IVT	21	18	5/7	13/14
Sampson et al., 1994	65	IVT	78	59	20/33	39/45
Selbing et al., 1993	66	IVT	35	31	NM	NM
Newnham et al., 1992	67	IVT	20	16	4/6	12/14
Weiner et al., 1991	68	IVT	48	46	11/13	35/35
Harman et al., 1990	43	IVT	44	40	18/21	22/23
Lemery et al., 1989	69	IVT	15	10	2/4	8/8
Nicolini et al., 1989	46	IVT/IPT	31	26	NM	NM
Pattison & Roberts, 1989	70	IVT, IVT/IPT	20	18	1/2	17/18
Poissonnier et al., 1989	71	IVT/IPT	107	84	29/47	55/60
Ronkin et al., 1989	72	IVT	8	8	2/2	6/6
Barss et al., 1988	73	IVT/IPT	14	12	5/6	7/8
Grannum et al., 1988	74	IVT	26	21	16/20	5/6
Orsini et al., 1988	75	IVT	15	10	4/8	6/7
Berkowitz et al., 1988	76	IVT	9	7	0/1	7/8
Parer, 1988	77	IVT	5	4	NM	NM
Socol et al., 1987	78	IVT	3	3	3/3	0/0
Berkowitz et al., 1986	35	IVT	8	6	2/4	4/4
Doyle et al., 1986	79	IVT	8	5	0/2	5/6
Nicolaides et al., 1986	80	IVT	18	17	9/10	8/8
de Crespigny et al., 1985	53	IVT	4	3	1/2	2/2
Bang et al., 1982	33	IVT	1	1	1/1	0/0
Survival				83%	70%	92%

Notes:

IVT is intravascular transfusion (direct or exchange); IVT/IPT is combined intravascular (direct or exchange) with intraperitoneal transfusion; NM indicates not mentioned in the article.

Table 10.4 Long-term studies of infants after intrauterine transfusion

Authors	Reference	Number of patients	Number of infants with cerebral palsy	Number of infants with hearing loss	Number of infants with severe developmental delay
Doyle et al., 1993	89	38	1	0	1*
Janssens et al., 1997	61	69	3	3	5#
Hudon et al., 1998	90	40	1	1	1
Grab et al., 1999	59	30	0	0	0
Totals		177	5 (2.8%)	4 (2.3%)	7 (3.9%)

Notes:

* Includes the infant with cerebral palsy in this series.

Includes three infants with cerebral palsy from this series.

Normal outcome = 93%.

tested 21 infants just prior to discharge. Two infants had mild peripheral sensitivity loss with recovery noted in one at 5 months of age; the other child was lost to follow-up. A third child exhibited severe bilateral deafness. These authors proposed that hearing loss appeared to be 5–10-fold increased over the general population in infants requiring in utero therapy for HDFN.

The issue of enhanced survival of the sick fetus and the relationship to long-term outcome has been addressed in two investigations. Using a two sample analysis, Janssens and coworkers[61] failed to find a correlation between either the presence of hydrops or the number of intrauterine transfusions and poor neonatal neurological outcome. Using a multivariate analysis, our group could find no relationship between global developmental scores and the number of intrauterine transfusions, lowest fetal haematocrit or presence of hydrops. These data are reassuring in counselling the couple that presents with the severely anaemic fetus. They can be reassured that a normal neurological outcome can be expected in over 90% of surviving infants even if hydrops fetalis is noted at the time of the first intrauterine transfusion.

10.4 Red cells for transfusion

Red cells used for intrauterine transfusion must undergo the same rigorous testing that occurs for any allogenic donation. In the USA, this includes a confidential written questionnaire that enquires about illicit substance abuse and high-risk sexual behaviour. Serum testing for antibodies to syphilis, hepatitis B core antigen, human immunodeficiency viruses (HIV I and II), hepatitis C virus (HCV), human lymphotropic viruses (HTLV I and II), as well as testing for the p24 antigen of the hepatitis C virus, hepatitis B surface antigen (HbsAg) and alanine aspartate transferase, is undertaken. Additional testing by nucleic acid amplification for HIV and HCV is currently being performed as part of a study which includes the vast majority of donations collected in the USA. In the UK, all donors are screened for HbsAg as well as antibodies against HIV, HCV and syphilis. Red cells to be used for intrauterine transfusion are often leukocyte reduced or are from donors who are seronegative for cytomegalovirus (CMV) to decrease the risk of transmitting the virus. A relatively fresh unit of blood is preferred to stored blood. Standards in the UK require that red cells used for intrauterine transfusion have been stored for less than 5 days. A recent review noted that six cases of graft-versus-host reaction have been reported in infants who underwent intrauterine transfusion.[92] Bohm and coworkers[93] proposed that this was due to the induction of immune tolerance to engrafting lymphocytes that gain entry to the fetal circulation through large volume intrauterine transfusions. The British Blood Transfusion Task Force[94] and the American Association of Blood Banks Standards[95] require that red cell units for intrauterine transfusion undergo gamma irradiation to prevent graft-versus-host reaction. In addition, leukodepletion is a requirement in the UK and, although not routinely practised in the USA, is often used to reduce the risk of transmitting CMV and will likely be universally accepted in the near future.

Maternal blood donation is an excellent source of red cells for intrauterine transfusion and the procedure is well tolerated. In a series of 21 patients, up to 6 units of blood per patient were harvested for intrauterine transfusion.[96] Supplementation with prenatal vitamins, folate and ferrous sulphate prevented maternal anaemia in all cases. No serious maternal or fetal effects were noted. Theoretical advantages to the use of maternal blood include a decreased risk for sensitization to new red cell antigens, longer half-life due to the fresh source of cells and decreased risk for transmission of viral agents. Vietor and coworkers[97] investigated the source of new red cell antibodies in 91 patients undergoing 280 intrauterine transfusions. Twenty-six per cent of the women developed new antibodies. In 14 cases, the source of the sensitizing antigen could be determined; in one-fifth of the cases, donor red cells carried the involved antigen. It would therefore appear that, in 5% of cases, the use of maternal blood as the source of red cells for intrauterine transfusion would prevent the development of new anti-red cell antibodies. Only one investigation has compared the effect of maternal and donor red cells on the fetus.[98] Seventy-six intrauterine transfusions in which maternal blood was used were compared with 213 intrauterine transfusions in which donor red cells were employed. The rate of haematocrit decline was significantly lower in the group receiving maternal red cells, although this difference did not manifest until after 33 weeks' gestation. In addition, infants who received maternal blood required fewer neonatal transfusions (mean of 0.38 versus 1.48) as compared with those who received donor cells. The authors conjectured that this finding could be related to increased maternal reticulocytosis after repeated donations. Such reticulocytosis would result in a younger population of red cells that would exhibit a longer half-life in the fetus. They concluded that maternal red cells were preferred over donor red cells because they offered the potential advantage of decreasing the total number of intrauterine transfusions necessary for the treatment of a particular fetus. To date, no study has compared the risk of fetal viral infection in maternal versus donor red cells.

In a maternal blood donation programme, the patient can, if intrauterine transfusions are likely, donate a unit of red cells after the first trimester. The unit can be separated into two smaller aliquots and refrigerated for up to 32 days. If not used by this date, the unit can then be frozen for use for a period of up to 10 years. Patients should be supplemented with additional iron therapy (324 mg ferrous sulphate twice daily) as well as additional folate (1 mg daily). Additional considerations related to pregnancy include positioning the patient in the left lateral recumbent position during the donation and replacing the donated volume with isotonic intravenous fluids. Fetal monitoring during the procedure is unnecessary.[99] A standard volume of 450 ± 45 ml is taken as subsequent washing and packing will markedly reduce the final volume available for transfusion. Maternal blood requires some additional processing before use for intrauterine transfusion. The blood is washed several times to remove the offending antibody. Since the mother and fetus will share HLA antigens at many loci, the possibility of a graft-versus-host reaction is higher than with the use of a nonrelated donor unit. In order to avoid this complication, the authors routinely leukoreduce the unit using specialized filters in addition to the standard irradiation with 25 Gy of gamma radiation to the central portion of the donor bag. The use of maternal blood in the CMV-seropositive patient is controversial. Dormant CMV is noted to reside in the polymorphonuclear leukocytes. Both leukoreduction and washing have been demonstrated to be effective mechanisms in the prevention of the transmission of CMV.[100] For this reason, the authors proceed with the use of maternal CMV-seropositive blood after careful counselling of the patient. Finally, the use of ABO-incompatible maternal red cells for intrauterine transfusion has raised concern. With fetal typing now available at the first fetal blood sampling, situations may arise in which the patient is found to be type A or B and the fetus is typed as O. We have used maternal blood in two such cases with no deleterious effects noted in the fetus. Follow-up at 3 years of age in one of these infants revealed anti-A and anti-B titres that were appropriate for age.

10.5 Experimental therapy

Although intrauterine transfusion remains the mainstay of treatment for cases of HDFN, various methods have been attempted in order to address the offending antibodies directly. Such techniques have included immunoabsorption, oral tolerance, chemotherapeutic antibody suppression and paternal leukocyte sensitization.

10.5.1 Immunoabsorption

Yoshida and coworkers[101] reported a single case of immunoabsorption in a patient with anti-P antibodies and four recurrent losses. Maternal plasma obtained by a flow cell separator was mixed with P-positive donor red cells in an effort to bind the anti-red cell antibodies. The mixture was centrifuged and the plasma returned to the patient. A series of procedures was performed on 215 l of maternal plasma between the sixth and 14th week of the pregnancy. The patient subsequently delivered a viable infant. Robinson[102] attempted a similar procedure in a patient with anti-D in which 2 l of the patient's plasma was absorbed with D-positive red cells and reinfused at 20, 21 and 22 weeks' gestation. Unfortunately, at 23 weeks, the patient's anti-D titre showed a marked increase associated with a fetal demise 2 weeks later. The author conjectured that red cell fragments contaminating the absorption process may have contributed to the rise in antibody. Soluble D antigen has recently been described that can be fixed to polystyrene beads.[103] This raises the possibility of the future development of an immunoabsorbent column that could be placed in a plasmapheresis circuit for the removal of anti-D.

10.5.2 Oral tolerance

Studies to date attempting oral desensitization to red cell antigens have revealed conflicting results. In 1979, Bierme and associates[104] investigated the use of oral D antigen in seven severely alloimmunized women. All previous pregnancies had resulted in intrauterine death even though intrauterine transfusions were used in four cases. Anti-D titres were noted to remain stable in all cases. In six of the seven treated cases, a D-positive infant was born at 35 weeks' gestation in good condition. In an attempt to duplicate these results, American investigators treated four patients with a history of severe HDFN with oral erythrocytes using the method of Bierme.[105] All four cases resulted in either fetal or neonatal death; hydrops fetalis was noted in all cases. In a rebuttal letter to the editor, Bierme's group[106] reported a larger series of 16 pregnancies with 12 live births using oral erythrocyte therapy in conjunction with oral promethazine. The authors proposed that a therapeutic trial should be undertaken. Three years later, Barnes and coworkers[107] reported a study into the effects of oral erythrocyte membrane therapy in nonpregnant patients. Six previously sensitized women were administered a 2 g/day dose of a lyophilized preparation of erythrocyte membranes for 4 weeks. One-half of the patients received an erythrocyte preparation prepared from D-negative red cells and one-half received D-positive red cell preparations. In three subjects, there was no change in antibody levels, while, in the remaining three, there was a clear elevation in antibody titres. In this latter group, two of the three had received D-positive oral antigen. These findings led the authors to conclude that their oral preparation was not tolerogenic but, in fact, immunogenic. No further reports can be found in peer-reviewed literature regarding this therapy; it appears to have been abandoned as a potential treatment with the advent of more effective methods of intrauterine transfusion.

10.5.3 Chemotherapeutic agents

In vitro, promethazine interferes with the ability of human fetal macrophages to phagocytose red cells sensitized with anti-D.[108] This has led several investigators to use this agent in an effort to ameliorate the effects of maternal anti-red cell antibodies in HDFN. Gusdon[109] treated 72 patients with alloimmunization to D with doses of 3.7–5.0 mg/kg/day divided in four doses beginning as early as 14 weeks' gestation.

The lowest dose was used in patients with a first affected pregnancy while the highest dose was used in patients with a history of previous intrauterine transfusion or fetal death. When compared with previous pregnancy, there was a marked improvement in outcome. Three perinatal deaths occurred in the pregnancies treated with promethazine as compared with eight deaths in previous pregnancies ($p < 0.05$). The infants from 28% of the treated pregnancies required neonatal exchange transfusion as compared with 44% of infants from previous pregnancies ($p < 0.05$). A similar investigation in 21 pregnancies was undertaken by a second group,[110] where general impression was that promethazine was not beneficial in view of the continued need for intrauterine transfusions. However, a therapeutic effect was possibly seen in some pregnancies with previous neonatal demise.

Steroids have been attempted in the treatment of HDFN, but no case series have been published.[111] Agents such as betamethasone and dexamethasone that cross the placenta have been associated with decreases in the absorbance density (ΔOD_{450}) of amniotic fluid.[112] However, these changes have not been associated with a decrease in the severity of HDFN, but, instead, are probably related to alterations in fetal bilirubin metabolism.[111]

10.5.4 Sensitization to paternal leukocyte antigens

In vitro data and clinical case reports suggest that maternal alloantibodies to paternal leukocytes may result in a blocking phenomenon which protects sensitized fetal red cells from haemolysis in utero (Section 1.3.2.8). Neppert and coworkers[113,114] reported that human sera with HLA-A, -B, -C and -DR antibodies inhibited the binding and phagocytosis of IgG-sensitized red cells by monocytes. The authors proposed that anti-HLA antibodies might inhibit the fetal reticuloendothelial system. This would explain the lack of clinical disease in some rare cases with a strongly positive direct antiglobulin test (Section 3.6) at birth.[115] In 1992, Dooren and coworkers[116] studied 12 pregnant women with anti-D in whom the in vitro antibody-dependent monocyte-mediated cytotoxicity assay (Section 8.4.2) predicted severe fetal disease, but the neonatal clinical course was benign. When donor monocytes were replaced in the assay by paternal cells (monocytes that should share HLA antigens with the neonate), seven of the repeat assays revealed a lack of lysis of the sensitized red cells. Six of the seven cases involved maternal monocyte-reactive antibodies of the paternal HLA-DR specificity. Three reports of clinical cases have appeared in the literature in which maternal HLA-antibodies were thought to be the explanation for unexpectedly mild outcomes.[117,118] In two cases, the specificity of the maternal antibody was HLA-DR while, in the remaining case, the antibody was directed against the HLA-A10 and DR13 antigens. New data suggest that these alloantibodies prevent the binding of anti-D-sensitized fetal red cells to FcγR-bearing splenic phagocytes, thus reducing the severity of HDFN.[119,120]

The authors have shown in a rabbit model for HDFN that alloimmunization to paternal leukocytes produces fetal haemoglobin levels in an affected litter that approach normal.

The potential limitations of using paternal leukocytes to elicit these blocking antibodies for the treatment for severe red cell alloimmunization are substantial. Any contaminating red cells could substantially boost maternal antibody levels. In addition, maternal sensitization to paternal HLA antigens could produce alloimmune thrombocytopenia.

10.6 Timing of delivery

When intraperitoneal transfusions were used as the sole means of in utero therapy, fetuses were routinely delivered at 32 weeks' gestation. Hyaline membrane disease and the need for neonatal exchange transfusions for the treatment of hyperbilirubinaemia were common. As experience with intravascular transfusions became widespread, pregnancies were delivered at later gestational ages. Most authorities will now perform the final intrauterine transfusion at up to 35 weeks' gestation, with delivery anticipated at 37–38 weeks. Such practice allows maturation of both the pulmonary and hepatic enzyme systems, virtually eliminating the need for neonatal exchange transfusions. After a viable gestational age is attained, performing the transfusion in immediate proximity to the labour and delivery suite appears prudent, so that operative delivery can be undertaken if fetal distress should occur.

10.7 Conclusion

Intrauterine transfusion remains the most effective treatment in the management of most cases of HDFN. In cases of previous perinatal loss in the early second trimester, intravenous immune globulin alone or in combination with plasmapheresis may represent a means for achieving a successful outcome in these pregnancies. Clearly, a multicentre trial should be undertaken to address this group of patients who continue to experience a high rate of perinatal loss. Possible future advances in therapy include selective immunotherapy to block or suppress maternal anti-red cell antibodies. If successful, such therapies could retire intrauterine transfusion into the annals of historical medicine.

10.8 References

1 Besalduch J, Forteza A, Duran MA, Reyero J & Caso M (1991). Rh hemolytic disease of the newborn treated with high-dose intravenous immunoglobulin and plasmapheresis. *Transfusion*, **31**, 380–1.

2 Odendaal HJ, Tribe R, Kriel CJ, Meyer M & Thom JC (1991). Successful treatment of severe Rh iso-immunization with immunosuppression and plasmapheresis. *Vox Sanguinis*, **60**, 169–73.

3 Al-Omari WR (1989). Improved fetal survival with small volume plasmapheresis in Rhesus disease. *International Journal of Gynaecology and Obstetrics*, **30**, 237–40.

4 Berlin G, Selbing A & Ryden G (1985). Rhesus haemolytic disease treated with high-dose intravenous immunoglobulin. *Lancet*, **1**, 1153.

5 Eklund J (1985). Intensive plasma exchange as an adjunct to management of severe rhesus disease. *Acta Obstetricia Gynecologica Scandinavica*, **64**, 7–10.

6 Van't Veer-Korthof ET, Niterink JS, van Nieuwkoop JA & Eernisse JG (1981). IgG subclasses in rhesus-D immunization. Effects of weekly small volume plasmapheresis. *Vox Sanguinis*, **41**, 207–11.

7 Hauth JC, Brekken AL & Pollack W (1981). Plasmapheresis as an adjunct to management of Rh isoimmunization. *Obstetrics and Gynecology*, **57**, 132–5.

8 Robinson AE & Tovey LA (1980). Intensive plasma exchange in the management of severe Rh disease. *British Journal of Haematology*, **45**, 621–31.

9 James V, Weston J, Scott IV, Doughty R, Tomlinson J & Whitfield M (1979). Intensive plasma exchange in rhesus isoimmunization. *Vox Sanguinis*, **37**, 290–5.

10 Gunston KD, Woods DL & Leader LR (1979). Corticosteroids, real-time ultrasound scanning and plasmapheresis in severe rhesus disease. *South African Medical Journal*, **56**, 666.

11 Graham-Pole J, Barr W & Willoughby ML (1977). Continuous-flow plasmapheresis in management of severe Rhesus disease. *British Medical Journal*, **77**, 1185–8.

12 Tilz GP, Weiss PA, Teubl I, Lanzer G & Vollmann H (1977). Successful plasma exchange in rhesus incompatibility. *Lancet*, **2**, 203.

13 Fraser ID, Bothamley JE, Bennett MO & Airth GR (1976). Intensive antenatal plasmapheresis in severe rhesus isoimmunization. *Lancet*, **1**, 6–8.

14 Pole JR, Barr W & Willoughby ML (1974). Continuous-flow exchange-plasmapheresis in severe rhesus isoimmunization. *Lancet*, **1**, 1051.

15 Fias I, Dombi E, Wenhardt E & Horvath I (1973). Plasmapheresis in Rh isoimmunization. *Lancet*, **1**, 1519–20.

16 Kovacs L, Keseru TL & Imre G (1973). Plasmapheresis in Rh isoimmunization. *Lancet*, **1**, 253.

17 Clarke CA, Elson CJ, Bradley J, Donohoe WT, Lehane D & Hughes-Jones NC (1970). Intensive plasmapheresis as a therapeutic measure in Rhesus-immunized women. *Lancet*, **1**, 793–8.

18 Bowman JM, Peddle LJ & Anderson C (1968). Plasmapheresis in severe Rh iso-immunization. *Vox Sanguinis*, **15**, 272–7.

19 Powell LC Jr (1968). Intense plasmapheresis in the pregnant Rh-sensitized woman. *American Journal of Obstetrics and Gynecology*, **101**, 153–70.

20 Bystryn JC, Graf MW & Uhr JW (1970). Regulation of antibody formation by serum antibody. II. Removal of specific antibody by means of exchange transfusion. *Journal of Experimental Medicine*, **132**, 1279–87.

21 Schur PH, Alpert E & Alper C (1973). Gamma G subgroups in human fetal, cord, and maternal sera. *Clinical Immunology and Immunopathology*, **2**, 62–6.

22 Margulies M, Voto LS & Mathet E (1991). High-dose intravenous IgG for the treatment of severe Rhesus alloimmunization. *Vox Sanguinis*, **61**, 181–9.

23 Voto LS, Mathet ER, Zapaterio JL, Orti J, Lede RL & Margulies M (1997). High-dose gammaglobulin (IVIG) followed by intrauterine transfusions (IUT): a new alternative for the treatment of severe fetal hemolytic disease. *Journal of Perinatal Medicine*, **25**, 85–8.

24 Dooren MC, van Kamp IL, Scherpenisse JW et al. (1994). No beneficial effect of low-dose fetal intravenous gammaglobulin administration in combination with intravascular transfusions in severe Rh D haemolytic disease. *Vox Sanguinis*, **66**, 253–7.

25 Rubo J, Albrecht K, Lasch P et al. (1992). High-dose intravenous immune globulin therapy for hyperbilirubinemia caused by Rh hemolytic disease. *Journal of Pediatrics*, **121**, 93–7.

26 Alonso JG, Decaro J, Marrero A, Lavalle E, Martell M & Cuadro JC (1994). Repeated direct fetal intravascular high-dose immunoglobulin therapy for the treatment of Rh hemolytic disease. *Journal of Perinatal Medicine*, **22**, 415–19.

27 Gottvall T & Selbing A (1995). Alloimmunization during pregnancy treated with high dose intravenous immunoglobulin. Effects on fetal hemoglobin concentration and anti-D concentrations in the mother and fetus. *Acta Obstetricia Gynecologica Scandinavica*, **74**, 777–83.

28 Yu Z & Lennon VA (1999). Mechanism of intravenous immune globulin therapy in antibody-mediated autoimmune diseases. *New England Journal of Medicine*, **340**, 227–8.

29 Plasma Exchange/Sandoglobulin Guillain-Barre Syndrome Trial Group (1997). Randomised trial of plasma exchange, intravenous immunoglobulin, and combined treatments in Guillain-Barre syndrome. *Lancet*, **349**, 225–30.

30 Moise KJ Jr & Carpenter RJ Jr (1993). Chorionic villus sampling for Rh typing: clinical implications. *American Journal of Obstetrics and Gynecology*, **168**, 1002–3.

31 Liley AW (1963). Intrauterine transfusion of foetus in haemolytic disease. *British Medical Journal*, **2**, 1107–9.

32 Rodeck CH, Kemp JR, Holman CA, Whitmore DN, Karnicki J & Austin MA (1981). Direct intravascular fetal blood transfusion by fetoscopy in severe Rhesus isoimmunization. *Lancet*, **1**, 625–7.

33 Bang J, Bock JE & Trolle D (1982). Ultrasound-guided fetal intravenous transfusion for severe rhesus haemolytic disease. *British Medical Journal*, **284**, 373–4.

34 Grannum PA, Copel JA, Plaxe SC, Scioscia AL & Hobbins JC (1986). In utero exchange transfusion by direct intravascular injection in severe erythroblastosis fetalis. *New England Journal of Medicine*, **314**, 1431–4.

35 Berkowitz RL, Chitkara U, Goldberg JD, Wilkins I, Chervenak FA & Lynch L (1986). Intrauterine intravascular transfusions for severe red blood cell isoimmunization: ultrasound-guided percutaneous approach. *American Journal of Obstetrics and Gynecology*, **155**, 574–81.

36 Weiner CP, Wenstrom KD, Sipes SL & Williamson RA (1991). Risk factors for cordocentesis and fetal intravascular transfusion. *American Journal of Obstetrics and Gynecology*, **165**, 1020–5.

37 Nicolini U, Santolaya J, Ojo OE et al. (1988). The fetal intrahepatic umbilical vein as an alternative to cord needling for prenatal diagnosis and therapy. *Prenatal Diagnosis*, **8**, 665–71.

38 Giannakoulopoulos X, Sepulveda W, Kourtis P, Glover V & Fisk NM (1994). Fetal plasma cortisol and beta-endorphin response to intrauterine needling. *Lancet*, **344**, 77–81.

39 Giannakoulopoulos X, Teixeira J, Fisk N & Glover V (1999). Human fetal and maternal noradrenaline responses to invasive procedures. *Pediatric Research*, **45**, 494–9.

40 Westgren M, Selbing A & Stangenberg M (1988). Fetal intracardiac transfusions in patients with severe rhesus isoimmunization. *British Medical Journal*, **296**, 885–6.

41 Antsaklis AI, Papantoniou NE, Mesogitis SA, Koutra PT, Vintzileos AM & Aravantinos DI (1992). Cardiocentesis: an alternative method of fetal blood sampling for the prenatal diagnosis of hemoglobinopathies. *Obstetrics and Gynecology*, **79**, 630–3.

42 Lewis M, Bowman JM, Pollock J & Lowen B (1973). Absorption of red cells from the peritoneal cavity of an hydropic twin. *Transfusion*, **13**, 37–40.

43 Harman CR, Bowman JM, Manning FA & Menticoglou SM (1990). Intrauterine transfusion – intraperitoneal versus intravascular approach: a case-control comparison. *American Journal of Obstetrics and Gynecology*, **162**, 1053–9.

44 Bowman JM (1978). The management of Rh-isoimmunization. *Obstetrics and Gynecology*, **52**, 1–16.

45 Moise KJ Jr, Carpenter RJ Jr, Kirshon B, Deter RL, Sala JD & Cano LE (1989). Comparison of four types of intrauterine transfusion: effect on fetal hematocrit. *Fetal Therapy*, **4**, 126–37.

46 Nicolini U, Kochenour NK, Greco P, Letsky E & Rodeck CH (1989). When to perform the next intra-uterine transfusion in patients with Rh allo-immunization: combined intravascular and intraperitoneal transfusion allows longer intervals. *Fetal Therapy*, **4**, 14–20.

47 Lepercq J, Poissonnier MH, Coutanceau MJ, Chavinie J & Brossard Y (1999). Management and outcome of fetomaternal Rh alloimmunization in twin pregnancies. *Fetal Diagnosis and Therapy*, **14**, 26–30.

48 Welch R, Rampling MW, Anwar A, Talbert DG & Rodeck CH (1994). Changes in hemorheology with fetal intravascular transfusion. *American Journal of Obstetrics and Gynecology*, **170**, 726–32.

49 Mandelbrot L, Daffos F, Forestier F, MacAleese J & Descombey D (1988). Assessment of fetal blood volume for computer-assisted management of in utero transfusion. *Fetal Therapy*, **3**, 60–6.

50 Giannina G, Moise KJ Jr & Dorman K (1998). A simple method to estimate the volume for fetal intravascular transfusion. *Fetal Diagnosis and Therapy*, **13**, 94–7.

51 Hallak M, Moise KJ Jr, Hesketh DE, Cano LE & Carpenter RJ Jr (1992). Intravascular transfusion of fetuses with rhesus incompatibility: prediction of fetal outcome by changes in umbilical venous pressure. *Obstetrics and Gynecology*, **80**, 286–90.

52 Radunovic N, Lockwood CJ, Alvarez M, Plecas D, Chitkara U & Berkowitz RL (1992). The severely anemic and hydropic isoimmune fetus: changes in fetal hematocrit associated with intrauterine death. *Obstetrics and Gynecology*, **79**, 390–3.

53 de Crespigny LC, Robinson HP, Quinn M, Doyle L, Ross A & Cauchi M (1985). Ultrasound-guided fetal blood transfusion for severe rhesus isoimmunization. *Obstetrics and Gynecology*, **66**, 529–32.

54 Moise KJ Jr, Carpenter RJ Jr, Deter RL, Kirshon B & Diaz SF (1987). The use of fetal neuro-

muscular blockade during intrauterine procedures. *American Journal of Obstetrics and Gynecology*, **157**, 874–9.

55 Moise KJ Jr, Deter RL, Kirshon B, Adam K, Patton DE & Carpenter RJ Jr (1989). Intravenous pancuronium bromide for fetal neuromuscular blockade during intrauterine transfusion for red-cell alloimmunization. *Obstetrics and Gynecology*, **74**, 905–8.

56 Bernstein HH, Chitkara U, Plosker H, Gettes M & Berkowitz RL (1988). Use of atracurium besylate to arrest fetal activity during intrauterine intravascular transfusions. *Obstetrics and Gynecology*, **72**, 813–16.

57 Daffos F, Forestier F, Mac Aleese J et al. (1988). Fetal curarization for prenatal magnetic resonance imaging. *Prenatal Diagnosis*, **8**, 312–14.

58 Pielet BW, Socol ML, MacGregor SN, Dooley SL & Minogue J (1988). Fetal heart rate changes after fetal intravascular treatment with pancuronium bromide. *American Journal of Obstetrics and Gynecology*, **159**, 640–3.

59 Grab D, Paulus WE, Bommer A, Buck G & Terinde R (1999). Treatment of fetal erythroblastosis by intravascular transfusions: outcome at 6 years. *Obstetrics and Gynecology*, **93**, 165–8.

60 Babinszki A, Lapinski RH & Berkowitz RL (1998). Prognostic factors and management in pregnancies complicated with severe Kell alloimmunization: experiences of the last 13 years. *American Journal of Perinatology*, **15**, 695–701.

61 Janssens HM, de Haan MJ, van Kamp IL, Brand R, Kanhai HH & Veen S (1997). Outcome for children treated with fetal intravascular transfusions because of severe blood group antagonism. *Journal of Pediatrics*, **131**, 373–80.

62 Inglis SR, Lysikiewicz A, Sonnenblick AL, Streltzoff JL, Bussel JB & Chervenak FA (1996). Advantages of larger volume, less frequent intrauterine red blood cell transfusions for maternal red cell alloimmunization. *American Journal of Perinatology*, **13**, 27–33.

63 Merchant R, Lulla C, Gupte S & Krishnani R (1994). Fetal outcome following intrauterine intravascular transfusion for rhesus alloimmunization. *Indian Pediatrics*, **32**, 971–7.

64 Plockinger B, Strumpflen I, Deutinger J & Bernaschek G (1994). Diagnosis and treatment of fetal anemia due to isoimmunization. *Archives of Gynecology and Obstetrics*, **255**, 195–200.

65 Sampson AJ, Permezel M, Doyle LW, de Crespigny L, Ngu A & Robinson H (1994). Ultrasound-guided fetal intravascular transfusions for severe erythroblastosis, 1984–1993. *Australian and New Zealand Journal of Obstetrics and Gynaecology*, **34**, 125–30.

66 Selbing A, Stangenberg M, Westgren M & Rahman F (1993). Intrauterine intravascular transfusions in fetal erythroblastosis: the influence of net transfusion volume on fetal survival. *Acta Obstetricia Gynecologica Scandinavica*, **72**, 20–3.

67 Newnham JP, Phillips JM & Stock R (1992). Intrauterine intravascular transfusion for fetal haemolytic anaemia: the Western Australian experience. *Medical Journal of Australia*, **157**, 660–1, 664–5.

68 Weiner CP, Williamson RA, Wenstrom KD et al. (1991). Management of fetal hemolytic disease by cordocentesis. II. Outcome of treatment. *American Journal of Obstetrics and Gynecology*, **165**, 1302–7.

69 Lemery D, Urbain MF, Van Lieferinghen P, Micorek JC & Jacquetin B (1989). Intra-uterine exchange transfusion under ultrasound guidance. *European Journal of Obstetrics, Gynecology and Reproductive Biology*, **33**, 161–8.

70 Pattison N & Roberts A (1989). The management of severe erythroblastosis fetalis by fetal transfusion: survival of transfused adult erythrocytes in the fetus. *Obstetrics and Gynecology*, **74**, 901–4.

71 Poissonnier MH, Brossard Y, Demedeiros N et al. (1989). Two hundred intrauterine exchange transfusions in severe blood incompatibilities. *American Journal of Obstetrics and Gynecology*, **161**, 709–13.

72 Ronkin S, Chayen B, Wapner RJ et al. (1989). Intravascular exchange and bolus transfusion in the severely isoimmunized fetus. *American Journal of Obstetrics and Gynecology*, **160**, 407–11.

73 Barss VA, Benacerraf BR, Frigoletto FD et al. (1988). Management of isoimmunized pregnancy by use of intravascular techniques. *American Journal of Obstetrics and Gynecology*, **159**, 932–7.

74 Grannum PA, Copel JA, Moya FR et al. (1988). The reversal of hydrops fetalis by intravascular intrauterine transfusion in severe isoimmune fetal anemia. *American Journal of Obstetrics and Gynecology*, **158**, 914–19.

75 Orsini LF, Pilu G, Calderoni P et al. (1988). Intravascular intrauterine transfusion for severe erythroblastosis fetalis using different techniques. *Fetal Therapy*, **3**, 50–9.

76 Berkowitz RL, Chitkara U, Wilkins IA, Lynch L, Plosker H & Bernstein HH (1988). Intravascular monitoring and management of erythroblastosis fetalis. *American Journal of Obstetrics and Gynecology*, **158**, 783–95.

77 Parer JT (1988). Severe Rh isoimmunization – current methods of in utero diagnosis and treatment. *American Journal of Obstetrics and Gynecology*, **158**, 1323–9.

78 Socol ML, MacGregor SN, Pielet BW, Tamura RK & Sabbagha RE (1987). Percutaneous umbilical transfusion in severe rhesus isoimmunization: resolution of fetal hydrops. *American Journal of Obstetrics and Gynecology*, **157**, 1369–75.

79 Doyle LW, Cauchi M, de Crespigny LC et al. (1986). Fetal intravascular transfusion for severe erythroblastosis: effects on haematology and survival. *Australian and New Zealand Journal of Obstetrics and Gynaecology*, **26**, 192–5.

80 Nicolaides KH, Soothill PW, Rodeck CH & Clewell W (1986). Rh disease: intravascular fetal blood transfusion by cordocentesis. *Fetal Therapy*, **1**, 185–92.

81 Saade GR, Moise KJ, Belfort MA, Hesketh DE & Carpenter RJ (1993). Fetal and neonatal hematologic parameters in red cell alloimmunization: predicting the need for late neonatal transfusions. *Fetal Diagnosis and Therapy*, **8**, 161–4.

82 Koenig JM, Ashton RD, De Vore GR & Christensen RD (1989). Late hyporegenerative anemia in Rh hemolytic disease. *Journal of Pediatrics*, **115**, 315–18.

83 Ovali F, Samanci N & Dagoglu T (1996). Management of late anemia in rhesus hemolytic disease: use of recombinant human erythropoietin (a pilot study). *Pediatric Research*, **39**, 831–4.

84 Millard DD, Gidding SS, Socol ML et al. (1990). Effects of intravascular, intrauterine transfusion on prenatal and postnatal hemolysis and erythropoiesis in severe fetal isoimmunization. *Journal of Pediatrics*, **117**, 447–54.

85 Maier RF, Obladen M, Scigalla P et al. (1994). The effect of epoetin beta (recombinant human erythropoietin) on the need for transfusion in very-low-birth-weight infants. *New England Journal of Medicine*, **330**, 1173–78.

86 Shannon KM, Mentzer WC, Abels RI et al. (1991). Recombinant human erythropoietin in the anemia of prematurity: results of a placebo-controlled pilot study. *Journal of Pediatrics*, **118**, 949–55.

87 Nasrat HA, Nicolini U, Nicolaidis P, Letsky EA, Gau G & Rodeck CH (1991). The effect of intrauterine intravascular blood transfusion on iron metabolism in fetuses with Rh alloimmunization. *Obstetrics and Gynecology*, **77**, 558–62.

88 Hardyment AF, Salvador HS, Towell ME, Carpenter CW, Jan JE & Tingle AJ (1979). Follow-up of intrauterine transfused surviving children. *American Journal of Obstetrics and Gynecology*, **133**, 235–41.

89 Doyle LW, Kelly EA, Rickards AL, Ford GW & Callanan C (1993). Sensorineural outcome at 2 years for survivors of erythroblastosis treated with fetal intravascular transfusions. *Obstetrics and Gynecology*, **81**, 931–5.

90 Hudon L, Moise KJ Jr, Hegemier SE et al. (1998). Long-term neurodevelopmental outcome after intrauterine transfusion for the treatment of fetal hemolytic disease. *American Journal of Obstetrics and Gynecology*, **179**, 858–63.

91 Newman TB & Maisels MJ (1992). Evaluation and treatment of jaundice in the term newborn: a kinder, gentler approach. *Pediatrics*, **89**, 809–18.

92 Harte G, Payton D, Carmody F, O'Regan P & Thong YH (1997). Graft versus host disease following intrauterine and exchange transfusions for rhesus haemolytic disease. *Australian and New Zealand Journal of Obstetrics and Gynaecology*, **37**, 319–22.

93 Bohm N, Kleine W & Enzel U (1977). Graft-versus-host disease in two newborns after repeated blood transfusions because of rhesus incompatibility. *Beiträge zur Pathologe*, **160**, 381–400.

94 British Committee for Standards in Haematology Blood Transfusion Task Force (1996). Guidelines on gamma irradiation of blood components for the prevention of transfusion-associated graft-versus-host disease. *Transfusion Medicine*, **6**, 261–71.

95 Vengelen-Tyler V (1999). *American Association of Blood Banks Technical Manual*. Bethesda, MD: American Association of Blood Banks.

96 Gonsoulin WJ, Moise KJ Jr, Milam JD, Sala JD, Weber VW & Carpenter RJ Jr (1990). Serial maternal blood donations for intrauterine transfusion. *Obstetrics and Gynecology*, **75**, 158–62.

97 Vietor HE, Kanhai HH & Brand A (1994). Induction of additional red cell alloantibodies after intrauterine transfusions. *Transfusion*, **34**, 970–4.

98 El-Azeem SA, Samuels P, Rose RL, Kennedy M & O'Shaughnessy RW (1997). The effect of the source of transfused blood on the rate of consumption of transfused red blood cells in pregnancies affected by red blood cell alloimmunization. *American Journal of Obstetrics and Gynecology*, **177**, 753–7.

99 Herbert WN, Owen HG & Collins ML (1988). Autologous blood storage in obstetrics. *Obstetrics and Gynecology*, **72**, 166–70.

100 Pamphilon DH, Rider JR, Barbara JA & Williamson LM (1999). Prevention of transfusion-transmitted cytomegalovirus infection. *Transfusion Medicine*, **9**, 115–23.

101 Yoshida H, Ito K, Emi N, Kanzaki H & Matsuura S (1984). A new therapeutic antibody removal method using antigen-positive red cells. II. Application to a P-incompatible pregnant woman. *Vox Sanguinis*, **47**, 216–33.

102 Robinson EA (1981). Unsuccessful use of absorbed autologous plasma in Rh-incompatible pregnancy. *New England Journal of Medicine*, **305**, 1346.

103 Yared MA, Moise KJ & Rodkey LS (1997). Stable solid-phase Rh antigen. *Transfusion Medicine*, **7**, 311–17.

104 Bierme SJ, Blanc M, Abbal M & Fournie A (1979). Oral Rh treatment for severely immunized mothers. *Lancet*, **1**, 604–5.

105 Gold WR Jr, Queenan JT, Woody J & Sacher RA (1983). Oral desensitization in Rh disease. *American Journal of Obstetrics and Gynecology*, **146**, 980–1.

106 Parinaud J, Bierme S, Fournie A, Grandjean H, Blanc M & Pontonnier G (1984). Oral Rh treatment for severely immunized mothers. *American Journal of Obstetrics and Gynecology*, **150**, 902.

107 Barnes RM, Duguid JK, Roberts FM et al. (1987). Oral administration of erythrocyte membrane antigen does not suppress anti-Rh(D) antibody responses in humans. *Clinical and Experimental Immunology*, **67**, 220–6.

108 Gusdon JP Jr, Caudle MR, Herbst GA & Iannuzzi NP (1976). Phagocytosis and erythroblastosis. I. Modification of the neonatal response by promethazine hydrochloride. *American Journal of Obstetrics and Gynecology*, **125**, 224–6.

109 Gusdon JP Jr (1981). The treatment of erythroblastosis with promethazine hydrochloride. *Journal of Reproductive Medicine*, **26**, 454–8.

110 Stenchever MA (1978). Promethazine hydrochloride: use in patients with Rh isoimmunization. *American Journal of Obstetrics and Gynecology*, **130**, 665–8.

111 Caudle MR & Scott JR (1982). The potential role of immunosuppression, plasmapheresis, and desensitization as treatment modalities for Rh immunization. *Clinics in Obstetrics and Gynecology*, **25**, 313–19.

112 Caritis SN, Mueller-Heuback E & Edelstone DI (1977). Effect of betamethasone on analysis of amniotic fluid in the rhesus-sensitized pregnancy. *American Journal of Obstetrics and Gynecology*, **127**, 529–32.

113 Neppert J, Pohl E & Mueller-Eckhardt C (1986). Inhibition of immune phagocytosis by human sera with HLA A, B, C and DR but not with DQ or EM type reactivity. *Vox Sanguinis*, **51**, 122–6.

114 Faust A & Neppert J (1987). Detection of antibodies specific for HLA-A, B, C, DR, DQ and DP by the erythrocyte antibody rosette inhibition (EAI) and immune phagocytosis inhibition (IPI) tests. *Journal of Immunological Methods*, **102**, 71–5.

115 Neppert J (1987). Rhesus-Du and -D incompatibility in the newborn without haemolytic disease: inhibition of immune phagocytosis? *Vox Sanguinis*, **53**, 239.

116 Dooren MC, Kuijpers RW, Joekes EC et al. (1992). Protection against immune haemolytic disease of newborn infants by maternal monocyte-reactive IgG alloantibodies (anti-HLA-DR). *Lancet*, **339**, 1067–70.

117 Dooren MC, van Kamp IL, Kanhai HH, Gravenhorst JB, von dem Borne AE & Engelfriet CP (1993). Evidence for the protective effect of maternal FcR-blocking IgG alloantibodies HLA-DR in Rh D-haemolytic disease of the newborn. *Vox Sanguinis*, **65**, 55–8.

118 Eichler H, Zieger W, Neppert J, Kerowgan M, Melchert F & Goldmann SF (1995). Mild course of fetal RhD haemolytic disease due to maternal alloimmunization to paternal HLA class I and II antigens. *Vox Sanguinis*, **68**, 243–7.

119 Shepard SL, Noble AL, Filbey D & Hadley AG (1996). Inhibition of the monocyte chemi-luminescent response to anti-D-sensitized red cells by Fc gamma RI-blocking antibodies which ameliorate the severity of haemolytic disease of the newborn. *Vox Sanguinis*, **70**, 157–63.

120 Wiener E, Mawas F, Dellow RA, Singh I & Rodeck CH (1995). A major role of class I Fc gamma receptors in immunoglobulin G anti-D-mediated red blood cell destruction by fetal mononuclear phagocytes. *Obstetrics and Gynecology*, **86**, 157–62.

11

Neonatal therapy for haemolytic disease of the newborn

Glynn Russell and Nic Goulden
The Children's Hospital, Bristol, UK

Improvements in preventative and therapeutic fetal medicine, such as the better timing of delivery guided by Liley's charts, fetal blood transfusion and the widespread use of anti-D immunoglobulin, have had dramatic effects on morbidity and mortality due to HDFN. Advances in neonatal intensive care have further contributed to this reduction. This chapter reviews therapies which may be used to treat hydrops, anaemia and jaundice in affected neonates.

11.1 Features of haemolytic disease in the neonate

There are three main clinically significant conditions seen during the first 28 days after birth caused by maternal blood group alloantibodies transferred to the fetus. These are hydrops, jaundice and anaemia.

11.1.1 Hydrops

The most severely affected fetuses present with hydrops manifesting as generalized tissue oedema, pleural effusions and ascites. Although the pathogenesis of these features is not clear, presumably neonates born with hydrops suffer the end result of fetal heart failure due to both hypoxic myocardial dysfunction and increased intravascular fluid retention (Section 9.3.1). Fetal liver dysfunction may also contribute to the oedema because the extensive erythropoiesis causes disruption to the portal circulation and impaired albumin synthesis. Antenatal treatment is aimed at the correction of the anaemia by fetal blood transfusion (Section 10.3), but, when a neonate is born with hydrops, early neonatal death may result from the inability to resuscitate the severely hydropic and anaemic baby at delivery. Later postnatal death may result from other consequences of hydrops, such as pulmonary hypoplasia, the complications of prematurity or even complications of treatment such as exchange transfusion. However, better neonatal intensive care has improved the survival of hydropic neonates. Although, of course, the prognosis is closely related to gestational age at delivery, the overall survival of alloimmune hydrops is between 65% and 85%.[1,2]

11.1.2 Neonatal jaundice

Early neonatal jaundice (usually detected within 24 hours of birth) may be accompanied by haemolytic anaemia, thrombocytopenia and, sometimes, neutropenia. Treatment by phototherapy and exchange transfusion is aimed primarily at avoiding the accumulation of toxic levels of bilirubin.[3] The placenta before delivery clears bilirubin, but a rapid rise of serum bilirubin after birth may cause the deposition of lipid-soluble unconjugated bilirubin in the basal nuclei of brain.[4] Bilirubin toxicity classically manifests in the short term as kernicterus with an acute encephalopathy and, in the long term, as athetoid cerebral palsy and/or sensorineural deafness.[5,6]

11.1.3 Persistent anaemia

Anaemia may persist beyond the early neonatal period as a consequence of haemolysis secondary to antibodies that continue to circulate. Exchange transfusion reduces the concentration of circulating antibodies only slightly because much of the antibody is distributed in the extravascular space.[7,8] If repeated neonatal (and/or fetal) blood transfusions have been performed, erythropoietin may be suppressed by the relatively normal or high haemoglobin concentrations. Erythropoietin levels may take weeks or months to recover and this contributes to the consequent anaemia.[9] Suppression of erythropoiesis secondary to the effects of anti-Kell antibodies may also cause persistent anaemia (Section 2.5.3).

11.2 Laboratory diagnosis

The diagnosis of alloimmune haemolysis in the neonate usually relies on paired parental and neonatal ABO, Rh and K typing, but, on occasion, typing for less common antigens will be appropriate. A direct antiglobulin test on the neonatal blood (Section 3.6) will normally reveal the presence of red cell-bound IgG, although this may not be the case after intrauterine transfusion or in neonatally transfused cases if antigen-positive red cells are cleared due to rapid haemolysis. The antibody responsible for haemolysis should be identified by testing maternal serum, but, if this is unavailable, an eluate from neonatal red cells or neonatal serum may be used. In most cases, it is possible to identify the antibody rapidly by testing against a panel of reagent cells (Section 3.4). In some cases, more than one antibody may be present and, in this situation, an examination of an eluate from neonatal red cells may reveal which antibody specificity is involved in the haemolytic process (Section 3.6). Occasionally, the presence of antibodies against high-frequency antigens may lead to a positive reaction against all panel cells tested and then an extended panel of rare red cells lacking these antigens may be required to elucidate the specificity. Sometimes, the maternal antibody screen may be negative in the presence of a positive direct antiglobulin test on the neonatal blood. This usually reflects the presence of antibodies to a low-frequency antigen inherited from the father.

11.3 General neonatal management

11.3.1 Communication

Good communication between fetal medicine, obstetric, neonatal and blood transfusion staff is essential to ensure effective neonatal treatment, but this is not always easy to achieve. Many of the complications of the disease and its fetal treatment are unpredictable. For example, a complication during a fetal transfusion may necessitate an immediate delivery. This can result in a premature, anaemic and acutely unwell baby being delivered at less than 10 minutes' notice. Another challenge may follow successful fetal transfusion therapy when the woman is likely to be delivered at 36–38 weeks in her local hospital. Should difficulties then arise, a different team of neonatologists may be involved. It is therefore important to keep informed all the people who could possibly be relevant to any given case. This may require a large number of communications, the majority of which may subsequently prove to have been unnecessary.

Despite the problems described above, when delivery is planned in advance, there are steps which can and should be achieved in a coordinated manner. There should be a careful consideration of antenatal corticosteroid treatment. Also, blood should be made available to the neonatologist by crossmatching against the mother's blood before the delivery. It is a good idea for the woman to be given the chance to meet the neonatologists and to visit the neonatal intensive care unit before delivery whenever possible. This can provide useful reassurance to the patient before birth, but it also makes communication easier after birth should neonatal complications arise.

11.3.2 Resuscitation

The need for full cardiopulmonary resuscitation should be anticipated, especially if hydrops is present. A secure airway and effective respiration with supplemental oxygen should be established. If severe hydrops is present, endotracheal intubation and ventilation will be needed and sometimes each may be achieved only with considerable difficulty. Facial and airway oedema may make endotracheal intubation difficult. Drainage of tense ascites and pleural fluid is also necessary in some cases to allow adequate ventilation. Pulmonary compliance may be poor because of tissue oedema and also because of surfactant deficiency if the baby is preterm or has hydrops. Chest wall oedema may restrict effective spontaneous respiration and necessitate high peak inflation pressures if mechanical ventilation is needed. The chest wall oedema limits chest auscultation and makes cardiac compression more difficult to achieve.

Vascular access should be gained via the umbilical vein and blood samples taken for acid base balance, albumin concentration, glucose concentration, haematocrit, full blood count, direct antiglobulin test, blood crossmatch (if not already done) and bilirubin concentration. As described earlier, if haemolytic disease is anticipated before delivery, blood crossmatched against the mother should be available for transfusion. In any event, fresh group O, D-negative, cytomegalovirus (CMV)-negative blood (1 adult unit) should be available for emergency use (Section 11.5.1).

11.4 Treatment of hydrops

Hydrops is usually associated with significant anaemia and poor cardiopulmonary function and so admission to a neonatal intensive care unit for respiratory and inotropic cardiac support with continuous monitoring is needed.[10,11] Continuous blood pressure monitoring is mandatory and, if possible, central venous pressure monitoring through an umbilical venous catheter placed in the right atrium should assist in managing circulating blood volume and cardiac function. The circulating blood volume is usually normal and, in most cases, the central venous pressure is not elevated. Inappropriate infusion of blood and fluids may, however, cause a rapid deterioration in cardiac function.[7] Hypoalbuminaemia is common, but there is no evidence that albumin infusions are helpful. Meticulous fluid, electrolyte and glucose management is obligatory. For example, crystalloid infusion rates should be restricted to 60 ml/kg/day and glucose infusion concentration increased to prevent hypoglycaemia.

11.5 Treatment of anaemia

11.5.1 Blood transfusion

Correction of anaemia is important and achieved by repeated small blood transfusions or a small-volume (30–50 ml/kg body weight) exchange blood transfusion in severe hydrops to increase the haemoglobin concentration. Neonates are at particular risk of a number of metabolic, infectious and immunological side-effects following blood transfusion. Each of these is considered in relation to the consequences of transfusion in a neonate suffering from HDFN.

11.5.1.1 Selection of compatible blood

Maternal serological investigation allows the selection of antigen-negative red cells for transfusion. In most cases the antigen involved will be either D, c, K, Fy(a), A or B (Sections 2.5 and 2.6). For this reason, Blood Centres in the UK routinely hold stocks of group O, D-negative, c-negative, K-negative blood. In cases where less commonly encountered antibodies are implicated, the advice of an expert transfusion physician should be sought. It is important to note that, even when a clearly defined antigen specificity has been documented and appropriate antigen-negative cells selected, cross matching is still mandatory. Ideally, the initial crossmatch should be against maternal plasma. In the absence of maternal plasma, an eluate from neonatal red cells and neonatal serum can be used.

11.5.1.2 Red cell concentrates

In recent years, the demand for plasma-derived products has been so great that transfusion services have moved away from the storage of whole blood. Packed red cell concentrates resuspended in optimal additive solutions are now the norm and commonly have a haematocrit of 50–70%. Whereas the infusion of small volumes (10 ml/kg) of this product as a top-up is unlikely to adversely affect the recipient, a conventional double volume exchange transfusion involves the infusion of 180 ml/kg of stored blood over a 60–90-minute period. In order to maintain whole blood viscosity, the haematocrit of the infused product should be 55–60%. In the UK, plasma-reduced whole blood (haematocrit 55–60%) is normally supplied for exchange transfusion. An alternative approach involves the 'reconstitution' of whole blood by mixing red cell concentrate and fresh frozen plasma.

11.5.1.3 Anticoagulant

Heparinized fresh whole blood has been widely used in the past but may increase the risk of bleeding and is no longer recommended.[7] Blood is collected into citrate–phosphate–dextrose anticoagulant and, in theory, infusion of citrate could lead to rebound hypoglycaemia, hypocalcaemia and acidosis. In practice, this appears not to be an issue after top-up transfusion in an otherwise well baby. Prophylactic administration of calcium gluconate during exchange transfusion with blood containing citrate remains controversial. Nevertheless, many units continue to administer prophylactic calcium. This may be particularly relevant in babies who have other medical conditions complicating their haemolytic process.

The shelf life of packed red cells can be extended when they are suspended in additive solutions. Commonly used additive solutions include SAG-M and AS-1, both of which contain glucose and mannitol. Infusions of these additives may lead to rebound hypoglycaemia and fluid balance problems, but, once again, this is unlikely after small-volume top-up transfusion. Nevertheless, exchange transfusion with these products is not recommended.

11.5.1.4 Storage

Blood stored at 4 °C under optimal conditions has a shelf life of 35 days.[12] During storage, potassium leaches from the red cells into the suspension medium and, after 35 days in AS-1, the potassium concentration reaches approximately 50 mmol/l. Storage also leads to complete depletion of 2,3-diphosphoglycerate (2,3-DPG) by 21 days. In spite of these changes, a top-up transfusion of 10 ml/kg of red cells up to 35 days old does not carry a significant risk to the neonate.[13] The advantage of such products is that they can be subdivided into small aliquots (so-called paedi-packs) and used for multiple top-up transfusions over a 5-week period, thus limiting exposure of the patient to a single donor. By contrast, blood for large-volume transfusion should be less than 5 days old, in order to minimize the effects of potassium loss and 2,3-DPG depletion.[13]

11.5.1.5 Leukodepletion and irradiation

CMV can be transmitted by blood derived from healthy but latently infected adult donors. Transfusion-acquired CMV disease may be life-threatening, particularly in immunocompromised recipients, but transmission can be prevented by reducing the transfused white cell dose to less than 1×10^6 by leukodepletion with a cell filter.[14] Filtration at the bedside is not recommended, as this may be unreliable and leukodepletion at the transfusion centre with attendant quality control is preferred. In the UK, all red cells and platelets are now leukodepleted. Prospective studies have suggested that CMV disease is most likely in very low birthweight children born to CMV-seronegative mothers. Current guidelines therefore recommend that all babies receive CMV-negative leukodepleted blood products.[13]

Despite leukodepletion, all red cell and platelet products contain viable mononuclear cells. Following transfusion, these are killed by the immune system of the recipient and cause no clinical problem in an immunocompetent patient. However, if very large volumes of fresh allogeneic mononuclear cells are infused, as in an intrauterine or exchange transfusion, then the stem cells contained within this population may engraft in the recipient.[15] Rarely, this may lead to lethal transfusion-associated graft-versus-host disease, which is more likely in immunodeficient recipients and in rare cases where blood is transfused from first-degree relatives who may share an HLA type with the recipient – which is an increased risk in units in which maternal blood is used for fetal transfusion.[13] Irradiation of blood (giving 2500 cGy as the minimum dose to any part of the pack, with no part receiving more than 5000 cGy) prevents proliferation of transfused mononuclear cells and can be considered to be universally effective. In the neonatal treatment of HDFN, irradiated blood products are recommended in the following situations:

(1) *Transfusion after fetal transfusion*. It is generally accepted that transfusion in utero is immunosuppressive, predisposing the neonate to an increased risk of

graft-versus-host disease. The use of irradiated cellular blood products for neonatal transfusion is mandatory in these cases.[13]

(2) *Exchange transfusion.* Without fetal transfusion, graft-versus-host disease is uncommon, but exchange transfusions involving large volumes of cells may increase the risk and so irradiation is recommended, provided this does not delay transfusion.[13]

11.5.2 Influence of fetal transfusions

Janssens and coworkers reported their experience of 92 fetuses treated between 1987 and 1993.[2] There was a significant negative correlation between the number of fetal transfusions received and the number of postnatal exchange transfusions required (91% of neonates received one or more exchange transfusions). Weiner and coworkers reported a similar observation, although only 20% of neonates required exchange transfusion in their study.[1] Thus, transfusion in utero appears to reduce significantly the requirement for transfusion postnatally.

Babies who are born at an adequate gestation for lung maturity, with an adequate haemoglobin and with the majority of fetal blood having been replaced by donor blood (such that the percentage of fetal blood cells is about 1%) normally require little specific management in the experience of the authors. Jaundice is usually mild and phototherapy alone is usually sufficient, although a top-up blood transfusion may be required to achieve a haemoglobin concentration of about 12–14 g/dl.

Babies who are born without complete suppression of fetal haemopoiesis will be at greater risk of both neonatal anaemia and hyperbilirubinaemia. This group needs to be closely monitored and some of these babies require exchange transfusion, phototherapy and top-up transfusions. Babies who have received no fetal transfusion need to be managed according to the traditional indications for exchange transfusion (Section 11.6.2.1). In addition, hydrops is more likely and needs to be managed accordingly.

11.5.3 Indications for transfusion

The degree of anaemia at which neonatal blood transfusion is indicated is unclear. It has been suggested that late transfusion is rarely needed for haemoglobin concentrations as low as 5–6 g/dl unless the patient is symptomatic (breathless, lethargic, feeding poorly or not thriving).[16] The clinical condition of the patient should be the primary determinant of the need for transfusion. Supplemental iron therapy should not be prescribed routinely unless the serum ferritin has fallen to low levels; repeated transfusions and ongoing haemolysis ensure that total body iron stores are usually significantly increased. Folate, at a dose of 100 μg/day, is recommended by some.[17]

Anaemia may last for 3 months or more following birth because of the persistence of antibodies and suppression of erythropoiesis. Babies who have had repeated transfusions with adult blood seem to tolerate low haemoglobin concentrations – perhaps because of the more efficient oxygen delivery of haemoglobin A compared with haemoglobin F.[18] A conservative blood transfusion policy allows the haemoglobin concentration to fall without further blood transfusions to avoid further donor exposure and to allow the natural stimulus for endogenous erythropoietin to occur.

The role of recombinant erythropoietin is not known. In the absence of fetal transfusions, endogenous erythropoietin is normal despite the reticulocytopenia.[19] However, in a small randomized trial of 20 babies with HDFN due to anti-D, erythropoietin treatment (200 IU/kg, three times a week for 6 weeks) significantly reduced the need for top-up blood transfusions for persistent anaemia (1.8 transfusions versus 4.2 transfusions in the control group).[20]

11.6 Treatment of neonatal jaundice

The rise in serum bilirubin that occurs when the placenta is removed and the haemolytic process continues is the main clinical problem that requires treatment in the absence of hydrops. The two established treatments available are phototherapy and exchange blood transfusion.

11.6.1 Phototherapy

Phototherapy is normally the first intervention in hyperbilirubinaemia, with exchange transfusion only being used if there is failure to control the bilirubin. The method uses light in the range of 425–475 nm wavelength and is effective in reducing serum bilirubin concentration by converting it into isomer forms or photoxidation products which are excreted in bile and urine. Phototherapy has been shown to reduce the requirement for exchange transfusion, but studies have not had the power to show an effect on neurodevelopmental outcome.[21,22] In haemolytic anaemia, phototherapy is typically used in conjunction with exchange transfusion to maintain the serum bilirubin concentration at safe levels. Low gestational age, hypoxia and acidosis are considered to be factors which reduce the level of bilirubin which may be considered safe for particular babies (see guidelines below).

11.6.2 Exchange blood transfusion
11.6.2.1 Indications for exchange blood transfusion

This procedure is indicated for the rapid correction of severe anaemia in seriously affected neonates (Section 11.5) and in the treatment of hyperbilirubinaemia or rapidly rising bilirubin concentrations, especially if phototherapy has failed. All the issues of blood transfusion in neonates discussed above (Section 11.5.1) also apply if this technique is being used to treat jaundice. In babies who have not had blood transfusions as fetuses, one or more exchange transfusions may be needed to correct the anaemia and to control the rise in bilirubin – or to reduce the level of bilirubin if it has already reached levels thought to be risking neurotoxicity. Exchange transfusion is also useful for correcting severe anaemia even in the absence of hyperbilirubinaemia, and may help to limit further serious rises in bilirubin by removing sensitized red cells from the circulation. Since the number of exchange transfusions performed has dramatically reduced in recent years,[1] the experience, and so perhaps skill, of neonatal practitioners in this procedure has probably fallen, with the potential for increasing the risks of the procedure.

Exchange transfusion has been shown to reduce the incidence of kernicterus.[23,24] The only randomized controlled trial of exchange transfusion ('double volume' or twice the average circulating blood volume of 80 ml/kg) was conducted in 1952.[25] There were fewer deaths and fewer cases of kernicterus in the group who received exchange transfusions compared with the group who received simple blood transfusions for anaemia. The incidence of kernicterus has fallen dramatically in the years that have followed.[24]

Indications for exchange transfusion are controversial and wide variation in practice exists.[26] Such variation in practice also seems to exist in the care of babies who have received multiple intrauterine transfusions, with reported incidences of postnatal exchange transfusions ranging from 20% to 91%.[1,2]

Traditionally, exchange transfusions have been considered to be indicated either within 12 hours of birth for anaemia and high bilirubin concentrations, or later, to control the rise in postnatal bilirubin despite phototherapy. Delayed exchange transfusions are performed when bilirubin concentrations have reached presumed toxic levels (Table 11.1) or when the rate of rise predicts that a toxic range will be reached. A rate of rise (despite phototherapy) of 0.5 mg/dl/hour or 10 μmol/l/hour is now commonly regarded as an indication for exchange transfusion.[7] Such a rise may predict more accurately the need for exchange transfusion than cord blood haemoglobin concentration (less than 13 g/dl) or serum bilirubin concentration (80 μmol/l).

11.6.2.2 Technical aspects of exchange transfusion

The original technique of exchange transfusion as described by Diamond in 1947 involves the insertion of an umbilical venous catheter and the withdrawal of aliquots of baby's blood (5–20 ml) and the infusion of the same volume of donor blood through a system of inline taps. An isovolaemic technique has been described which involves withdrawing blood at a constant rate from an arterial line and the constant infusion at the same rate of the donor blood via a vein.[28] This isovolaemic technique seems to result in greater haemodynamic stability.[28] The volumes of

Table 11.1 Management of hyperbilirubinaemia in the healthy term newborn

| | Total serum bilirubin level mg/dl (μmol/l) | | | |
Age (hours)	Consider phototherapy	Phototherapy	Exchange transfusion if intensive phototherapy fails	Exchange transfusion and phototherapy
≤24	—	—	—	—
25–48	≥12 (170)	≥15 (260)	≥20 (340)	≥25 (430)
49–72	≥15 (260)	≥18 (310)	≥25 (430)	≥30 (510)
>72	≥17 (290)	≥20 (340)	≥25 (430)	≥30 (510)

Source: From the American Academy of Pediatrics, 1994.[27]

blood used in an exchange transfusion range from 'single' volume (80 ml/kg) to double volume (160 ml/kg). The single-volume exchange is generally used for correcting anaemia and the double volume for the treatment of hyperbilirubinaemia. The effect of the double-volume exchange is to replace 80–90% of the baby's blood. This results in the removal of most of the sensitized erythrocytes and also the plasma which contains the circulating antibodies and bilirubin. The double-volume procedure usually takes 1.5–2 hours to complete.

11.6.2.3 Complications and risks

Following exchange transfusion for hyperbilirubinaemia, it is well recognized that there may be a rebound in serum bilirubin.[7] A reduction in serum bilirubin of about 50% occurs at the end of the procedure, but, within 30 minutes, the bilirubin concentration may increase to 60% of the pre-exchange level because of active haemolysis and equilibration between tissues and plasma.[7,29]

Exchange transfusion is associated with significant risks.[30] A mortality rate of 2–3 per 1000 has been reported, but the rate may be higher in sick, low birthweight babies.[30,31] Vascular complications may also develop from catheter damage, haemorrhage, incorrect volume infusion, bacteraemia, viral infections, emboli (air or thrombotic), necrotizing enterocolitis or rebound hypoglycaemia. The latter is caused by the increased secretion of insulin in response to the dextrose present in the transfused blood.

11.6.3 An integrated approach to treating neonatal jaundice

The are many published guidelines for the use of phototherapy and exchange blood transfusion.[27,32–35] Although phototherapy and exchange transfusion have been shown to reduce hyperbilirubinaemia effectively, there is still no certainty as to the bilirubin level at which intervention should occur.[36] The current levels used in practice are derived from limited scientific data and are based more on consen-

Table 11.2 Approaches to the treatment of hyperbilirubinaemia in term infants (≥37 weeks' gestation)

Treatment	Total bilirubin level mg/dl (μmol/l)	
	No haemolysis and infant well	Haemolysis likely or infant sick
Phototherapy	17–22 (290–325)	13–15 (220–255)
Exchange transfusion	25–29 (425–500)	17–22 (290–375)

Source: Adapted from Newman and Maisels, 1992.[32]

Table 11.3 Approaches to the use of phototherapy and exchange transfusion in low birthweight infants

Birthweight	Total bilirubin level mg/dl (μmol/l)	
	Phototherapy	Exchange transfusion
<1500	5–8 (85–140)	13–16 (220–275)
1500–1999	8–12 (140–200)	16–18 (275–300)
2000–2499	11–14 (190–240)	18–20 (300–340)

Source: Adapted from Newman and Maisels, 1992.[34]

Table 11.4 Use of phototherapy in full-term infants with ABO haemolytic disease

Age (hours)	Total bilirubin level mg/dl (μmol/l)
<12	10 (170)
12–17	12 (200)
18–23	14 (240)
≥24	15 (255)

Source: Adapted from Osborn et al. (1984).[37]

sus. No single serum level will be appropriate for all babies. Additional factors which increase the risk of bilirubin toxicity need to be considered when deciding on the form and timing of treatment. Factors that increase the risk of toxicity are thought to relate to haemolysis, acidosis, asphyxia, low gestation and birthweight, and drugs which alter bilirubin binding (e.g. aminoglycoside antibiotics and frusemide).

Various approaches to the treatment of hyperbilirubinaemia taken from various guidelines are summarized in Tables 11.1, 11.2, 11.3 and 11.4, but these need to be applied with careful consideration of the additional risk factors present. No guidelines exist for neonatal intervention following fetal transfusion.

A newer approach has been the administration of high-dose intravenous immuno-globulin. This is thought to block Fc receptors on macrophages and so reduce the lysis of sensitized red cells. Voto and coworkers demonstrated in a blinded random-ized trial of 40 babies with HDFN due to anti-D that the treated group had signifi-cantly decreased duration of hospitalization, less haemolysis and less marked increases in bilirubin. They received less treatment with exchange transfusions and simple blood transfusions as a result.[38]

11.7 Experimental treatments

New approaches for the treatment of neonatal jaundice include high-dose synthetic blood group trisaccharides in ABO haemolytic disease and haem oxygenase inhib-itors. Trisaccharides determining the A and B blood groups (Section 2.6.1) have been synthesized and shown to neutralize specific antibodies and to accelerate their dissociation from red cells.[39] A trial of A and B trisaccharides has been conducted in babies with severe or moderately severe HDFN due to anti-A or anti-B.[39] Thirteen babies (10 group A and three group B) were treated. The severity and duration of hyperbilirubinaemia and the need for exchange transfusion was com-pared with 21 similar babies previously treated with conventional means (photo-therapy and exchange transfusion when indicated). Serum bilirubin concentrations were significantly lower in the treated babies who also required fewer exchange transfusions. In addition, a subgroup of babies tested for anti-A antibody were found to have higher antibody levels after treatment than before, suggesting that the mechanism of action was indeed by displacement of antibodies from the surface of sensitized red cells. A randomized controlled trial is awaited.

Haem oxygenase is an enzyme which catalyses the conversion of haem to biliver-din in the production of bilirubin from haemoglobin breakdown. By inhibiting this step, the production of bilirubin could be reduced. Early human trials in ABO incompatibility confirmed that bilirubin levels were lower in patients treated with tin protoporphyrin.[40] However, there are significant concerns about the safety of these agents and therefore little progress has been made.[29,40,41]

11.8 References

1 Weiner CP, Williamson RA, Wenstrom KD et al. (1991). Management of hemolytic disease by cordocentesis. II. Outcome of treatment. *American Journal of Obstetrics and Gynecology*, 165, 1302–7.

2 Janssens HM, de Haan MJJ, van Kamp IL, Brand R, Kanhai HHH & Veen S (1997). Outcome for children treated with fetal intravascular transfusions because of severe blood group antag-onism. *Journal of Pediatrics*, 131, 373–80.

3 Brown AK, Kim MH, Wu PYK & Btylaa DA (1985). Efficacy of phototherapy in prevention and management of neonatal hyperbilirubinaemia. *Pediatrics*, **75**, 393–400.

4 Hsia DY-Y, Allen FH, Gelliss SS & Drummond LK (1952). Erythroblastosis fetalis, VIII: studies on serum bilirubin in relation to kernicterus. *New England Journal of Medicine*, **247**, 668–71.

5 Doyle LW, Kelly EA, Rickards AL, Ford GW & Callanan C (1993). Sensorineural outcome at 2 years for survivors of erythroblastosis treated with fetal intravascular transfusions. *Obstetrics and Gynecology*, **81**, 931–5.

6 Hudon L, Moise KJ, Hegemier SE et al. (1998). Long-term neurodevelopmental outcome after intrauterine transfusion for the treatment of fetal hemolytic disease. *American Journal of Obstetrics and Gynecology*, **179**, 858–63.

7 Bowman JM (1999). Alloimmune hemolytic disease of the fetus and newborn. In: *Wintrobe's Clinical Hematology*, eds. GR Lee, J Foeister, J Lukers, F Paraskevas, JP Greer & GM Odgers, pp. 1210–32. Baltimore, MD: Williams and Wilkins.

8 Ebbesen F (1979). Late anemia in infants with rhesus haemolytic disease treated with intensive phototherapy. *European Journal of Pediatrics*, **130**, 285–90.

9 Millard DD, Gidding SS, Socol ML et al. (1990). Effects of intravascular, intrauterine transfusion on prenatal and postnatal hemolysis and erythropoiesis in severe fetal isoimmunization. *Journal of Pediatrics*, **117**, 447–54.

10 Bowman JM (1977). Neonatal management. In *Modern Management of the Rh Problem*, 2nd edn, ed. JT Queenan, pp. 200–39. New York: Harper and Row.

11 Carlton DP, McGillivray BC & Schreiber MD (1989). Nonimmune hydrops fetalis: a multidisciplinary approach. *Clinics of Perinatology*, **16**, 834–51.

12 The United Kingdom Blood Transfusion Services/National Institute for Biological Standards and Controls Joint Executive Liaison Committee (2000). *Guidelines for the Blood Transfusion Services in the United Kingdom*, 4th edn. Norwich: The Stationary Office.

13 British Committee for Standards in Haematology Blood Transfusion Task Force (1994). Guidelines for the administration of blood products: transfusion of infants and neonates. *Transfusion Medicine*, **4**, 63–9.

14 Pamphilon DH, Rider JR, Barbara JA & Williamson LM (1999). Prevention of transfusion-transmitted cytomegalovirus infection. *Transfusion Medicine*, **9**, 115–23.

15 Parkman R, Mosier D, Umansky I, Cochran W, Carpenter CB & Rosen FS (1974). Graft-versus-host disease after intrauterine and exchange transfusions for hemolytic disease of the newborn. *New England Journal of Medicine*, **290**, 359–63.

16 Oski FA & Naiman JL (1982). Eythroblastosis fetalis. In *Hematologic Problems in the Newborn*, 4th edn, p. 283. Philadelphia, PN: WB Saunders.

17 Lasker MR, Eddleman K & Tool AH (1995). Neonatal hepatitis and excessive hepatic iron deposition following intrauterine transfusion. *American Journal of Perinatology*, **12**, 14–17.

18 Delivoria-Papadopoulos M, Roncervie N & Oski FI (1971). Postnatal changes in oxygen transport on term, premature and sick infants: the role of red cell 2:3 diphosphoglycerate and adult hemoglobin. *Pediatric Research*, **5**, 235–45.

19 Scaradavou A, Inglis S, Peterson P, Dunne J, Chervenack F & Bussel J (1993). Suppression of

erythropoiesis by intrauterine transfusions in hemolytic disease of the newborn: use of erythropoietin to treat the late anemia. *Journal of Pediatrics*, **123**, 279–84.

20 Ovali F, Samanci N & Dagoglu T (1996). Management of late anemia in Rhesus hemolytic disease: use of recombinant human erythropoietin (a pilot study). *Pediatric Research*, **39**, 831–4.

21 Sisson TRC, Kendall N, Glauser S, Knutson S & Bunyaviroch E (1971). Phototherapy of jaundice in newborn infants. I. ABO blood group incompatibility. *Journal of Pediatrics*, **79**, 904–9.

22 National Institute of Child Health and Human Development (1985). Randomized controlled trial of phototherapy for neonatal hyperbilirubinaemia. *Pediatrics*, **75** (suppl), 385–441.

23 Maisels MJ (1994). Jaundice. In *Neonatology: Pathophysiology and Management of the Newborn*, eds. GB Avery, MA Fletcher & MG MacDonald. Philadelphia, PN: JB Lippincott.

24 Allen FH, Diamond LK & Vaughan VC (1950). Erythroblastosis fetalis: VI. Prevention of kernicterus. *American Journal of Diseases of Childhood*, **80**, 779–89.

25 Mollison PL & Walker W (1952). Controlled trials of the treatment of haemolytic disease of the newborn. *Lancet*, **262**, 429–39.

26 Stern SCM, Cockburn SH & de Silva PM (1998). Current practice in neonatal exchange transfusions: a retrospective audit based at one transfusion centre. *Transfusion Medicine*, **8**, 97–101.

27 American Academy of Pediatrics (1994). Practice Parameter: management of hyperbilirubinaemia in the healthy term newborn. *Pediatrics*, **94**, 558–65.

28 Martin JR (1973). A double catheter technique for exchange transfusion in the newborn infant. *New Zealand Medical Journal*, **77**, 167–9.

29 Valaes T (1963). Bilirubin distribution and dynamics of bilirubin removal by exchange transfusion. *Acta Paediatrica Scandinavica*, **52**, 149

30 Keenan WJ, Novak KK, Sutherland JM, Bryla DA & Fetterly KL (1985). Morbidity and mortality associated with exchange transfusion. *Pediatrics*, **75**, 417–21.

31 Jackson JC (1997). Adverse events associated with exchange transfusion in healthy and ill newborns. *Pediatrics*, **99**, E7.

32 Newman TB & Maisels MJ (1992). Evaluation and treatment of jaundice in the term newborn: a kinder, gentler approach. *Pediatrics*, **89**, 809–18.

33 Dodd K (1993). Neonatal jaundice – a lighter touch. *Archives of Diseases of Childhood*, **68**, 529–32.

34 Ahlfors CE (1994). Criteria for exchange transfusion in jaundiced newborns. *Pediatrics*, **93**, 488–94.

35 Newman TB & Maisels MJ (1993). Neonatal hyperbilirubinemia and long term outcome: another look at the Collaborative Perinatal Project. *Pediatrics*, **92**, 651–7.

36 Peterec SM (1995). Management of neonatal Rh disease. *Clinics in Perinatology*, **22**, 561–92.

37 Osborn LM, Lenarsky C, Oakes RC & Reiff MI (1984). Phototherapy in full-term infants with hemolytic disease secondary to ABO incompatibility. *Pediatrics*, **74**, 371–4.

38 Voto LS, Sexer H, Ferreiro G et al. (1995). Neonatal administration of high dose intravenous immunoglobulin in rhesus hemolytic disease. *Journal of Perinatal Medicine*, **23**, 443–51.

39 Romano EL, Soyano A, Montano RF et al. (1994). Treatment of ABO hemolytic disease with synthetic blood group trisaccharides. *Vox Sanguinis*, **66**, 194–9.

40 Kappas A, Drummond GS, Manola T, Petmezaki S & Valaes T (1988). Sn-protoporphyrin use in the management of hyperbilirubinemia in term newborns with direct Coombs-positive ABO incompatibility. *Pediatrics*, **81**, 485–97.

41 Fort FL & Gold J (1989). Phototoxicity of tin protoporphyrin, tin mesoporphyrin, and tin diiododeuteroporphyrin under neonatal phototherapy conditions. *Pediatrics*, **84**, 1031–7.

The diagnosis of alloimmune thrombocytopenia

Andrew G Hadley

International Blood Group Reference Laboratory, Bristol, UK

12.1 Clinical aspects of diagnosis

Alloimmune thrombocytopenia is caused by maternal antibodies which cross the placenta and bring about the immune destruction of fetal platelets (Section 1.1.3 and 1.3.3). The syndrome occurs in about one in 1500 births (Section 4.2). Fetal alloimmune thrombocytopenia may start early in pregnancy. There is no spontaneous remission of thrombocytopenia in utero and, in the absence of therapy, platelet counts usually fall as gestation progresses. Almost 50% of affected fetuses have a platelet count of less than $20 \times 10^9/l$.[1] In the absence of screening programmes, alloimmune thrombocytopenia is usually recognized at birth when the majority of affected cases have petechiae, purpura or overt bleeding.[2] Approximately 28% of these affected infants show evidence of central nervous system haemorrhage and up to one-half of these haemorrhages occur prenatally.[3–5] In utero intracranial haemorrhages may be associated with severe neurological sequelae, porencephaly and optic hypoplasia.[6]

Clinically, alloimmune thrombocytopenia is a diagnosis of exclusion. Typically, infants have no signs of disseminated intravascular coagulation, infection or congenital anomalies – each of which may be associated with thrombocytopenia. Typically, the mother has no history of autoimmune disease, thrombocytopenia or ingestion of drugs which may cause thrombocytopenia – since any of these would suggest a different diagnosis. At delivery, standard laboratory tests show that the neonatal platelet count is low (Section 12.4.1), and the haemoglobin concentration may be low if bleeding has occurred. Maternal platelet counts are normal; this distinguishes alloimmune thrombocytopenia from fetal thrombocytopenia associated with maternal autoimmune thrombocytopenia. Bone marrow biopsy of the infant in alloimmune thrombocytopenia usually reveals normal levels of megakaryocytes, but, rarely, they may be reduced.[7] Cranial ultrasound and computerized tomographic scans may reveal dilated cerebral ventricles and evidence of intraventricular haemorrhage.[8,9]

Once suspected on clinical grounds, a provisional diagnosis of alloimmune thrombocytopenia should be confirmed by establishing the presence of platelet-specific alloantibodies in the maternal serum which react with fetal platelets. Prospective studies have shown that the frequency of neonatal thrombocytopenia in unselected newborns is around 0.9% and an alloimmune aetiology can be demonstrated in about 30% of these cases.[10,11] The remainder of this chapter reviews the platelet antigens and antibodies which have been implicated in alloimmune thrombocytopenia and the laboratory assays which may be used to detect and characterize the causative antibodies.

12.2 Platelet antigen systems

Platelet alloantigens have been identified by many groups around the world over the past 30 years and this has resulted in the evolution of different terminologies. Since 1990, the Human Platelet Antigen (HPA) nomenclature has been almost universally adopted[12] and the platelet antigens which have been assigned to this system are listed in Table 12.1. Currently, five systems (HPA-1 to HPA-5) and eight low-frequency alloantigens (HPA-6bw to HPA-13bw) have been assigned. Platelet antigens which elicit the alloantibodies involved in fetal thrombocytopenia are carried on membrane glycoproteins involved in cell adhesion and haemostasis. As shown in Table 12.1, several platelet membrane proteins are encoded by allelic genes.

12.2.1 Platelet antigens on glycoprotein IIb/IIIa

The glycoprotein IIb/IIIa (CD41/CD61) is a heterodimer; glycoprotein IIb constitutes the α subunit and glycoprotein IIIa constitutes the β subunit of the complex. Glycoprotein IIb/IIIa is the major platelet integrin, present at approximately 50 000 copies per platelet. Upon platelet activation, glycoprotein IIb/IIIa is involved in platelet aggregation by binding adhesive proteins such as fibrinogen, fibronectin and von Willebrand factor. A bleeding disorder called Glanzmann's thrombasthenia results when glycoprotein IIb/IIIa is absent or dysfunctional.

Glycoprotein IIIa is the most polymorphic molecule on the platelet surface apart from HLA class I. The molecular genetic basis of eight of the antigens on glycoprotein IIIa has been determined. Seven of the antigens (HPA-1b, -4b, -6w, -7w, -8w, -10w and -11w) are encoded by relatively rare single nucleotide substitutions in the common wild-type form of glycoprotein IIIa (see Table 12.1 for references). The exception to date is the Oe^a antigen which results from the deletion of three nucleotides from the gene encoding the HPA-1b form of the glycoprotein. The HPA-1a/1b polymorphism is the most frequent cause of alloimmunization and is responsible for most cases of alloimmune thrombocytopenia. The immune response to the HPA-1a antigen has been characterized at a molecular level (Section 1.1.3).

12.2.2 Platelet antigens on glycoprotein Ia/IIa

There are approximately 2000 copies of glycoprotein Ia/IIa (CD49/CD29) per platelet. Glycoprotein Ia/IIa is a receptor for collagen and laminin, and a mild bleeding disorder may result when the complex is absent.[48] The molecular genetic basis for two alloantigen systems (HPA-5 and -13w) which reside on glycoprotein Ia have been determined; both result from single nucleotide substitutions (Table 12.1).

12.2.3 Platelet antigens on glycoprotein Ib/IX/V

Glycoprotein Ib/IX/V (CD42) binds von Willebrand factor and mediates the adhesion of platelets to exposed vascular subendothelium under conditions of high shear stress. Glycoprotein Ib comprises two disulphide-bonded subunits, glycoprotein Ibα (CD42b) and glycoprotein Ibβ (CD42c). Glycoprotein Ib is noncovalently associated with one glycoprotein IX molecule (CD42a) and glycoprotein V (CD42d). There are approximately 25 000 glycoprotein Ib/IX molecules and 12 000 glycoprotein V molecules per platelet. The absence of the complex results in an inherited bleeding disorder called Bernard–Soulier syndrome.

Three antigen systems (HPA-2, HPA-12w and Pe^a) on the glycoprotein Ib/IX/V complex have been described (Table 12.1).

12.3 Platelet antibody specificities involved in alloimmune thrombocytopenia

All the well-characterized platelet-specific alloantigens have been associated with alloimmune thrombocytopenia. Table 12.1 provides a list of reports describing at least one case of alloimmune thrombocytopenia due to each of the antigens.

In Caucasians, anti-HPA-1a is implicated in about 75% of cases of alloimmune thrombocytopenia (Table 12.2). This is due in part to the relative immunogenicity of the HPA-1a antigen and to the phenotypic frequency of the antigen; 98% of Caucasians are positive for HPA-1a which means that 2% of pregnant women may potentially produce anti-HPA-1a. In fact, far fewer than 2% of women are immunized because the ability to form anti-HPA-1a is associated with the HLA DR3*0101 genotype (Section 4.2.2).

Antibodies to HPA-5b are responsible for approximately 20% of cases of alloimmune thrombocytopenia among Caucasians (Table 12.2). As there are relatively few antigen sites per platelet (Section 12.2.2) the thrombocytopenia due to anti-HPA-5b tends to be mild. Although antibodies to HPA-1a are most commonly implicated in alloimmune thrombocytopenia in Caucasians, HPA-1b is very rare among Blacks and Orientals and so anti-HPA-1a antibodies are also rare.[24,50] Therefore, among Orientals, anti-HPA-4a and anti-HPA-4b cause alloimmune thrombocytopenia more frequently than do other platelet antibodies.

Table 12.1 Characteristics of the platelet-specific antigens implicated in alloimmune thrombocytopenia

System	Antigen	Alternative names	Glycoprotein	Nucleotide change	Amino acid change	Reference on antigen characterization	References describing alloimmune thrombocytopenia
HPA-1	HPA-1a	Zw^a, Pl^{A1}	GPIIIa	T^{196}	Leucine[33]	13	14
	HPA-1b	Zw^b, Pl^{A2}		C^{196}	Proline[33]		15
HPA-2	HPA-2a	Ko^b	GPIb	C^{524}	Threonine[145]	16	17
	HPA-2b	Ko^a Sib^a		T^{524}	Methionine[145]		18
HPA-3	HPA-3a	Bak^a, Lek^a	GPIIb	T^{2622}	Isoleucine[843]	19	20
	HPA-3b	Bak^b		G^{2622}	Serine[843]		21
HPA-4	HPA-4a	Yuk^b, Pen^a	GPIIIa	G^{526}	Arginine[143]	22	23
	HPA-4b	Yuk^a, Pen^b		A^{526}	Glutamine[143]		24
HPA-5	HPA-5a	Br^b, Zav^b	GPIa	G^{1648}	Glutamic acid[505]	25	27
	HPA-5b	Br^a, Zav^a, Hc^a		A^{1648}	Lysine[505]	26	28
HPA-6w	HPA-6bw	Ca^a, Tu^a	GPIIIa	G^{1564}	Arginine[489]	29	30
				A^{1564}	Glutamine[489]		
HPA-7w	HPA-7bw	Mo	GPIIIa	C^{1267}	Proline[407]	31	31
				G^{1267}	Alanine[407]		
HPA-8w	HPA-8bw	Sr^a	GPIIIa	T^{2004}	Arginine[636]	32	33
				C^{2004}	Cysteine[636]		
HPA-9w	HPA-9bw	Max^a	GPIIb	G^{2603}	Valine[837]	34	34
				A^{2603}	Methionine[837]		
HPA-10w	HPA-10bw	La^a	GPIIIa	G^{281}	Arginine[62]	35	35
				A^{281}	Glutamine[62]		
HPA-11w	HPA-11bw	Gro^a	GPIIIa	G^{1996}	Arginine[633]	36	37
				A^{1996}	Histidine[633]		

HPA-12w	Iy[a]	GPIb	G^{141} A^{141}	Glycine[15] Glutamic acid[15]	38	39
HPA-13w	Sit[a]	GPIa	C^{2531} T^{2531}	Threonine[799] Methionine[799]	40	40
	Oe[a]	GPIIIa	$AAG^{1929-1931}$ deletion	Lysine[611] deletion	41	42
	Va[a]	GPIIb/IIIa	—	—	43	43
	Gov[a] Gov[b]	CD109	—	—	44	45
	Pe[a]	GPIb	—	—	46	46
	Dy[a]	38kD GP	—	—	47	47

Table 12.2 Antibodies implicated in alloimmune thrombocytopenia in a Caucasian population

Specificity	% cases (n=415)
HPA-1a	73
HPA-5b	19
HPA-1a + HPA-5b	3
HPA-3a	2
HPA-2b	1
HPA-1b	1
HPA-5a	<1
HPA-8b	<1
HPA-12bw	<1
HPA-13bw	<1
HPA-4b	<1
Oeᵃ	<1

Source: Data from Kroll et al.[49]

There are isolated reports which have ascribed neonatal thrombocytopenia to the presence of maternal anti-HLA antibodies.[51,52] The mechanism of platelet destruction in these cases is uncertain because it is not clear how antibodies specific for antigens which are expressed on a variety of fetal tissues would localize to the fetal platelets. It may be that the thrombocytopenia in these rare cases is caused by platelet-specific antibodies which have not been detected by the techniques presently available. Indeed, epidemiological studies have shown that the platelet counts of fetuses delivered by women with anti-HLA antibodies are not statistically lower than counts in fetuses of women without anti-HLA antibodies.[53]

12.4 Laboratory diagnosis of alloimmune thrombocytopenia

12.4.1 Haematology

The neonatal full blood count usually reveals isolated thrombocytopenia from birth. In infants with alloimmune thrombocytopenia due to anti-HPA-1a, initial platelet counts are less than 10×10^9/l in approximately 30% of cases, and $10–30 \times 10^9$/l in approximately 25% of cases.[14] Platelet counts may decrease further during the first 48 hours after delivery, reaching counts of less than 10×10^9/l in approximately 50% of cases.

The mother's platelet count is usually normal. However, approximately 8% of all pregnant women develop mild thrombocytopenia ($100–150 \times 10^9$/l) during the second and third trimester of pregnancy.[54] The infants of these women do not appear to be at any additional risk of developing thrombocytopenia. However, it is difficult to distinguish this gestational thrombocytopenia from autoimmune thrombocytopenia and so it should not be assumed that the thrombocytopenia in infants delivered by mothers with mild thrombocytopenia is due to autoantibodies. It is therefore important to test for the presence of maternal alloantibodies, even in the cases of maternal thrombocytopenia.

12.4.2 Assays for the detection of antiplatelet antibodies

Once suspected on clinical grounds, a provisional diagnosis of alloimmune thrombocytopenia should be confirmed by demonstrating the presence of platelet-specific alloantibodies in the maternal serum. It is also useful to perform platelet antigen typing to show that the mother's platelets lack the antigen to which antibodies have been formed. Phenotyping or genotyping of the father or infant may also be performed to demonstrate that the infant's platelets express the antigen to which the mother has been immunized. Finally, a crossmatch of maternal serum against paternal platelets should be performed to ensure the detection of antibodies to low-frequency antigens. Knowledge of the ethnic background of the family is useful because phenotypic frequencies vary between ethnic groups. In addition to testing maternal serum, female siblings of the mother are at increased risk and should be tested prospectively before the birth of their first child in order to identify potential cases of alloimmune thrombocytopenia.

It should be emphasized that therapy, particularly the transfusion of HPA-1a-negative, HPA-5b-negative platelets, should not be postponed if there is delay or difficulty in confirming the provisional diagnosis of alloimmune thrombocytopenia.

12.4.2.1 The platelet immunofluorescence test

The platelet indirect immunofluorescence test (PIFT) is probably the most widely used technique for demonstrating the presence of platelet-binding immunoglobulins in serum or plasma.[55] In this test, platelets are incubated with maternal serum and then washed. The platelets are then incubated with an anti-IgG reagent which is conjugated with a fluorochrome such as fluorescein isothiocyanate (which emits green fluorescence) or phycoerythrin (which emits red fluorescence). Platelet fluorescence is then assessed using a microscope equipped with UV illumination or, preferably, measured using a flow cytometer. Elevated levels of platelet membrane-associated fluorescence indicate the presence of platelet-binding antibodies.

12.4.2.2 Platelet glycoprotein-specific assays

Platelets express HLA class I antigens in addition to the glycoproteins implicated in alloimmune thrombocytopenia. Thus, the indirect immunofluorescence test is not

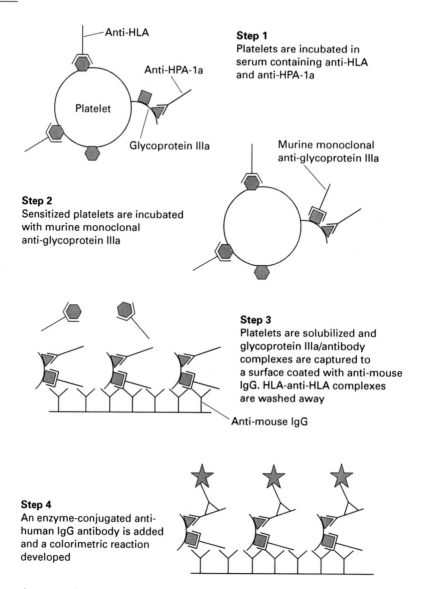

Step 1
Platelets are incubated in
serum containing anti-HLA
and anti-HPA-1a

Step 2
Sensitized platelets are incubated
with murine monoclonal
anti-glycoprotein IIIa

Step 3
Platelets are solubilized and
glycoprotein IIIa/antibody
complexes are captured to
a surface coated with anti-mouse
IgG. HLA-anti-HLA complexes
are washed away

Step 4
An enzyme-conjugated anti-
human IgG antibody is added
and a colorimetric reaction
developed

Figure 12.1   Diagrammatic representation of the monoclonal antibody immobilization of platelet antigens assay.

able to distinguish platelet-specific antibodies from anti-HLA antibodies. For this reason, the indirect immunofluorescence test is often performed together with a glycoprotein-specific assay. The basis for one such assay, the monoclonal antibody immobilization of platelet antigens assay (MAIPA),[56] is shown diagrammatically in Figure 12.1. Platelets of known phenotype are first incubated with maternal serum and then washed. Sensitized platelets are then incubated with a (murine) mono-clonal antibody which is specific for one of the platelet glycoproteins implicated in alloimmune thrombocytopenia. Following a wash step, the platelets are solubilized using a detergent and the lysates are added to wells of a microtitre plate coated with antimouse IgG antibodies. In this way, complexes of maternal antiplatelet glyco-protein antibody/platelet glycoprotein/monoclonal antibody are specifically immo-bilized in wells of the microtitre plate. Since anti-HLA antibodies complexed with HLA antigens are not immobilized, they are removed by washing. The presence of glycoprotein-specific (immobilized) maternal antibody is then determined by the addition of an enzyme-conjugated anti-human IgG reagent to catalyse a colorimet-ric reaction upon the addition of a suitable substrate. Antibody specificity may be deduced by determining the reactivity of antibodies with a selected panel of typed platelets.

Assays using monoclonal antibodies to immobilize platelet antigens are specific and sensitive, but are relatively laborious and are generally performed only in spe-cialist laboratories. Increasingly, kits for detecting platelet antibodies are becoming commercially available. These kits usually employ isolated platelet glycoproteins immobilized in wells of a microtitre plate. They are, therefore, convenient and rapid, eliminating the need for panels of typed platelets to determine antibody specificity. However, they may not be as sensitive as the MAIPA assay described above and may not detect all antibodies implicated in alloimmune thrombocyto-penia.[57]

12.4.3 DNA-based genotyping

Determining which alloantigens are expressed on platelets from a particular individ-ual is important in order to select panels of typed platelets which can then be used to characterize platelet-specific antibodies in maternal sera. Platelet typing is also important to establish an incompatibility between a mother and her fetus or infant. International workshops have revealed relatively poor levels of agreement between laboratories using serological techniques for platelet typing.[58] Moreover, antisera containing platelet-specific antibodies to many of the platelet antigens are scarce.

Since the molecular genetic basis for most of the platelet antigens is now known, DNA-based genotyping techniques are the methods of choice for platelet typing. These methods are based on the polymerase chain reaction (PCR) (Section 7.2). Several assays have been described,[49] but many laboratories have chosen to use techniques based on allele-specific PCR.[59,60] In this approach, primers are designed to anneal to the 3′ end of the allele to be detected, so that a mismatch on the alter-native allele does not result in DNA amplification and no PCR product results. This approach is useful when applied to typing the diallelic platelet antigens most com-monly implicated in alloimmune thrombocytopenia. However, it is less useful for antigens with very low frequencies when it is not possible to validate the stringency of the PCR reaction. Recently, Epstein–Barr virus-transformed B-lymphoblastoid cell lines have been developed as a reference source of DNA for platelet antigen genotyping.[61]

Fetal genotyping may be used to establish the phenotype of a fetus by analysing the fetal DNA present in samples of amniotic fluid or chorionic villus. This is particularly useful in the clinical management of alloimmunized pregnant women who have had a previously affected fetus but where the father is heterozygous for the implicated alloantigen. In this way, it is possible to establish whether or not the fetus is antigen positive and at risk of developing alloimmune thrombocytopenia.

12.4.4 Antibody characteristics and disease severity

12.4.4.1 Antibody specificity

It is generally accepted that antibodies to HPA-5b usually result in a less severe form of alloimmune thrombocytopenia than do antibodies to HPA-1a.[62] This has been attributed to the lower expression of the glycoprotein carrying HPA-5 system antigens; there are about 2000 copies of glycoprotein Ia per platelet compared with 50000 copies of glycoprotein IIb/IIIa which carries the HPA-1 system antigens. However, the clinical course of fetal thrombocytopenia due to HPA-5 system antibodies is not always mild and severe cases of fetal thrombocytopenia due to anti-HPA-5a and anti-HPA-5b have been described.[63,64] This variability might be related to an inherited predisposition in some individuals to express relatively high levels of glycoprotein Ia.

12.4.4.2 Antibody concentration

Some recent reports have suggested that the concentration of maternal anti-HPA-1a antibodies may be predictive of disease severity. Williamson et al.[65] reported a study of 46 women with anti-HPA-1a where severe thrombocytopenia was associated with third trimester anti-HPA-1a titres in the MAIPA assay (Section 12.4.2.2) of over 32. In contrast, severe thrombocytopenia was not observed in babies of women with anti-HPA-1a antibodies which were transient or only detectable post-natally. Similarly, in a study of 28 women with anti-HPA-1a, Husebekk et al.[66] found that antibody levels tended to rise towards the end of gestation and, in all but two cases, antibody levels measured in an ELISA technique were predictive for the severity of thrombocytopenia in the newborn. However, there are several reports of severe fetal thrombocytopenia where anti-HPA-1a antibodies only became detectable in the maternal plasma several weeks after delivery.[67]

12.5 Future perspectives

An ongoing challenge in the clinical management of platelet-alloimmunized women is the difficulty in predicting the severity of fetal thrombocytopenia using assays which measure the levels of antibodies in maternal plasma. One approach may be to measure the biological activity of platelet-specific antibodies, as has been done successfully to predict the severity of HDFN (Section 8.4.4). Preliminary data suggest that the chemiluminescence test might be used to measure the metabolic response of human monocytes to sensitized platelets and that the extent of the response may correspond with the severity of fetal thrombocytopenia.[68,69]

Several groups have recently described the production of soluble recombinant platelet glycoproteins. For example, Peterson et al.[70] used a baculovirus expression system to produce soluble glycoprotein IIb/IIIa complexes. These complexes assumed an active ligand-binding conformation and contained epitopes for a range of glycoprotein-specific monoclonal and human antibodies. Thus, it seems likely that recombinant glycoproteins will herald the introduction of improved techniques for the detection of platelet-specific antibodies. An important feature of this technology is the ability to introduce new alloantigens by site-directed mutagenesis. This should facilitate the detection of antibodies to rare platelet-specific alloantigens as well as obviate the need to maintain panels of typed platelets.

12.6 References

1 Bussel JB, Zabusky MR, Berkowitz RL & McFarland JG (1997). Fetal alloimmune thrombocytopenia. *New England Journal of Medicine*, **337**, 22–6.

2 Deaver JE, Leppert PC & Zaroulis CG (1986). Neonatal alloimmune thrombocytopenic purpura. *American Journal of Perinatology*, **3**, 127–31.

3 Herman JH, Jumbelic ML, Ancona RJ & Kickler TS (1986). In utero cerebral hemorrhage in alloimmune thrombocytopenia. *American Journal of Pediatric Hematology and Oncology*, **8**, 312–17.

4 de Vries LS, Connell J, Bydder GM et al. (1988). Recurrent intracranial haemorrhages in utero in an infant with alloimmune thrombocytopenia. Case report. *British Journal of Obstetrics and Gynaecology*, **95**, 299–302.

5 Giovangrandi Y, Daffos F, Kaplan C, Forestier F, Mac Aleese J & Moirot M (1990). Very early intracranial haemorrhage in alloimmune thrombocytopenia. *Lancet*, **336**, 310.

6 Sitarz AL, Driscoll JM Jr & Wolff JA (1976). Management of isoimmune neonatal thrombocytopenia. *American Journal of Obstetrics and Gynecology*, **124**, 39–42.

7 Bizzaro N & Dianese G (1988). Neonatal alloimmune amegakaryocytosis. Case report. *Vox Sanguinis*, **54**, 112–14.

8 Friedman JM & Aster RH (1985). Neonatal alloimmune thrombocytopenic purpura and congenital porencephaly in two siblings associated with a 'new' maternal antiplatelet antibody. *Blood*, **65**, 1412–15.

9 Burrows RF, Caco CC & Kelton JG (1988). Neonatal alloimmune thrombocytopenia: spontaneous in utero intracranial hemorrhage. *American Journal of Hematology*, **28**, 98–102.

10 Dreyfus M, Kaplan C, Verdy E, Schlegel N, Durand-Zaleski I & Tchernia G (1997). Frequency

of immune thrombocytopenia in newborns: a prospective study. Immune Thrombocytopenia Working Group. *Blood*, **89**, 4402–6.

11 de Moerloose P, Boehlen F, Extermann P & Hohfeld P (1998). Neonatal thrombocytopenia: incidence and characterization of maternal antiplatelet antibodies by MAIPA assay. *British Journal of Haematology*, **100**, 735–40.

12 von dem Borne AEG Kr & Decary F (1990). Nomenclature of platelet specific antigens. *British Journal of Haematology*, **74**, 239–40.

13 Newman PJ, Derbes RS & Aster RH (1989). The human platelet alloantigens, PlA1 and PlA2, are associated with a leucine33/proline33 amino acid polymorphism in membrane glycoprotein IIIa, and are distinguishable by DNA typing. *Journal of Clinical Investigation*, **83**, 1778–81.

14 Mueller-Eckhardt C, Kiefel V, Grubert A et al. (1989). 348 cases of suspected neonatal alloimmune thrombocytopenia. *Lancet*, **i**, 363–6.

15 Mueller-Eckhardt C, Becker T, Weisheit M, Witz C & Santoso S (1986). Neonatal alloimmune thrombocytopenia due to fetomaternal Zw[b] incompatibility. *Vox Sanguinis*, **50**, 94–6.

16 Kuijpers RW, Faber NM, Cuypers HT, Ouwehand WH & von dem Borne AE (1992). NH2-terminal globular domain of human platelet glycoprotein Ib alpha has a methionine 145/threonine145 amino acid polymorphism, which is associated with the HPA-2 (Ko) alloantigens. *Journal of Clinical Investigation*, **89**, 381–4.

17 Kuijpers RW, van den Anker JN, Baerts W & von dem Borne AE (1994). A case of severe neonatal thrombocytopenia with schizencephaly associated with anti-HPA-1b and anti-HPA-2a. *British Journal of Haematology*, **87**, 576–9.

18 Kroll H, Muntean W, Kiefel V et al. (1994). Anti Ko(a) as a cause of neonatal alloimmune thrombocytopenia. *Beiträge zur Infusionstherapie und Transfusionsmedizin*, **32**, 244–6.

19 Lyman S, Aster RH, Visentin GP & Newman PJ (1990). Polymorphism of human platelet membrane glycoprotein IIb associated with the Bak[a]/Bak[b] alloantigen system. *Blood*, **75**, 2343–8.

20 von dem Borne AE, von Riesz E, Verheugt FW et al. (1980). Bak[a], a new platelet-specific antigen involved in neonatal allo-immune thrombocytopenia. *Vox Sanguinis*, **39**, 113–20.

21 McGrath K, Minchinton R, Cunningham I & Ayberk H (1989). Platelet anti-Bak[b] antibody associated with neonatal alloimmune thrombocytopenia. *Vox Sanguinis*, **57**, 182–4.

22 Wang R, Furihata K, McFarland JG, Friedman K, Aster RH & Newman PJ (1992). An amino acid polymorphism within the RGD binding domain of platelet membrane glycoprotein IIIa is responsible for the formation of the Pen[a]/Pen[b] alloantigen system. *Journal of Clinical Investigation*, **90**, 2038–43.

23 Matsui K, Ohsaki E, Goto A, Koresawa M, Kigasawa H & Shibata Y (1995). Perinatal intracranial hemorrhage due to severe neonatal alloimmune thrombocytopenic purpura (NAITP) associated with anti-Yukb (HPA-4a) antibodies. *Brain Development*, **17**, 352–5.

24 Shibata Y, Matsuda I, Miyaji T & Ichikawa Y (1986). Yuk[a], a new platelet antigen involved in two cases of neonatal alloimmune thrombocytopenia. *Vox Sanguinis*, **50**, 177–80

25 Santoso S, Kalb R, Walka M, Kiefel V, Mueller-Eckhardt C & Newman PJ (1993). The human platelet alloantigens Br(a) and Br(b) are associated with a single amino acid polymorphism on glycoprotein Ia (integrin subunit alpha 2). *Journal of Clinical Investigation*, **92**, 2427–32.

26 Simsek S, Gallardo D, Ribera A & von dem Borne AE (1994). The human platelet alloantigens, HPA-5(a+, b−) and HPA-5(a−, b+), are associated with a Glu505/Lys505 polymorphism of glycoprotein Ia (the alpha 2 subunit of VLA-2). *British Journal of Haematology*, 86, 671–4.

27 Bettaieb A, Fromont P, Rodet M, Godeau B, Duedari N & Bierling P (1991). Br^b, a platelet alloantigen involved in neonatal alloimmune thrombocytopenia. *Vox Sanguinis*, 60, 230–4.

28 Kiefel V, Santoso S, Katzmann B & Mueller-Eckhardt C (1988). A new platelet-specific alloantigen Br^a. Report of 4 cases with neonatal alloimmune thrombocytopenia. *Vox Sanguinis*, 54, 101–6.

29 Wang R, McFarland JG, Kekomaki R & Newman PJ (1993). Amino acid 489 is encoded by a mutational 'hot spot' on the beta 3 integrin chain: the CA/TU human platelet alloantigen system. *Blood*, 82, 3386–91.

30 McFarland JG, Blanchette V, Collins J, Newman PJ, Wang R & Aster RH (1993). Neonatal alloimmune thrombocytopenia due to a new platelet-specific alloantibody. *Blood*, 15, 3318–23.

31 Kuijpers RW, Simsek S, Faber NM, Goldschmeding R, van Wermerkerken RK & von dem Borne AE (1993). Single point mutation in human glycoprotein IIIa is associated with a new platelet-specific alloantigen (Mo) involved in neonatal alloimmune thrombocytopenia. *Blood*, 81, 70–6.

32 Santoso S, Kalb R, Kroll H et al. (1994). A point mutation leads to an unpaired cysteine residue and a molecular weight polymorphism of a functional platelet beta 3 integrin subunit. The Sr^a alloantigen system of GPIIIa. *Journal of Biological Chemistry*, 18, 8439–44.

33 Kroll H, Kiefel V, Santoso S & Mueller-Eckhardt C (1990). Sr^a, a private platelet antigen on glycoprotein IIIa associated with neonatal alloimmune thrombocytopenia. *Blood*, 76, 2296–302.

34 Noris P, Simsek S, de Bruijne-Admiraal LG et al. (1995). Max(a), a new low-frequency platelet-specific antigen localized on glycoprotein IIb, is associated with neonatal alloimmune thrombocytopenia. *Blood*, 86, 1019–26.

35 Peyruchaud O, Bourre F, Morel-Kopp MC et al. (1997). HPA-10w(b) (La(a)): genetic determination of a new platelet-specific alloantigen on glycoprotein IIIa and its expression in COS-7 cells. *Blood*, 89, 2422–8.

36 Simsek S, Folman C, van der Schoot CE & von dem Borne AE (1997). The Arg633His substitution responsible for the private platelet antigen Gro(a) unravelled by SSCP analysis and direct sequencing. *British Journal of Haematology*, 97, 330–5.

37 Simsek S, Vlekke AB, Kuijpers RW, Goldschmeding R, von dem Borne AE (1994). A new private platelet antigen, Gro^a, localized on glycoprotein IIIa, involved in neonatal alloimmune thrombocytopenia. *Vox Sanguinis*, 67, 302–6.

38 Sachs UJ, Kiefel V, Bohringer M, Afshar-Kharghan V, Kroll H & Santoso S (2000). Single amino acid substitution in human platelet glycoprotein Ib-beta is responsible for the formation of the platelet-specific alloantigen Iy(a). *Blood*, 95, 1849–55.

39 Kiefel V, Vicariot M, Giovangrandi Y et al. (1995). Alloimmunization against Iy, a low-frequency antigen on platelet glycoprotein Ib/IX as a cause of severe neonatal alloimmune thrombocytopenic purpura. *Vox Sanguinis*, 69, 250–4.

40 Santoso S, Amrhein J, Hofmann HA et al. (1999). A point mutation Thr(799)Met on the

alpha(2) integrin leads to the formation of new human platelet alloantigen Sit(a) and affects collagen-induced aggregation. *Blood*, **94**, 4103–11.

41 Santoso S, Pylypiw R, Wilke IG, Kroll H & Kiefel V (1998). One amino acid deletion of the PlA2 allelic form of GPIIIa leads to the formation of the new platelet alloantigen, Oe(a). *Transfusion Medicine*, **8**, 257a.

42 Kroll H, Santoso S, Bohringer M et al. (1995). Neonatal alloimmune thrombocytopenia caused by immunization against Oe[a], a new low frequency alloantigen on platelet glycoprotein IIIa. *Blood*, **86**, 540a.

43 Kekomäki R, Raivio P & Kero P (1992). A new low-frequency platelet alloantigen, Va[a], on glycoprotein IIbIIIa associated with neonatal alloimmune thrombocytopenia. *Transfusion Medicine*, **2**, 27–33.

44 Smith JW, Hayward CP, Horsewood P, Warkentin TE, Denomme GA & Kelton JG (1995). Characterization and localization of the Gova/b alloantigens to the glycosylphosphatidylinositol-anchored protein CDw109 on human platelets. *Blood*, **86**, 2807–14.

45 Bordin JO, Kelton JG, Warner MN et al. (1997). Maternal immunization to Gov system alloantigens on human platelets. *Transfusion*, **37**, 823–8.

46 Kekomäki R, Partanen J, Pitkänen S, Ilanmaa E, Ämmälä P & Teramo K (1993). Glycoprotein Ib/IX-specific alloimmunization in an HPA-2b-homozygous mother in association with neonatal thrombocytopenia. *Thrombosis and Haemostasis*, **69**, 99.

47 Smith JW, Horsewood P, McCusker PJ, Rombough IR & Kelton JG (1998). Severe neonatal alloimmune thrombocytopenia due to a novel low-frequency alloantigen Dy[a]. *Blood*, **92** (suppl 1), 180a.

48 Nieuwenhuis HK, Akkerman JW, Houdijk WP & Sixma JJ (1985). Human blood platelets showing no response to collagen fail to express surface glycoprotein Ia. *Nature*, **318**, 470–2.

49 Kroll H, Kiefel V & Santoso S (1998). Clinical aspects and typing of platelet alloantigens. *Vox Sanguinis*, **74** (suppl 2), 345–54.

50 Ramsey G & Salamon DJ (1986). Frequency of Pl[A1] in blacks. *Transfusion*, **26**, 531–2.

51 del Rosario ML, Fox ER, Kickler TS & Kao KJ (1998). Neonatal alloimmune thrombocytopenia associated with maternal anti-HLA antibody: a case report. *Journal of Pediatric Hematology and Oncology*, **20**, 252–6.

52 Tanaka T, Umesaki N, Nishio J et al. (2000). Neonatal thrombocytopenia induced by maternal anti-HLA antibodies: a potential side effect of allogenic leukocyte immunization for unexplained recurrent aborters. *Journal of Reproductive Immunology*, **46**, 51–7

53 King KE, Kao KJ, Bray PF et al. (1996). The role of HLA antibodies in neonatal thrombocytopenia: a prospective study. *Tissue Antigens*, **47**, 206–11.

54 Burrows RF & Kelton JG (1988). Incidentally detected thrombocytopenia in healthy mothers and their infants. *New England Journal of Medicine*, **21**, 142–5

55 von dem Borne AE, van Leeuwen EF, von Riesz LE, van Boxtel CJ & Engelfriet CP (1981). Neonatal alloimmune thrombocytopenia: detection and characterization of the responsible antibodies by the platelet immunofluorescence test. *Blood*, **57**, 649–56.

56 Kiefel V, Santoso S, Weisheit M & Mueller-Eckhardt C (1987). Monoclonal antibody-specific immobilization of platelet antigens (MAIPA): a new tool for the identification of platelet-reactive antibodies. *Blood*, **70**, 1722–6.

57 Lucas GF & Rogers SE (1999). Evaluation of an enzyme-linked immunosorbent assay kit (GTI PakPlus) for the detection of antibodies against human platelet antigens. *Transfusion Medicine*, 9, 63–7.

58 Teramura G & Slichter SJ (1996). Report on the Sixth International Society of Blood Transfusion Platelet Serology Workshop. *Transfusion*, 36, 75–81.

59 Metcalfe P & Waters AH (1993). HPA-1 typing by PCR amplification with sequence-specific primers (PCR-SSP): a rapid and simple technique. *British Journal of Haematology*, 85, 227–9.

60 Cavanagh G, Dunn A, Chapman CE & Metcalfe P (1997). HPA genotyping by PCR sequence specific priming (PCR-SSP): a streamlined method for rapid routine investigations. *Transfusion Medicine*, 7, 41–5.

61 Carl B, Kroll H, Bux J, Bein G & Santoso S (2000). B-lymphoblastoid cell lines as a source of reference DNA for human platelet and neutrophil antigen genotyping. *Transfusion*, 40, 62–8.

62 Kaplan C, Morel-Kopp MC, Kroll H et al. (1991). HPA-5b (Br(a)) neonatal alloimmune thrombocytopenia: clinical and immunological analysis of 39 cases. *British Journal of Haematology*, 78, 425–9

63 Kanhai HH, Porcelijn L, van Zoeren D et al. (1996). Antenatal care in pregnancies at risk of alloimmune thrombocytopenia: report of 19 cases in 16 families. *European Journal of Obstetrics, Gynecology and Reproductive Biology*, 68, 67–73.

64 Kekomäki S, Koskela S, Laes M, Teramo K & Kekomäki R (2000). Neonatal thrombocytopenia in two of six human platelet alloantigen (HPA) 5a-positive children of an HPA-5a-immunized mother. *Transfusion Medicine*, 10, 81–5.

65 Williamson LM, Hackett G, Rennie J et al. (1998). The natural history of fetomaternal alloimmunization to the platelet-specific antigen HPA-1a (Pl^{A1}, Zwa) as determined by antenatal screening. *Blood*, 92, 2280–7.

66 Husebekk A, Jaegtvik S, Aune B, Oian P, Dahl LB & Skogen BR (1999). Maternal level of anti-HPA-1a antibodies predicts the severity of neonatal alloimmune thrombocytopenia. *Blood*, 94, 14a.

67 Schabel A, Konig AL, Brand U, Schnaidt M & Sugg U (1996). Severe neonatal alloimmune thrombocytopenia with delayed antibody detection. *Beiträge zur Infusionstherapie und Transfusionsmedizin*, 33, 156–9

68 Lucas GF, Hadley AG & Holburn AM (1987). Anti-platelet opsonic activity in alloimmune and autoimmune thrombocytopenia. *Clinical and Laboratory Haematology*, 9, 59–66.

69 Kelsch R, Bertelsbeck U, Cassens U, Garritsen B, Kehrel W & Sibrowski W (1997). Detection of platelet glycoprotein IIB/IIIA-reactive antibodies through a monocyte chemiluminescent response assay. *Blood*, 90, 40a.

70 Peterson JA, Visentin GP, Newman PJ & Aster RH (1998). A recombinant soluble form of the integrin alpha IIb beta 3 (GPIIb-IIIa) assumes an active, ligand-binding conformation and is recognized by GPIIb-IIIa-specific monoclonal, allo-, auto-, and drug-dependent platelet antibodies. *Blood*, 92, 2053–63.

The immunological diagnosis of alloimmune neutropenia

Geoff Lucas

International Blood Group Reference Laboratory, Bristol, UK

13.1 Introduction

Alloimmune neutropenia is caused by the placental transfer of maternal antibodies which recognize neutrophil antigens inherited by the fetus from the father. Alloimmune neutropenia is characterized by a severe but transient neutropenia and is the neutrophil equivalent of haemolytic disease of the fetus and newborn and alloimmune thrombocytopenia. Neutrophils have a fundamental role in innate immunity and the inflammatory response, so neutropenic patients often present with local or systemic infections. The diagnosis of alloimmune neutropenia is dependent on demonstrating the presence of maternal antibodies which react with the infant's neutrophils. The target antigens are only expressed on mature polymorphonuclear neutrophils and these have been shown to be controlled by a number of different genetic loci.

13.2 Pathophysiology and clinical history

13.2.1 Immunogenicity of fetal neutrophils

The reported incidence of immunization against neutrophil alloantigens during pregnancy varies from 0.1% to 20%.[1-3] Estimates of the incidence of alloimmune neutropenia are considerably lower, at less than 0.1% and 0.2%, for the German and US populations, respectively.[4-6] The relatively low numbers of circulating neutrophils compared with red cells and platelets implies that maternal alloimmunization against fetal neutrophil-specific antigens resulting from fetomaternal haemorrhage might be infrequent. However, it is possible that significant numbers of granulocytes reach the maternal circulation by active migration through tissues in a process known as diapedesis.

13.2.2 Clinical manifestations and haematological findings

Alloimmune neutropenia is a rare clinical condition with a number of characteristic features. The disorder usually has a benign course with infants developing mild infections, predominantly of the skin and mucosal membranes, often with gram-positive bacteria. However, life-threatening infections resulting in pneumonia and meningitis can also develop and a mortality of approximately 5% of affected infants has been reported.[5] In common with alloimmune thrombocytopenia, the condition may occur in the first-born infant.[6,7] Haematological investigation reveals a severe neutropenia (usually less than 0.5×10^9/l) which may persist for between 3 and 28 weeks;[6,7] the neutropenia may be accompanied by monocytosis. Neutrophil counts immediately after birth may be normal, with the neutropenia developing in the following few days. An explanation of this phenomenon is that the phagocytic system for the destruction of sensitized neutrophils may mature after birth, removing opsonised neutrophils from the circulation. There is evidence that the appropriate antigens are expressed on neonatal neutrophils in the first days of life.[8] The persistence of the cytopenia in alloimmune neutropenia compared with alloimmune thrombocytopenia is a remarkable feature of this condition and probably occurs because the target antigens in alloimmune neutropenia are expressed on a relatively small mass of mature precursor forms in the bone marrow or circulating neutrophils. Consequently, there is selective destruction of these mature forms while the immature precursor forms in the bone marrow remain unaffected. This is consistent with the bone marrow picture, which is typically either normal or hypercellular with a left-shift in appearance.[6,7] As in the other alloimmune cytopenias, the duration of neutropenia in the infant is also dependent on the rate of production and turnover of target cells and the half-life of the maternal IgG alloantibodies.

It is likely that alloimmune neutropenia is often undiagnosed, especially if the infant is asymptomatic at birth, since differential white cell counts are rarely performed at delivery and because clinical awareness of the condition may be low. The clinical underdiagnosis is complicated by a general lack of appropriate serological expertise. Even when alloimmune neutropenia is recognized, clinical management is usually conservative since the condition is self-resolving. Parents should be advised that affected infants should be protected from potentially infectious agents and that greater attention be given to hygiene during the period of neutropenia. The use of prophylactic antibiotics may be appropriate and both intravenous IgG[6] and granulocyte colony-stimulating factor[9,10] may be of benefit in severely affected cases.

13.2.3 Differential diagnosis

Other disease processes, drugs and environmental factors may all result in neutropenia or impair the functional integrity of neutrophils and hence increase susceptibility to infection.[11] In addition, a number of different causes of neutropenia are specifically recognized in early childhood. These may be divided into disorders

Table 13.1 Neutropenic syndromes of early childhood

Failures of production or altered release from bone marrow
Cyclic neutropenia
Infantile genetic agranulocytosis (Kostmann's syndrome)
Familial benign chronic neutropenia
Reticular dysgenesis
Aplastic anaemia
Lazy leukocyte syndrome
Myelokathexis

Excessive neutrophil consumption or destruction
Neutropenias secondary to bacterial and viral infections
Immune-mediated neutropenias – transitory congenital neutropenia
                                autoimmune neutropenia of infancy
                                alloimmune neutropenia

---

arising from defective neutrophil production or release from the bone marrow, and into those disorders caused by excessive neutrophil destruction or consumption (Table 13.1). Two other conditions which result from antibody-mediated neutrophil destruction, namely transitory congenital neutropenia and autoimmune neutropenia of infancy, are worthy of further discussion since they may complicate the differential diagnosis of alloimmune neutropenia at both clinical and laboratory levels.

13.2.3.1 Transitory congenital neutropenia

Transient neutropenia can be observed in infants born to mothers with autoimmune neutropenia. In this condition, maternal transfer of antineutrophil autoantibodies results in neonatal neutropenia. The mother is also neutropenic and the antibodies can be shown to react with maternal neutrophils.[12]

13.2.3.2 Autoimmune neutropenia of infancy

The clinical and serological characteristics of autoimmune neutropenia of infancy, originally documented as chronic benign neutropenia,[13] have been confirmed in a number of studies.[14–16] Autoimmune neutropenia of infancy is characterized by an isolated neutropenia often associated with an accompanying monocytosis. Onset of the disease usually occurs between the ages of 4 months and 2 years, but has been observed 1 month after birth.[13,16] The incidence of the disorder has been estimated as approximately one in 100 000.[17] Autoimmune neutropenia of infancy is a self-resolving condition in which spontaneous remission occurs in 95% of patients between 7 and 24 months of age. Serological studies reveal the presence of granulo-cyte-specific IgG or IgM autoantibodies and, although the incidence in the reported studies varies considerably,[16,18] anti-HNA-1a antibodies (Section 13.3.2.1) are often identified. Despite an absence of transfusions, antibody reactivity against lympho-cytes is also observed in some patients. The course of the disease, which is associated with infections of the skin, middle ear, throat and respiratory and digestive tracts, is generally relatively benign. Clinical management consists largely of the use of prophylactic antibiotics. The disorder has been attributed to a suppressor T-lymphocyte deficiency and the production of anti-HNA-1a antibodies has been linked to the HLA-DR2 haplotype.[19] The temporal overlap in the presentation of alloimmune neutropenia and autoimmune neutropenia of infancy, combined with the similarity of clinical features, may pose a clinical problem in diagnosis, especially if alloimmune neutropenia is suspected some months after birth or if autoimmune neutropenia of infancy presents early. However, in the laboratory, autoimmune neutro-penia of infancy can be readily differentiated from alloimmune neutropenia by the lack of anti-neutrophil autoantibodies in the maternal serum.

13.3 The structure and function of antigens involved in alloimmune neutropenia

Granulocyte membrane antigens may be divided into three types:

(1) The granulocyte-specific antigens, many of which have been localized to Fcγ receptor IIIb (CD16).

(2) The 'shared' antigens which often have a limited distribution among other cell types, usually other leukocytes. Some of the 'shared antigens' have been local-ized to CD11/18.

(3) The 'common' antigens which have a wider tissue distribution, being found on several blood and tissue cells. The 'common' antigens include the I and P blood group systems, Le^x and sialyl-Le^x (CD15) and HLA class I. These antigens are not involved in alloimmune neutropenia and so will not be discussed further.

13.3.1 Nomenclature

The nomenclature originally proposed for these antigens used the letter N, to indi-cate neutrophil specificity (even though many studies used granulocytes rather than purified neutrophils), followed by a capital letter to designate the locus of the gene controlling the production of the antigen, followed by a number designating a specific allele at that locus, e.g. NA1.[7] Subsequently, a number of antigens, many of which have a wider distribution, have been described which do not follow this convention. A different nomenclature (the human neutrophil antigens – HNA – system) has recently been proposed which includes both granulocyte-specific and more widely distributed antigens.[20] Those antigens, which have not been incorporated into the proposed system, because of insufficient scientific information, will continue to be referred to by the original acronym. The HNA nomenclature is used throughout this chapter, but the old acronyms are also presented in Tables 13.2 and 13.3, since the majority of publications to date have used this system.

13.3.2 Granulocyte-specific antigens

13.3.2.1 Polymorphisms of Fcγ receptor IIIb (CD16)

Five antigens termed HNA-1a, HNA-1b, HNA-1c, LAN and SAR are located on Fcγ receptor IIIb. The human Fcγ receptor IIIb (CD16) molecule is a member of the immunoglobulin superfamily which is distinct from, but closely related to, other human receptors for the Fc domain of IgG (Fcγ receptors).[45] Fcγ receptor IIIb is a protein composed of approximately 190 amino acids encoded by the *FcγRIIIB* gene located on human chromosome 1.[46] The molecule has an extracellular region comprising two disulphide-bonded 'immunoglobulin-like' domains and is linked to the plasma membrane via a glycosylphosphatidylinositol anchor. Fcγ receptor IIIb has a low affinity for IgG and is selectively expressed on neutrophils.[46] In immunoprecipitation and SDS-polyacrylamide gel electrophoresis studies, Fcγ receptor IIIb migrates as a broad band with a molecular weight between 50 kD and 80 kD. This variation in apparent molecular weight is the result of differences in glycosylation between FcγRIIIb^{HNA-1a} (HNA-1a) and FcγRIIIb^{HNA-1b} (HNA-1b).[47] The differences in glycosylation arise from amino acid differences between HNA-1a and HNA-1b at positions 65 and 82, which result in two additional glycosylation sites in HNA-1b.[30] At the DNA level, there are five nucleotide differences between the *FcγRIIIB*$^{HNA-1a}$ and *FcγRIIIB*$^{HNA-1b}$ genes, but only four of these substitutions give rise to changes in amino acids (Figure 13.1 and Table 13.2). Large-scale studies of the incidence of granulocyte-specific antigens in different ethnic groups have not been performed, but preliminary data have suggested that the frequency of the HNA-1a antigen is more common in Japanese, Chinese and Korean populations than in Caucasians.[50–52] An antigen referred to as NC1 has been reported,[38] but evidence now suggests that NC1 is identical to HNA-1b.[39]

The HNA-1c antigen is associated with a single base mutation in the *FcγRIIIB* gene. The nucleotide sequence of the HNA-1c allele is identical to the *FcγRIIIB*$^{HNA-1b}$ sequence except for the substitution of an adenine for cytosine at position 266. This nucleotide substitution results in an amino acid substitution of alanine by aspartic acid at position 78 of FcγRIIIb[32] (Figure 13.1). Gene duplication appears to have led to many HNA-1c-positive individuals having three rather than two *FcγRIIIB* genes.[53] Normally, there are between 100 000 and 200 000 copies of Fcγ receptor IIIb per neutrophil,[31] but individuals with three *FcγRIIIB* genes express proportionately greater amounts of Fcγ receptor IIIb.

Table 13.2 Granulocyte-specific alloantigens

HNA nomenclature	Original name of system	Original acronym for antigen	Caucasian phenotype frequency %	Caucasian gene frequency %	Glycoprotein	Nucleotide change	Amino acid change	References: description of antigen	References: genetic basis
HNA-1a	NA	NA1	46	0.35	FcγRIIIb	G^{108}	Arginine[36]	29	30, 31
						C^{114}	None		
						A^{197}	Asparagine[65]		
						G^{247}	Aspartic acid[82]		
						G^{319}	Valine[106]		
HNA-1b	NA	NA2	88	0.65	FcγRIIIb	C^{108}	Serine[36]	7	30, 31
						T^{114}	None		
						G^{197}	Serine[65]		
						A^{247}	Asparagine[82]		
						A^{319}	Isoleucine[106]		
HNA-1c	SH	SH+	5		FcγRIIIb	A^{266}	Aspartic acid[78]	32	32
		SH–				C^{266}	Alanine[78]	32	32
HNA-2a	NB	NB1	97	0.83	56–64kD	nk	nk	33	34, 35
		NB2	32	0.17	45–56kD	nk	nk	36	37
	NC	NC1*	91	0.72	nk	nk	nk	38	39
	ND	ND1	98.5	0.88	nk	nk	nk	40	—
	NE	NE1	23	0.12	nk	nk	nk	41	—
	LAN	LAN[a]	>99		FcγRIIIb	nk	nk	42	43
	SAR	SAR[a]	>99		FcγRIIIb	nk	nk	44	44

Notes:

The single nucleotide codes presented for HNA-1a and HNA-1b have been calculated from the data given in the original publication. nk is not known.

* NC1 has been shown to be identical to HNA-1b.[39]

Source: This table first appeared in an article entitled 'Platelet and granulocyte glycoprotein polymorphisms' by GF Lucas & PM Metcalfe (2000).

Transfusion Medicine, **10**, 157–74.

Table 13.3 Alloantigens expressed on granulocytes and other cell types (shared antigens)

HNA nomenclature	Original name of system	Original acronym for antigen	Caucasian phenotype frequency %	Caucasian gene frequency %	Glycoprotein	Nucleotide change	Amino acid change	References: description of antigen	References: genetic basis
	9	9a	58	0.35	nk	nk	nk	21, 22	
	Five	5a		0.181	nk	nk	nk	23	
HNA-3a		5b		0.66/0.819	70–95kD	nk	nk	23, 24	
HNA-4a	Mart	Mart^a(+)	99.1	0.906	CD11b	G^{302}	Arginine^{61}	25	26
		Mart^a(−)			CD11b	A^{302}	Histidine^{61}		26
HNA-5a	Ond	Ond^a(+)	>99	>0.91	CD11a	G^{2466}	Arginine^{766}	27	26
		Ond^a(−)			CD11a	C^{2466}	Threonine^{766}		26
	SL	SL^a	66	0.90	nk	nk	nk	28	

Notes:

nk is not known

Source: This table first appeared in an article entitled 'Platelet and granulocyte glycoprotein polymorphisms' by GF Lucas & PM Metcalfe (2000).

Transfusion Medicine, **10**, 157–74.

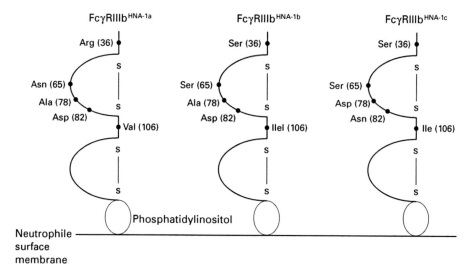

Figure 13.1   Schematic representation of the amino acid substitutions resulting in the HNA-1a, -1b and
-1c forms of Fcγ receptor IIIb, adapted from the illustration published by Salmon et al.[48]
The positions of the amino acids are noted according to the numbering system of
Ravetech and Perussia.[49]

LAN and SAR are high-frequency antigens which have been localized to Fcγ
receptor IIIb using antisera from women who gave birth to neutropenic infants.
The anti-LAN serum, from an Australian aboriginal woman, was reactive with neutrophils from over 99% of Caucasians.[42,43] The anti-SAR serum was from a Turkish
woman and reacted with neutrophils from all of 150 German blood donors tested.[44]
The LAN and SAR antigens are defined solely by human antisera; the molecular
localization of these antigens on Fcγ receptor IIIb is not known.

13.3.2.2 The HNA-2a antigen

The HNA-2a (NB1) antigen is expressed on granulocytes from 97% of the population.[33] HNA-2a is associated with a 56–64 kD glycosylphosphatidylinositol anchor-
linked glycoprotein[34,35] and is expressed on the plasma membrane surface and
intracellularly on the membranes of small vesicles and specific granules. Anti-NB2
antibodies do not react with this 56–64 kD glycoprotein. At present, it seems that
antibodies with the presumed anti-NB2 specificity do not recognize the antithetical antigen to HNA-2a.[54] This conclusion is supported by the finding that the NB2-
bearing glycoprotein has a smaller molecular weight of 46–56 kD.[37] Furthermore,
NB2 has a serological reactivity identical to 9a (human monocyte antigen, HMA-
1), but the gene frequencies for HNA-2a and 9a are inconsistent with simple allel-
ism between these antigens.[15,36]

13.3.2.3 The ND and NE antigens

In contrast to the HNA-1a, -1b, -1c and -2a, and LAN and SAR antigens, which were defined using alloantibodies, the ND1 antigen[40] and the NE1 antigen[41] were each defined by autoantibodies obtained from a single patient. The molecular basis and nature of the ND and NE antigens are unknown.

13.3.3 'Shared' antigens

13.3.3.1 Polymorphisms of CD11/18

The HNA-4a and HNA-5a antigens are located on the β2-integrins CD11b/18 and CD11a/CD18, respectively. These integrins belong to a family of heterodimers sharing the common β subunit CD18 (95 kD) noncovalently associated with one of three different α subunits – namely, CD11a (80 kD), CD11b (165 kD) or CD11c (150 kD). CD11a is expressed on all leukocytes while CD11b (C3bi receptor) and CD11c are expressed on granulocytes, monocytes and natural killer cells.

Studies using glycoprotein-specific monoclonal antibodies have shown that the HNA-5a antigen is located on CD11a whereas the HNA-4a antigen is located on CD11b. At the molecular level, both these antigens result from single nucleotide substitutions, causing amino acid dimorphisms of the corresponding α chains (Table 13.3).[26] The HNA-4a antigen has a calculated gene frequency of 0.906 and is expressed on granulocytes, monocytes and a subpopulation of T lymphocytes.[25] The HNA-5a antigen is detected in 91.8% of Dutch individuals and is expressed on granulocytes, monocytes, and T and B lymphocytes.[27]

13.3.3.2 The five system antigens

The biallelic five system antigens (now referred to as 5a and HNA-3a – see Table 13.3) were identified using antisera obtained from women immunized during pregnancy.[23] The five system antigens were originally thought to be expressed on granulocytes, platelets, lymphocytes, kidney, spleen and lymph node tissue. More recent evidence suggests that the five system may be granulocyte specific and that the previously reported wider tissue distribution was an artefact caused by the contamination of antisera with other alloantibodies, probably anti-HLA.[55] The genes encoding five system antigens have been localized to human chromosome 4.[56] The HNA-3a antigen has been localized to a granulocyte glycoprotein with a molecular weight of 70–95 kD.[24] Antisera to the 5a antigen are rare and, consequently, both the clinical significance and the molecular location of this antigen remain unknown.

13.3.3.3 The SL antigen

The SL antigen was originally defined by an antiserum from a mother who gave birth to a neutropenic infant. The antiserum reacted with granulocytes and T lymphocytes from 66% of individuals. The SL antigen is not associated with HNA-1a, -1b, -2a, -3a, -4a or -5a, NB2, NC1 or 9a antigens, or the Fcγ receptor IIIb molecule. The molecule carrying the SL antigen could not be identified by immunoblotting or immunoprecipitation studies.[28]

13.3.3.4 The 9a antigen

An antiserum from a multiparous blood donor defined a granulocyte-specific antigen known as 9a, which has a gene frequency of 0.41.[21] More recently, the 9a antigen has been reported to be related to NB2 and human monocyte antigen 1 and it should, therefore, be classified as a 'shared' antigen.[22] The molecular localization of the 9a antigen is not known.

13.3.3.5 Other antigens

A number of other granulocyte antigens have been described, but their involvement in alloimmune neutropenia has not been established. These include the granulocyte-specific HGA-3 system, which is comprised of five alleles.[57] Further investigation of this system has not been possible because of the rarity of antisera. Other studies have described two further granulocyte-specific antigen systems (GA, GB, GC and Gr1, Gr2), a granulocyte–monocyte antigen (HGA-1) and AYD, an antigen present on granulocytes, monocytes and endothelial cells.[15]

13.3.4 Antibody specificities involved in alloimmune neutropenia

Alloimmune neutropenia is usually caused by fetomaternal incompatibility with respect to the HNA-1a, -1b, -1c, -2a and -2b antigens,[5,6,32,58] but also may result from incompatibility with respect to high-frequency antigens[42,44] and, possibly, five system antigens.[24] Isoimmune neutropenia may also occur in the infants of women who lack Fcγ receptor IIIb and who become immunized against Fcγ receptor IIIb during pregnancy.[59,60]

13.3.5 The function of granulocyte antigens

Until recently, the importance of granulocyte antigens was restricted to their ability to induce the formation of antibodies. However, there is also evidence that certain granulocyte polymorphisms may affect cellular function and may be associated with an increased risk of disease. The HNA-1a and -1b antigens influence the function of Fcγ receptor IIIb; granulocytes from HNA-1a individuals exhibit greater levels of phagocytosis than granulocytes from HNA-1b individuals.[61] A further functional polymorphism is exhibited on granulocytes in which Fcγ receptor IIa exists as a high responder (HR) or low responder (LR) form, as determined by two amino acid substitutions.[45,46] The FcγRIIa[LR] phenotype enables effective interaction with IgG2 immune complexes and is associated with reduced infections by encapsulated bacteria such as *Haemophilus influenzae* and *Staphylococcus pneumoniae*, which elicit a predominantly IgG2 response. The FcγRIIa[LR] form may also confer resistance against *Neisseria meningitidis* infections.[62] The coexpression of Fcγ receptor IIa and Fcγ receptor IIIb on granulocytes raises the possibility that particular combinations of Fcγ receptor polymorphisms may influence susceptibility to bacterial infections and immune responses.

13.4 Laboratory diagnosis of alloimmune neutropenia

The laboratory diagnosis of alloimmune neutropenia involves the detection of granulocyte antibodies, phenotyping and genotyping studies, and, critically, performance of a crossmatch to demonstrate the reactivity of antibodies in maternal serum with paternal, fetal and/or neonatal neutrophils.

13.4.1 Assays for granulocyte antibodies

Granulocytes represent a small percentage of the circulating blood cells. They are difficult to isolate and must be freshly prepared for in vitro studies. Furthermore, granulocytes are functionally active cells which may aggregate upon stimulation and may up- or downregulate membrane surface antigens during isolation procedures, thereby influencing the number of antibody-binding sites. Granulocytes also have a number of different membrane surface antigens, including HLA class I antigens, which may complicate the results of antibody-binding studies involving human sera. As a result, a wide range of techniques have been developed for granulocyte antibody detection over the last 25 years, but only a small number have proved suitable for reliable routine use. A combination of two techniques, the granulocyte agglutination test (GAT) and the granulocyte immunofluorescence test (GIFT), is currently regarded as optimal for antibody detection[63] because neither technique used in isolation can detect all granulocyte antibodies.[1,5] The GAT relies on an interaction between viable granulocytes in the presence of sera containing IgG or IgM granulocyte-reactive antibodies over several hours.[64] The granulocytes migrate together to form aggregates in a time- and temperature-dependent process. The GAT appears to provide the most reliable method for detecting anti-5b antibodies.[63] The absence of a cell washing step after granulocytes have been sensitized in the GAT may increase the ability of this test to detect low affinity antibodies. The GAT does, however, require lengthy incubation periods for optimal sensitivity. Moreover, the degree of agglutination needs to be assessed microscopically.

The GIFT[1] measures membrane-bound antibodies by the use of anti-human immunoglobulin reagents labelled with a fluorescent compound such as fluorescein isothiocyanate. In the original method, granulocyte-associated fluorescence was assessed by microscopy. Many laboratories now use flow cytometry since this provides a semiquantitative endpoint, together with increased sensitivity and reliability. Furthermore, flow cytometry provides a ready distinction between intact granulocytes and those with disrupted cell membranes. The latter nonspecifically bind fluorescein-labelled antibodies and often cause problems of interpretation in microscopically assessed immunofluorescence assays.

The GAT and GIFT have a continuing and fundamental role in granulocyte serology. However, many human antisera contain antibodies which react with a number of granulocyte antigens rather than just one, and, consequently, both the GAT and GIFT are prone to interference from immune complexes and HLA class I antibodies (unless the sera are preabsorbed with platelets). The monoclonal antibody immobilization of granulocyte antigens (MAIGA) assay[43,65] utilizes monoclonal antibodies to capture solubilized target membrane glycoproteins that have bound human antibody. The principle behind this assay is identical to the monoclonal antibody immobilization of platelet antigens (MAIPA) assay (Section 12.4.2.2). These glycoprotein-specific assays avoid interference by HLA antibodies and immune complexes. Thus, the MAIGA enables the elucidation of complex mixtures of granulocyte-reactive antibodies with different specificities. The limited availability of monoclonal antibodies to capture all the relevant granulocyte glycoproteins restricts the application of the MAIGA assay, but granulocyte antibodies reactive with FcγRIIIb, HNA-2a and CD11/18 can be detected and identified.[26,43,44] The assay is unable to detect all antibodies because stearic hindrance by the monoclonal antibodies used to capture the granulocyte antigens can prevent the binding of the human antibodies in the patient's serum.

Several other techniques have recently been applied to the detection of granulocyte-specific antibodies and may be used in the diagnosis of alloimmune neutropenia. These include the granulocyte chemiluminescence test, immunoprecipitation, immunoblotting and the mixed passive haemagglutination assay. These techniques are often used to supplement the granulocyte agglutination, immunofluorescence or MAIGA assays and thereby improve the reliability of diagnosis. The granulocyte chemiluminescence test is a rapid functional assay which measures the interaction between human monocytes and opsonised granulocytes.[66] This test is analogous to an assay which measures the chemiluminescent response of monocytes to sensitized red cells (Section 8.4.4). The granulocyte chemiluminescence test provides a measure of the functional activity of granulocyte antibodies and has been shown to be of comparable sensitivity to the granulocyte immunofluorescence test in the detection of granulocyte-specific antibodies.[67] However, without preabsorption of sera with platelets, the granulocyte chemiluminescence test is unable to discriminate between HLA- and granulocyte-specific antibodies. Immunoprecipitation and immunoblotting have been used for the biochemical localization of antigens.

The recently described mixed passive haemagglutination assay has the advantage of utilizing extracted and immobilized granulocyte antigens which can be stored at $-80\,^{\circ}$C for at least a year.[68] The development of HNA-transfected cell lines[69] and the expression of recombinant molecules expressing granulocyte antigens will probably enhance and/or simplify antibody detection.

13.4.2 Role of crossmatching and parental typing

Crossmatching and typing are important elements in the investigation of suspected cases of alloimmune neutropenia. Crossmatching studies establish whether any maternal anti-granulocyte antibodies react with granulocytes from the father and/or infant – a prerequisite for the diagnosis of alloimmune neutropenia. Crossmatching can be especially important in cases where antibodies to low-frequency antigens are present, since a typing panel of granulocytes may not include cells with the corresponding antigen. Crossmatching may be performed using any of the techniques described in Section 13.4.1, although the interpretation of the results may be complicated by the presence of HLA class I antibodies and it may be necessary to use a MAIGA assay (Section 13.4.1).

13.4.3 Granulocyte antigen typing

13.4.3.1 Antigen typing using human antisera

Until recently, granulocyte antigen typing was restricted by the availability of appropriate human typing sera. Many human sera containing granulocyte-reactive alloantibodies also contain anti-HLA antibodies or other granulocyte-reactive antibodies and these can cause unreliable results in tests which utilize intact granulocytes. The advent of the MAIGA assay (Section 13.4.1) has circumvented this problem for many granulocyte antigens but, at present, phenotyping using the GAT or GIFT with human typing sera is the only available option for identifying the granulocyte-associated HNA-3a, -5a and -9a, and NB2 and SL antigens.

13.4.3.2 Monoclonal antibodies against granulocyte-specific antigens

Monoclonal antibodies with anti-HNA-1a, -1b and -2a specificities have been described which have specificities identical to human granulocyte-specific alloantisera and these can, therefore, be used for antigen typing. Monoclonal antibodies have the advantages of monospecificity and continuity of supply and can be readily conjugated to fluorescent or other molecules. All phenotyping techniques have the disadvantage of requiring freshly prepared granulocytes.

13.4.3.3 Molecular biology techniques for granulocyte antigen typing

The determination of the genetic basis of the HNA-1a/1b antigens[30] has enabled the development of a number of PCR-based techniques for these antigens.[70–72] In a

HNA sequence-specific
primers added to each
PCR reaction:

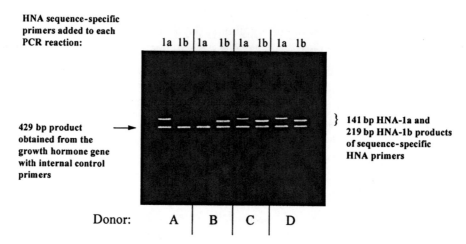

Figure 13.2   Results of HNA-1a and HNA-1b genotyping using a PCR with sequence-specific primers
for four individual donors. HNA-1a and -1b genotyping using the technique of Bux et al.[70]
The figure shows the results obtained with DNA extracted from an HNA-1a homozygous
individual (donor A), an HNA-1b homozygous individual (donor B) and two HNA-
1a/HNA-1b heterozygous individuals (donors C and D). PCR products visualized on a
1.5% w/v agarose gel using ethidium bromide staining and ultraviolet illumination.

comparative study of HNA-1a and -1b typing methods, results of the MAIGA assay
(Section 13.4.1) and a PCR assay using sequence-specific primers (Section 7.2.3)
were in complete concordance, but the GIFT produced an error rate of 15%.[70] A
PCR-based technique has also been described for the HNA-1c antigen[32] and, with
the description of the molecular basis of the HNA-4a and HNA-5a antigens,[26] it is
likely that DNA typing will also become available for these polymorphisms. An
example of the results obtained using sequence-specific primers in a PCR for typing
HNA-1a and HNA-1b is shown in Figure 13.2.

13.5 References

1 Verheugt FWA, von dem Borne AEGKr, Décary F & Engelfriet CP (1977). The detection of
granulocyte alloantibodies with an indirect immunofluorescence test. *British Journal of
Haematology*, 36, 533–44.

2 Clay ME & Kline WE (1984). The frequency of granulocyte-specific antibodies in postpartum sera and a family study of the 6B antigen. *Transfusion*, 24, 252–5.

3 Skacel PO, Stacey TE, Tidmarsh CEF & Contreras M (1989). Maternal alloimmunization to
HLA, platelet and granulocyte-specific antigens during pregnancy: its influence on cord
blood granulocyte and platelet counts. *British Journal of Haematology*, 71, 119–23.

4 Levine DH, Madyastha P, Wade TR & Levkoff AH (1982). Neonatal isoimmune neutropenia.
Pediatric Research, 16, 296A, 1304.

5 Lalezari P (1984). Alloimmune neonatal neutropenia. In *Research Monographs in Immunology*, Vol. 5: *Immunohaematology*, eds. CP Engelfriet, JJ von Loghem & AEGKr von dem Borne , pp. 178–86. Amsterdam: Elsevier.

6 Bux J, Jung D, Kauth T & Mueller-Eckhardt C (1992). Serological and clinical aspects of granulocyte antibodies leading to alloimmune neonatal alloimmune neutropenia. *Transfusion Medicine*, 2, 143–9.

7 Lalezari P & Radel E (1974). Neutrophil-specific antigens: immunology and clinical significance. *Seminars in Hematology*, 11, 281–90.

8 Madyastha PR, Glassman AB & Levine DH (1984). Incidence of neutrophil antigens on human cord neutrophils. *American Journal of Reproductive Immunology*, 6, 124–7.

9 Gilmore MM, Stroncek DF & Korones DN (1994). Treatment of alloimmune neonatal alloimmune neonatal neutropenia with granulocyte colony-stimulating factor. *Journal of Pediatrics*, 125, 948–51.

10 Rodwell RL, Gray PH, Taylor KM & Minchinton R (1996). Granulocyte colony stimulating factor treatment for alloimmune neonatal neutropenia. *Archives of Diseases of Childhood and Fetal Neonatology*, 75, 57–8.

11 Klebanoff SJ & Clark RA (eds.) (1978). *The Neutrophil: Function and Clinical Disorders*. Oxford: North-Holland.

12 Stefanini M, Mele RH & Skinner D (1958). Transitory congenital neutropenia: a new syndrome, a report of two cases. *American Journal of Medicine*, 25, 749–58.

13 Lalezari P, Jiang AF, Yegen L & Santorineou M (1975). Chronic autoimmune neutropenia due to anti-NA2 antibody. *New England Journal of Medicine*, 293, 744–7.

14 Lalezari P, Karshidi M & Petrosova M (1986). Autoimmune neutropenia of infancy. *Journal of Pediatrics*, 109, 764–9.

15 McCullough J, Clay M & Kline W (1987). Granulocyte antigens and antibodies. *Transfusion Medicine Reviews*, 1, 150–60.

16 Bux J, Behrens G, Jaeger G & Welte K (1998). Diagnosis and clinical course of autoimmune neutropenia in infancy: analysis of 240 cases. *Blood*, 91, 181–6.

17 Lyall EGH, Lucas GF & Eden OB (1992). Autoimmune neutropenia of infancy. *Journal of Clinical Pathology*, 45, 431–4.

18 Bruin MCA, von dem Borne AEGKr, Tamminga RYJ, Kleijer M, Buddelmeijer L & de Haas M (1999). Neutrophil antibody specificity in different types of childhood autoimmune neutropenia. *Blood*, 94, 1797–802.

19 Bux J, Mueller-Eckhardt G & Mueller-Eckhardt C (1991). Autoimmunization against the neutrophil-specific NA1 antigen is associated with HLA-DR2. *Human Immunology*, 30, 18–21.

20 Bux J (1999). Nomenclature of granulocyte alloantigens. *Transfusion*, 39, 662–3.

21 van Rood JJ, van Leeuwen A, Schippers AMJ et al. (1965). Leukocyte groups, the normal lymphocyte transfer test and homograft sensitivity. In *Histocompatibility Testing*, eds. DB Amos & JJ van Rood, pp. 37–50. Copenhagen: Munksgaard.

22 Jager MJ, Claas FHJ, Witvliet M & van Rood JJ (1986). Correspondence of the monocyte antigen HMA-1 to the non-HLA antigen 9a. *Immunogenetics*, 23, 71–7.

23 van Leeuwen A, Eernisse JG & van Rood JJ (1964). A new leucocyte group with two alleles: leucocyte group five. *Vox Sanguinis*, 9, 431–46.

24 de Haas M, Muniz-Diaz E, Alonso LG et al. (2000). Neutrophil antigen 5b is carried by a protein, migrating from 70 to 95 kD, and may be involved in neonatal alloimmune neutropenia. *Transfusion*, **40**, 222–7.

25 Kline WE, Press C, Clay M, Keashen-Schnell M, Hackel E & McCullough J (1986). Three sera defining a new granulocyte-monocyte-T-lymphocyte antigen. *Vox Sanguinis*, **50**, 181–6.

26 Simsek S, van der Schoot CE, Daams M et al. (1996). Molecular characterization of antigenic polymorphisms (Ond[a] and Mart[a]) of the beta 2 family recognized by human leukocyte alloantisera. *Blood*, **88**, 1350–8.

27 Décary F, Verheugt FWA, van Helden-Henningheim L et al. (1979). Recognition of non-HLA-ABC antigen present on B and T lymphocytes and monocytes only detectable with indirect immunofluorescence test. *Vox Sanguinis*, **36**, 150–8.

28 Stroncek DF, Ramsey G, Herr GP, Eiber G, Clay ME & Ketyer EC (1994). Identification of a new white cell antigen. *Transfusion*, **34**, 706–11.

29 Lalezari P & Bernard GE (1966). An isologous antigen-antibody reaction with human neutrophiles, related to neonatal neutropenia. *Journal of Clinical Investigation*, **45**, 1741–50.

30 Ory PA, Clark MR, Kwoh EE, Clarkson SB & Goldstein IM (1989). Sequences of complementary DNAs that encode the NA1 and NA2 forms of Fc receptor III on human neutrophils. *Journal of Clinical Investigation*, **84**, 1688–91.

31 Huizinga TWJ, Kleijer M, Tetteroo PAT, Roos D & von dem Borne AEGKr (1990). Biallelic neutrophil NA-antigen system is associated with a polymorphism on the phospho-inositol-linked Fcγ receptor III (CD16). *Blood*, **75**, 213–17.

32 Bux J, Stein E-L, Bierling P et al. (1997). Characterization of a new alloantigen (SH) on the human neutrophil Fcγ receptor IIIb. *Blood*, **89**, 1027–34.

33 Lalezari P, Murphy GB & Allen FH (1971). NB1, a new neutrophil-specific antigen involved in the pathogenesis of neonatal neutropenia. *Journal of Clinical Investigation*, **50**, 1108–15.

34 Stroncek DF, Skubitz KM & McCullough JJ (1990). Biochemical characterization of the neutrophil-specific antigen NB1. *Blood*, **75**, 744–55.

35 Goldschmeding R, van Dalen CM, Faber N et al. (1992). Further characterization of the NB1 antigen as a variably expressed 56–62kD GPI-linked glycoprotein of plasma membranes and specific granules of neutrophils. *British Journal of Haematology*, **81**, 336–45.

36 Lalezari P, Petrosova M & Jiang AF (1982). NB2, an allele of NB1 neutrophil specific antigen: relationship to 9[a]. *Transfusion*, **22**, 433, S123 (Abstract).

37 Wu GG, Curtis BR, Shao YL & Aster RH (1993). Investigation of human neutrophil antigens with a new nonradioactive immunoprecipitation technique: characterization of NB1 and NB2 antigenic targets. *Transfusion*, **33**, 78S S301 (Abstract).

38 Lalezari P, Thalenfield B & Weinstein WJ (1970). The third neutrophil antigen. In *Histocompatibility Testing*, ed. P. Terasaki, pp. 319–22. Baltimore, MD: Williams and Wilkins.

39 Bux J, Behrens G, Leist M & Mueller-Eckhardt C (1995). Evidence that the granulocyte-specific antigen NC1 is identical with NA2. *Vox Sanguinis*, **68**, 46–9.

40 Verheugt FWA, von dem Borne AEGKr, van Noord-Bokhorst JC, Nijenhuis LE & Engelfriet CP (1978). ND1, a new neutrophil granulocyte antigen. *Vox Sanguinis*, **35**, 13–17.

41 Claas FHJ, Langerak J, Sabbe LJM & van Rood JJ (1979). NE1: a new neutrophil specific antigen. *Tissue Antigens*, **13**, 129–34.

42 Rodwell RL, Tudehope DI, O'Regan PO, Minchinton R & Waters AH (1991). Alloimmune neonatal neutropenia in Australian aboriginals: an unrecognized disorder? *Transfusion Medicine*, **1**, 63–7.

43 Metcalfe P & Waters AH (1992). Location of the granulocyte-specific antigen LAN on the Fc-receptor III. *Transfusion Medicine*, **2**, 283–7.

44 Bux J, Hartmann C & Mueller-Eckhardt C (1994). Alloimmune neonatal neutropenia resulting from immunization to a high frequency antigen on the granulocyte Fcγ receptor III. *Transfusion*, **34**, 608–11.

45 de Haas M, Vossbeld PJM, von dem Borne AEGKr & Roos D (1995). Fcγ receptors of phagocytes. *Journal of Laboratory and Clinical Medicine*, **126**, 330–41.

46 van de Winkel JGJ & Capel PJA (1993). Human IgG Fc receptor heterogeneity: molecular aspects and clinical implications. *Immunology Today*, **14**, 215–21.

47 Werner G, von dem Borne AEGKr, Bos MJE et al. (1989). Localization of the human NA1 alloantigen on neutrophil Fc-γ-receptors. In *Leucocyte Typing II, White Cell Differentiation Antigens*, eds. EL Reinharz, BF Haynes, LM Nadler & ID Bernstein, pp. 109–121. New York: Springer.

48 Salmon JE, Edberg, JC & Kimberley RP (1996). FcγR on neutrophils. In *Human IgG Fc receptors*, eds. JGJ van de Winkel & PJA Capel, pp. 79–105. Austin, TX: RG Landes Co.

49 Ravetech JV & Perussia B (1989). Alternative membrane forms of FcγRIII (CD16) on human natural killer cells and neutrophils. *Journal of Experimental Medicine*, **170**, 481–97.

50 Ohto H & Matsuo Y (1989). Neutrophil-specific antigen and gene frequencies in Japanese. *Transfusion*, **29**, 654 (Letter).

51 Lin M, Chen CC, Wang CL & Lee HL (1994). Frequencies of neutrophil-specific antigens among Chinese in Taiwan. *Vox Sanguinis*, **66**, 247.

52 Han KS & Um TH (1997). Frequency of neutrophil-specific antigens among Koreans using the granulocyte indirect immunofluorescence test (GIFT). *Immunohematology*, **13**, 15–16.

53 Koene HR, Kleijer M, Roos D, de Haas M & von dem Borne AEGKr (1998). FcγRIIIB genes in NA(1+,2+)SH(+) individuals. *Blood*, **91**, 673–9.

54 Stroncek DF, Shankar RA, Plachta LB, Clay ME & Dalmasso AP (1993). Polyclonal antibodies against the NB1-bearing 58- to 64 kD glycoprotein of human neutrophils do not identify an NB2-bearing molecule. *Transfusion*, **33**, 399–404.

55 Kuijpers RWAM, Dooren MC, von dem Borne AEGK & Ouwehand WH (1991). Detection of human monocyte-reactive alloantibodies by flow cytometry after selective downmodulation of the Fc receptor I. *Blood*, **78**, 2150–6.

56 Geurts van Kessel AHM, Stoker K, Class FHJ, van Agthoven AJ & Hagemeijer A (1983). Assignment of the leucocyte group five surface antigens to human chromosome 4. *Tissue Antigens*, **21**, 213–18.

57 Thompson JS, Overlin VL, Herbrick JK et al. (1980). New granulocyte antigens demonstrated by microgranulocytotoxicity assay. *Journal of Clinical Investigation*, **65**, 1431–9.

58 Curtis BR, Ebert DD, Hessner MJ & Aster RH (1998). Neonatal alloimmune neutropenia due to anti-SH. *Transfusion Medicine*, **8**, 263 (Abstract).

59 Huizinga TWJ, Kuijpers R, Kleijer M et al. (1990). Maternal genomic neutrophil FcRIII deficiency leading to neonatal iso-immune neutropenia. *Blood*, **76**, 1927–32.

60 Stroncek DF, Skubitz KM, Plachta LB et al. (1991). Alloimmune neonatal neutropenia due to an antibody to the neutrophil Fc-γ receptor III with maternal deficiency of CD16 antigen. *Blood*, **77**, 1572–80.

61 Salmon JE, Edberg JC & Kimberley RP (1990). Fcγ receptor III on human neutrophils. Allelic variants have functionally distinct capacities. *Journal of Clinical Investigation*, **85**, 1287–95.

62 Bredius RGM, Derkx BHF, Fijen CA et al. (1994). Fcγ receptor IIa (CD32) polymorphism in fulminant meningococcal septic shock in children. *Journal of Infectious Diseases*, **170**, 848–53.

63 Bux J & Chapman J (1997). Report of the Second International Granulocyte Serology Workshop. *Transfusion*, **37**, 977–83.

64 Jiang A & Lalezari P (1975). A micro-technique for detection of leukocyte agglutinins. *Journal of Immunological Methods*, **7**, 103–8.

65 Bux J, Kober B, Kiefel V & Mueller-Eckhardt C (1993). Analysis of granulocyte-reactive antibodies using an immunoassay based upon monoclonal-antibody-specific immobilization of granulocyte antigens. *Transfusion Medicine*, **3**, 157–62.

66 Hadley AG & Holburn AM (1984). The detection of anti-granulocyte antibodies by chemiluminescence. *Clinical and Laboratory Haematology*, **6**, 351–61.

67 Lucas GF (1994). Prospective evaluation of the chemiluminescence test for the detection of granulocyte antibodies: comparison with the granulocyte immunofluorescence test. *Vox Sanguinis*, **66**, 141–7.

68 Araki N, Nose Y, Kohsaki M, Mito H & Ito K (1999). Anti-granulocyte antibody screening with extracted granulocyte antigens by a micro-mixed passive haemagglutination method. *Vox Sanguinis*, **77**, 44–51.

69 Bux J, Kissel K, Hofmann C & Santoso S (1998). Detection of NA1-, NA2- and SH-specific neutrophil antibodies using CHO transfectants. *Transfusion Medicine*, **8**, 262 (Abstract).

70 Bux J, Stein EL, Santoso S & Mueller-Eckhardt C (1995). NA gene frequencies in the German population, determined by polymerase chain reaction with sequence-specific primers. *Transfusion*, **35**, 54–7.

71 Stein EL, Bux J, Santoso S & Mueller-Eckhardt C (1994). Typing of the granulocyte-specific NA antigens by restriction fragment length polymorphism analysis. *British Journal of Haematology*, **87**, 428–30.

72 Satoh T, Kobayashi M, Kaneda M, Tanihiro M, Okada K & Ueda K (1994). Genotypical classification of neutrophil Fcγ receptor III by polymerase chain reaction-single-strand conformation polymorphism. *Blood*, **83**, 3312–15.

Fetal and neonatal treatment of alloimmune thrombocytopenia

Michael F. Murphy,[1,2] Rachel Rayment,[1] David Allen[1] and David Roberts[1,2]

[1] National Blood Service, Oxford, UK
[2] University of Oxford, Oxford, UK

14.1 Introduction

Alloimmune thrombocytopenia is the commonest cause of neonatal thrombocytopenia, occurring in one in 1000–2000 live births;[1–3] this is equivalent to 400–800 cases per year in the UK. The pathogenesis of alloimmune thrombocytopenia is similar to HDFN (Chapter 1):

- The mother is negative for a platelet alloantigen which the fetus has inherited from the father, and maternal alloimmunization occurs in a proportion of women who may have a genetic predisposition to become immunized (Section 1.3.3).
- Placental transfer of IgG antibodies may result in moderate to severe thrombocytopenia as early as 16 weeks' gestation.[4]
- The most clinically significant incompatibility is for HPA-1a, the frequency of this antigen being 97.5% in Caucasians (Section 12.3).[5,6]
- HPA-1a alloimmunization is HLA class II restricted; there is a strong association with HLA-DRw52a (HLA-DR3*0101),[7,8] which is present in one in three of Caucasian women. Although the negative predictive value of the absence of HLA-DR3*0101 for HPA-1a alloimmunization in HPA-1a-negative women is >99%, the positive predictive value of its presence for alloimmunization has been estimated to be only 35%, and not all alloimmunized mothers will have babies with thrombocytopenia (Section 4.2).[9]
- The antibody titre and isotype have not been shown to correlate consistently with the development or severity of disease (Section 12.4.4.2).[10]

Unlike HDFN, alloimmune thrombocytopenia often affects the first child, and subsequent children are usually more severely affected. Severe thrombocytopenia may cause major bleeding such as intracranial haemorrhage both after birth and in utero, resulting in significant morbidity and mortality. Considerable progress has been made in the laboratory aspects of platelet immunology, allowing more precise diagnosis of the condition (Section 12.4). The prognosis of the disease has improved, due to advances in both fetal and transfusion medicine, particularly for women with a previous history of an affected pregnancy. The question of antenatal screening for alloimmune thrombocytopenia has been raised (Section 4.3), but this cannot be implemented until there are better methods for predicting which fetuses of alloimmunized mothers are most severely affected, in order to justify the risks of antenatal intervention. At present, strategies for the antenatal management of alloimmune thrombocytopenia are focussed on women known to be at risk due to a history of previously affected pregnancies. In this chapter, the neonatal management of alloimmune thrombocytopenia and the antenatal management of subsequent pregnancies of women with an affected child will be considered.

14.2 Neonatal management of alloimmune thrombocytopenia

Since there is currently no routine antenatal screening, most cases of alloimmune thrombocytopenia are unexpected and are diagnosed after birth, commonly following the observation of purpura. However, more serious bleeding, such as intracranial haemorrhage, may occur, causing death or severe neurological sequelae in about 25% of affected infants.[11] Intracranial haemorrhage is most likely to occur during or soon after delivery, but it may occur spontaneously in utero in up to 10% of cases. The duration of thrombocytopenia is usually between 1 and 2 weeks, but prolonged thrombocytopenia of 6 weeks' duration may occur. The need for immediate treatment depends on the presence of bleeding and the severity of the thrombocytopenia. If treatment is required, it should not be delayed while confirmatory tests are performed.

In a survey of UK Haematology Departments,[12] the reported incidence of alloimmune thrombocytopenia was significantly lower than expected, suggesting under-recognition of the disorder. Unavailability of HPA-1a-negative platelets or a lack of facilities with which to prepare maternal platelets were cited as the major causes of delay in treatment of the neonate (Table 14.1).[12] These delays, along with a lack of awareness of the potential seriousness of the disease, have the potential to cause significant morbidity to the neonate.

14.2.1 Platelet transfusion

Treatment of an affected neonate should be with compatible antigen-negative platelets.[13,14] There is controversy over the transfusion of random donor platelets in neonates – at best, platelet survival is reduced[15] – but, in at least some cases, it appears to be ineffective in raising the platelet count even if combined with high-dose intravenous immunoglobulin (IVIG) (see Figure 14.1).[16] In one recent case managed by one of the authors (MF Murphy), an apparent response to a pool of

Table 14.1 Reasons for delay in providing therapy effective in raising the baby's platelet count

Responses from 93 (31%) of 301 Haematology Departments in the UK to a questionnaire about the postnatal management of alloimmune thrombocytopenia*

			Number of hospitals
(a)	Local effects, such as:		
	(i)	lack of awareness of the potential seriousness of the clinical situation	44
	(ii)	lack of urgency in obtaining results of platelet counts	22
	(iii)	delay in notifying haematologist	33
	(iv)	other (see below)	7
		'Other' local problems cited by hospitals included inexperience of clinical staff and a lack of awareness of the seriousness of alloimmune thrombocytopenia and the appropriate treatment, poor liaison between the paediatric and haematology teams, and delay in obtaining samples from the mother because she had left hospital	
(b)	Unavailability of HPA-1a-negative platelet concentrates		18
(c)	Unavailability of facilities for the preparation of a platelet concentrate from the mother		15
(d)	Unavailability of a rapid platelet serology service		21
(e)	Other problems (see below)		6

Some hospitals specifically commented on the lack of an apheresis facility at the local transfusion centre, and the unavailability of or delays in obtaining HPA-1a-negative platelets. Some hospitals noted that delays at several stages were additive and that delays vary with the time of day and at weekends

Source: Data from Murphy and coworkers.[12]

random platelets occurred because two of the four donors, whose platelets made up the pool, were by chance HPA-1a negative.

The maternal antibodies are directed against HPA-1a or HPA-5b in 78% and 19% of cases, respectively;[5,6] more recent data from over 600 cases from platelet immunology laboratories in Oxford and Cambridge show that maternal antibodies are directed against HPA-1a and HPA-5b in 81% and 10% of cases, respectively (Table 14.2). Approximately 2% of blood donors are negative for both these antigens and can be easily identified using established methods (Section 12.4). The National Blood Service in England has a registry of HPA-1a-negative and HPA-5b-negative platelet donors who donate regularly, and some Blood Centres keep a supply of these platelets (see below).

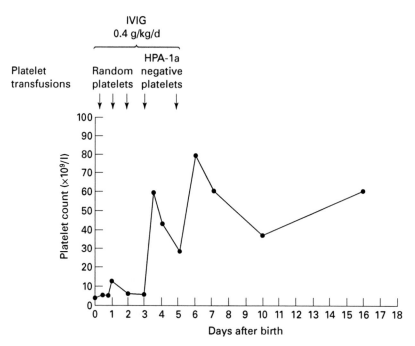

Figure 14.1. Platelet counts after birth in response to the initial treatment of a baby with alloimmune thrombocytopenia due to anti-HPA-1a with IVIG and random donor platelets, and later transfusion of HPA-1a-negative platelets. From Murphy and Allen (1997).[16]

Washed maternal platelets have been used in the treatment of alloimmune thrombocytopenia for many years, with demonstrable benefit.[17] There are, however, logistical problems with this approach:

- apheresis facilities for platelet collection may not be available at the time required;
- platelets need to be washed before use, which may result in platelet activation;
- the platelets need irradiation to prevent transfusion-associated graft-versus-host disease; and
- there is a risk of transmitting infection to the neonate.

14.2.2 Intravenous immunoglobulin

If antigen-negative or maternal platelets are not available, then IVIG is recommended.[18] There have been isolated case reports describing the successful administration of IVIG to affected neonates,[19] but only one formal study.[20] In this latter study, the response rate was 75%, but the increase in platelet count was delayed for 24–48 hours. IVIG is not thought to be helpful in cases with clinical signs of haemorrhage. It may be used as an adjunct to platelet transfusion if the recovery is prolonged, but should not replace immediate therapy with platelets as the baby will be at risk of significant haemorrhage. In urgent situations, where antigen-negative

Table 14.2 Investigation of cases of neonatal thrombocytopenia in the National Blood Service Oxford and Cambridge platelet immunology laboratories – frequencies of antibody specificities in 154 cases of alloimmune thrombocytopenia investigated over 3 years between 1997 and 1999

Antibody specificity	Incidence	%
HPA-1a	131/154	85.1
HPA-3a	3/154	1.9
HPA-3b	1/154	0.6
HPA-5b	16/154	10.4
Gov[a]	4/94	4.3
Gov[b]	1/94	1.1
Unidentified glycoprotein IIb/IIIa	6/154	3.9
Unidentified glycoprotein Ia/IIa	2/154	1.3
Unidentified glycoprotein Ib/IX	1/154	0.6

platelets are not available and the neonate is bleeding, then a combination of IVIG and random platelets should be given until compatible donor platelets are available.[16,21]

14.2.3 Monitoring of the effectiveness of neonatal treatment

The clinical condition of the infant should be carefully monitored and the platelet count measured at least once daily until it is obvious that it has reached a 'safe' level and is increasing spontaneously. If there has been severe thrombocytopenia, a cerebral ultrasound or nuclear magnetic resonance scan should be performed to detect clinically silent intracranial haemorrhage.

14.3 Antenatal management of alloimmune thrombocytopenia

The recurrence of thrombocytopenia in subsequent pregnancies is high (over 85%), the risk depending on whether the partner's platelet genotype is homozygous (HPA-1a/1a) or heterozygous (HPA-1a/1b) – indicating a risk of 100% and 50%, respectively.[22] Determination of the fetal platelet genotype can be carried out using material obtained by amniocentesis, chorionic villous or fetal blood sampling (Section 12.4.3). In the future, noninvasive typing may be possible from maternal blood (Section 7.4).

The severity of alloimmune thrombocytopenia usually increases in subsequent pregnancies. If a previous pregnancy was affected by intracranial haemorrhage, subsequent pregnancies are at significant risk of severe thrombocytopenia and intracranial haemorrhage, justifying antenatal intervention. As already discussed,

laboratory tests such as maternal antibody titres do not predict reliably the severity of thrombocytopenia, and the best predictive indicator for severe fetal thrombocytopenia is the occurrence of antenatal intracranial haemorrhage in a previously
affected pregnancy.[23]

It is more difficult to assess risk in cases where the previous infant had thrombocytopenia without significant haemorrhage. However, in the absence of any noninvasive test for the severity of alloimmune thrombocytopenia, most fetal medicine
units would recommend fetal blood sampling at around 20–22 weeks' gestation
where there was a pregnancy previously affected by alloimmune thrombocytopenia with moderate or severe thrombocytopenia (platelet count less than $50 \times 10^9/l$).

Although there is a risk of bleeding during delivery, nearly 50% of intracranial
haemorrhages occur in utero, usually between 30 and 35 weeks' gestation, but
sometimes as early as 20 weeks.[24,25] There may be more unusual presentations, and
alloimmune thrombocytopenia should be considered in cases such as hydrocephalus, unexplained fetal anaemia or recurrent miscarriages.[26]

Even if there is moderate thrombocytopenia, it appears to be appropriate to start
treatment since the fetal platelet count is likely to fall further in untreated fetuses.[23]
If the platelet count is normal or there is mild thrombocytopenia, fetal blood sampling may need to be repeated at regular intervals, possibly every 4 weeks, to detect
a significant fall in the fetal platelet count indicating the need for antenatal treatment.

Early delivery at around 34 weeks' gestation is usually carried out in pregnancies
severely affected by alloimmune thrombocytopenia; fetal lung maturity has
occurred, and the long-term outlook for premature newborns of this gestational
age is very good. Antenatal treatment appears to have improved the outcome of
severely affected cases of alloimmune thrombocytopenia, but there is little information on the long-term development of those children who have been treated in
utero.

14.3.1 Fetal blood sampling

The way to assess the severity of fetal thrombocytopenia is by fetal blood sampling.[27] This allows both the collection of blood (for the measurement of the platelet count and HPA genotyping) and the administration of intrauterine platelet
transfusion.

Fetal blood sampling for alloimmune thrombocytopenia is associated with at
least a 1% fetal loss and should, therefore, only be performed in specialist centres.
The procedure takes a few minutes; a few millilitres of fetal blood is obtained from
the umbilical cord prior to and following transfusion to assess the platelet count
and the subsequent increment. Most centres give a transfusion of platelets to cover
fetal blood sampling for alloimmune thrombocytopenia as platelet counting may

be performed some distance from the fetal medicine unit and because there is an expectation of severe thrombocytopenia. Transfusion may also be needed urgently in the event of bleeding. Platelet counts in pure samples are reliable, but contamination of the sample with maternal blood or amniotic fluid must be avoided – requiring significant skill and expertise. The normal range for the fetal platelet count is similar to adults, but it rises significantly with gestational age.

The risk of complications related to fetal blood sampling varies according to the underlying disorder, the gestational age and the experience of the operator,[28] but it has been estimated that, in low-risk pregnancies, the risk of early fetal loss is 0.6% and that the fetal spontaneous loss is 1.29%.[29] In the same study, no serious haemorrhage from the umbilical cord occurred in a series of 5194 fetal blood samplings including 247 fetuses with platelet counts of less than $150 \times 10^9/l$.

The risk of bleeding complications with fetal blood sampling is higher in pregnancies affected by alloimmune thrombocytopenia. Fetal and neonatal losses were reported in five pregnancies affected by alloimmune thrombocytopenia being assessed for their suitability for antenatal therapy in a large multicentre international study.[30] The five fetal and neonatal deaths were thought to be as a result of exsanguination, but no precise loss rate could be determined because they represented a collection of cases rather than a study of a defined population. They were compared with a group of 44 other affected fetuses who underwent the same procedure and survived (controls); the mean platelet count at the time of fetal blood sampling was lower in the fetuses who died than in the controls, and the incidence of antenatal intracranial haemorrhage in the previously affected pregnancy was greater in the siblings of the fetuses who died than in the controls. Once the authors of this study became aware of these five cases of exsanguination, they changed their practice to perform in utero platelet transfusions when the fetal platelet count was found to be less than $50 \times 10^9/l$. Since instituting this practice, no procedure-related losses occurred in 10 further cases where platelet transfusions were administered to severely thrombocytopenic fetuses, and they strongly recommend this approach. This latter experience agrees with the experience of the antenatal management of alloimmune thrombocytopenia of another group.[31]

14.3.2 Maternal treatment

Noninvasive antenatal therapies have been tried, with varying success. These include maternal administration of steroids, IVIG and combined steroids and IVIG.

14.3.2.1 Steroids

There are minimal data regarding the effectiveness of maternal administration of steroids alone (Table 14.3). Daffos et al.[32] reported an increase in the fetal platelet

Table 14.3 Results of antenatal treatment for alloimmune thrombocytopenia with steroids

Number of fetuses treated	Prednisolone (daily)	ICH	Platelet count $<50 \times 10^9$/l at delivery	Additional therapy	Study reference
1	10 mg from 23 weeks	0	0	Nil	32
4	10 mg from 22 to 26 weeks until delivery at 37–38 weeks	0	2	Prednisolone increased to 25 mg daily from 27 to 28 weeks in two cases IUT prior to delivery	11
2	25 mg from 21 weeks	0	1	IVIG 1 g/kg/week from 26 weeks until delivery at 38 weeks in one case IUT prior to delivery	11

Notes:
IUT is intrauterine platelet transfusion; ICH is intracranial haemorrhage.
See also Table 14.6 for the data on two studies using either maternal treatment or fetal platelet transfusions.

count after maternal treatment with prednisone (10 mg/day) from 23 weeks' gestation. However, in a larger series of cases, the same group found that treatment of the mother with steroids or IVIG was not reliably effective in raising the fetal platelet count, and a fetal platelet transfusion was given prior to delivery if the fetal platelet count remained low.[11]

There is considerable experience from North America with the combined use of steroids and IVIG, and one study has concluded that steroids do not add significantly to the effect of IVIG.[33] A study of antenatal management of alloimmune thrombocytopenia in Europe found a significant response to steroids in only one in 10 (10%) of cases treated with steroids alone.[34]

14.3.2.2 IVIG

There is conflicting evidence on the efficacy of IVIG (Table 14.4). Several reports document good responses to the maternal administration of IVIG (dose 1 g/kg body weight/week), both in the prevention of intracranial haemorrhage and in achieving a platelet count greater than 30×10^9/l at the end of pregnancy.[33,36,43] In the most recent study involving 54 pregnancies,[33] there was a mean increase in the fetal platelet count between the first and second fetal blood sample of 36×10^9/l and from first fetal blood sample to birth of 69×10^9/l; responses occurred in 62–85% of pregnancies depending on the criteria used to define a successful response (see below), and there were no intracranial haemorrhages.

To avoid unnecessary treatment of a pregnancy at risk, fetal blood sampling is necessary prior to treatment with IVIG. Subsequent monitoring of treatment is

Table 14.4 Results of antenatal treatment for alloimmune thrombocytopenia with IVIG

Number of fetuses treated	IVIG administration (to the mother except where indicated)	Steroid administration (daily)	Number with ICH	Number with platelet counts $<30\times10^9$/l at FBS or delivery	Salvage therapy in nonresponders	Study reference
1	0.8 mg/kg loading dose at 30 weeks, then 0.4 mg/kg/week from 31 weeks	Nil	1	1	None	35
27	1 g/kg/week from diagnosis of thrombocytopenia	Nil	2[1]	Not available[2]	IUT (n=1)	34
18	1 g/kg/week from diagnosis of thrombocytopenia at 20–22 weeks (one case received 0.5 mg/kg/week)	Nine mothers also received dexamethasone 1.5–5 mg or prednisolone 10 mg	0	2	None	36
1	1 g/kg/week from week 25	Nil	0	0	Platelet count at 27 weeks was low and weekly IUTs were given until delivery at 32 weeks	37
6	1 g/kg/week	Dexamethasone 1.5 mg (n=3)	0	1	Prednisolone 60 mg/day (n=2)	38
1	1 g/kg/week from 17 to 34 weeks	Nil	0	1	Failed IUT prior to delivery	39
1	1 g/kg/week from 20 weeks	Nil	1	0	IUTs from time of ICH at 32 weeks until delivery at 35 weeks	40
1	Intrauterine transfusion to fetus	Nil	0	0	Single IUT given prior to delivery	41
1	Intrauterine transfusion to fetus	Nil	0	0	IVIG to the mother	42
54	1 g/kg/week from diagnosis of thrombocytopenia at 20–22 weeks	Dexamethasone 1.5 mg (26) versus no treatment (28)	0	12[3]	Prednisolone 60 mg/day (n=10)	33

Notes:
[1] One death, one with neurological sequelae.
[2] In nine cases, where the platelet count fell with treatment, the median platelet count was 25×10^9/l.
[3] FBS (fetal blood sampling) 4–6 weeks after commencement of antenatal treatment. Twelve had a 'poor response'. Three were electively delivered; nine plus one additional patient were treated with salvage therapy, and five responded with an increase in the fetal platelet count and all five had platelet counts at birth over 30×10^9/l.
IUT is intrauterine platelet transfusion; ICH is intracranial haemorrhage.
See also Table 14.6 for the data on two studies using either maternal treatment or fetal platelet transfusions.

also by fetal blood sampling, which allows the introduction of serial platelet trans-fusions (see below), if the platelet count falls. However, a number of case reports[35,37–42] suggest that this therapy is ineffective in raising the fetal platelet count, and antenatal intracranial haemorrhage has occurred during maternal treat-ment with IVIG.[40] Other studies have found a tendency for good responses in the mildest affected cases of alloimmune thrombocytopenia, and failure in those most severely affected:

- one study found no effect of IVIG in three severely affected cases and mainten-ance or an increase in the fetal platelet count in three out of four mildly affected cases, the latter defined as a fetal platelet count of above $50 \times 10^9/l$ in the initial fetal blood sample;[31]
- another found good responses in two out of eight pregnancies treated, and the two responders were the mildest affected cases;[44] and
- a correlation between the response to IVIG treatment and the platelet count in the initial fetal blood sample has been noted by a North American group.[43]

In a larger study, European centres treating 37 pregnancies only found success with the use of maternal IVIG in seven of 27 (27%) cases, and steroids in one in 10 (10%).[34] Therapy was unsuccessful in nine of 27 (33%) cases with IVIG, and in seven of 10 cases treated with steroids. There was no significant change in the fetal platelet count in 11 of 27 (41%) cases treated with IVIG, and in two of 10 (20%) cases treated with steroids. Failure of response was associated with clinical outcome; haemorrhagic complications occurred in three pregnancies where there was no response to treatment:

- intracranial haemorrhage in two pregnancies, leading to neurological sequelae in one and death in the other; and
- cord haemorrhage leading to abortion.

The reported experience with IVIG is therefore quite different in North America and Europe. This may be due to differences in the selection of cases or in the dose, timing or type of IVIG used. However, the most likely explanation is variation in the crite-ria for determining an increase in the fetal platelet count. In the North American study,[33] a successful response at the time of the second fetal blood sample (usually 4–6 weeks after the first) was defined as an increase in the fetal platelet count com-pared with the first and a fetal platelet count over $20 \times 10^9/l$, or a decrease in the fetal platelet count of no more than $10 \times 10^9/l$ from the first fetal blood sample and a fetal platelet count of over $40 \times 10^9/l$. In the European collaborative study,[34] the treatment was considered to be successful if there was no intracranial haemorrhage, if there was a significant increase in the fetal platelet count assessed by regression analysis and if the platelet count was above $30 \times 10^9/l$ at the end of therapy. The most appro-priate criteria for a successful response are debatable. However, 18 of 27 (67%) cases in the European study could be considered to have had a good response if the pregnancies with a plateau in the fetal platelet count were reclassified as successful, and this would then produce a comparable result to the North American study.

It has been suggested that the direct injection of IVIG to the fetus by cordocentesis may be more effective than its indirect administration to the mother.[41] However, this method of administering IVIG has all the risks of fetal blood sampling discussed above, and was not found to be effective by another group.[42]

The mechanism of action of IVIG in the antenatal management of alloimmune thrombocytopenia is uncertain. Suggested modes of action include Fc receptor blockade of fetal reticuloendothelial cells, feedback inhibition of maternal antibody production, anti-idiotypic interactions, increased antibody catabolism and placental Fc receptor blockade.[45]

14.3.3 Fetal platelet transfusion

A number of studies have shown the value of platelet transfusions given by cordocentesis in raising the platelet count, but the platelet count is raised for only a few days. A single predelivery transfusion[17,25,46] may protect against bleeding at the time of delivery, but the fetus remains at risk of spontaneous intracranial haemorrhage earlier in pregnancy (Table 14.5). Weekly in utero platelet transfusions have been shown to be effective in preventing intracranial haemorrhage in severe cases of alloimmune thrombocytopenia.[17,31,41,47,48] The two largest series of cases managed with either steroids and/or IVIG or serial fetal platelet transfusions are summarized in Table 14.6.[31,44]

An example of the use of serial fetal platelet transfusions for alloimmune thrombocytopenia is shown in Figure 14.2. If the fetal platelet count is raised to $300–500 \times 10^9/l$ after each transfusion, it is usually no lower than $30 \times 10^9/l$ 1 week later.[48] This may be considered as a 'safe' level at which to maintain the fetal platelet count, and 7 days as an acceptable interval between transfusions in the high-risk pregnancies where serial transfusions are used. If the interval between transfusions is prolonged beyond 7 days, the nadir of the fetal platelet count is less than $30 \times 10^9/l$ (unpublished data). From 26 weeks' gestation, the procedure should be performed in the operating theatre where facilities are available to perform an emergency Caesarean section.

The volume of platelet hyperconcentrate to be transfused is calculated from a formula:

$$\frac{(\text{desired platelet increment} \times \text{feto-placental blood volume for gestational age}) \times R}{\text{platelet count of the concentrate, which is measured on each occasion}}$$

The fetoplacental volume for gestational age is calculated from standard charts. The immediate post-transfusion platelet increment was found to be 50% of that

Table 14.5 Results of antenatal treatment for alloimmune thrombocytopenia with fetal platelet transfusion

Number of fetuses treated	Platelet administration	Number with ICH	Additional therapy	Number with a platelet count $<30 \times 10^9/l$ at delivery	Study reference
1	IUT prior to delivery	0	Nil	0	46
7	One IUT at 38 weeks	0	IVIG 0.4 g/kg/5 days ($n=1$) weekly IUT from 35 weeks if platelet $<20 \times 10^9/l$ ($n=1$)	1	17
2	Weekly IUT from 26 and 27 weeks until delivery	0	IVIG from week 25 with persistent thrombocytopenia ($n=1$)	0	37
1	Weekly IUT from 26 weeks	0	Nil	0	47
1	Weekly IUT from 29 weeks until delivery at 34 weeks	0	Nil	0	48

Notes:

IUT is intrauterine platelet transfusion; ICH is intracerebral haemorrhage.

See also Table 14.6 for the data on two studies using either maternal treatment or fetal platelet transfusions.

Table 14.6 The antenatal treatment for alloimmune thrombocytopenia: results from two studies using either steroids and/or IVIG or fetal platelet transfusions

Study 1, Murphy and coworkers (1994)[31]

	Platelet therapy	IVIG therapy alone	Steroid therapy alone	Steroids plus IVIG
Number: 15[1]	4*	4**	2**	3**
Mode of treatment	Weekly IUT from 18 to 29 weeks until delivery at 33–35 weeks, apart from one case[2]	1 g/kg/week beginning at 21–34 weeks to 31–38 weeks	Prednisolone 20 mg/day from 16 to 26 weeks to 25–36 weeks	Prednisolone 20 mg/day 1 g IVIG/kg/week beginning 14–20 weeks up to 16–33 weeks
Number ICH	0	0	0	One at 16 weeks
Number deaths	0	1[3]	1[4]	One pregnancy terminated due to ICH at 16 weeks
Additional therapy	0	0	Fetal platelet count fell to 50×10^9/l at 34 weeks, and then weekly IUTs were given until delivery at 36 weeks	Neither of the two other cases responded to IVIG. Both received weekly IUT from 26 and 31 weeks up to delivery at 33–35 weeks

Notes:

* Severely affected babies with initial fetal platelet count $<20 \times 10^9$/l were treated with fetal platelet transfusions.

** Mildly affected fetuses with initial fetal platelet count $>50 \times 10^9$/l were initially treated either with steroids or IVIG alone, or a combination of steroids and IVIG.

[1] Two pregnancies were terminated following ICH prior to fetal blood sampling with no other treatment given.

[2] One patient referred at 36 weeks received a single platelet transfusion prior to delivery.

[3] Fall caused fetal death.

[4] FBS at 25 weeks showed a fetal platelet count of 10×10^9/l and resulted in cord haematoma causing fetal death.

ICH is intracerebral haemorrhage; IUT is intrauterine platelet transfusion.

Table 14.6 *(cont.)*

Study 2, Sainio and coworkers (1999)[44]

	Platelet therapy	IVIG therapy	IVIG plus steroids
Number: 15	6	8[1]	1**
Mode of treatment	Weekly IUT from 25 to 29 weeks to 33–36 weeks, apart from two cases*	1g/kg/week from 25–32 weeks to 35–39 weeks	Prednisolone 20 mg/day from 22 to 35 weeks IVIG–1 g/kg for 1 week only at 35 weeks
Number ICH	0	0	0
Additional therapy	0	Only two cases responded to IVIG The other six received IUT prior to delivery	IUT given prior to delivery (platelet count 18×10^9/l)

Notes:

* Two pregnancies were managed with a single transfusion; one immediately prior to delivery at 34 weeks, and the other at 28 weeks prior to delivery at 37 weeks.

** One mother had autoimmune thrombocytopenia in addition.

[1] One case also received prednisolone 30 mg/day from 24 to 29 weeks.

ICH is intracerebral haemorrhage; IUT is intrauterine platelet transfusion.

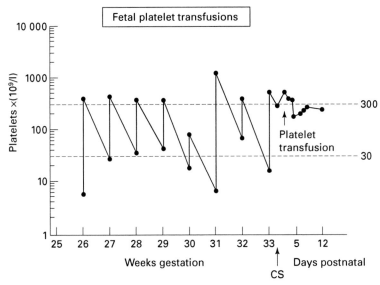

Figure 14.2   Seventh pregnancy of a patient who had had five miscarriages. The last of these was shown to have hydrops and hydrocephalus and a platelet count of only 17×10^9/l, and the serological findings supported a diagnosis of alloimmune thrombocytopenia due to anti-HPA-1a. The fetal platelet count was less than 10×10^9/l at 25 weeks' gestation in the sixth pregnancy, and a cord haematoma developed during fetal blood sampling resulting in fetal death. In the seventh pregnancy, prednisolone 20 mg/day and intravenous immunoglobulin 1 g/week were administered to the mother from 16 weeks until delivery. The figure shows pre- and post-transfusion platelet counts following serial fetal blood samplings and platelet transfusions. The fetal platelet count was less than 10×10^9/l at 26 weeks. The aim was to maintain the fetal platelet count above 30×10^9/l by raising the immediate post-transfusion platelet count to above 300×10^9/l after each transfusion. The fetal platelet count fell below 10×10^9/l on one occasion when there were problems in preparing the fetal platelet concentrate and the dose of platelets was inadequate. CS is Caesarean section.

expected, i.e. 50% platelet recovery, probably because of pooling in the fetoplacental circulation. The volume calculation takes account of this by introducing the factor $R = 2$, thus doubling the volume of platelets transfused.

14.3.4 Serial fetal platelet transfusions compared with maternal administration of high-dose IVIG

The data on the effectiveness and risks of these two approaches have been summarized in Table 14.6. The decision on which approach to use is a difficult one and is a balance between the more reliable means of increasing the fetal platelet count and the apparent lower risk of severe haemorrhage with the use of transfusions, set against the morbidity and mortality associated with an increased number of fetal blood samples.

Antenatal therapy appears to have improved the outcome of severely affected cases of alloimmune thrombocytopenia. Further prospective and collaborative studies are needed to determine the relative roles of fetal platelet transfusions and maternal administration of IVIG, both in the prevention of significant haemorrhage and in providing the optimal quality of life to the child.

14.3.5 Timing of the initial fetal blood sample

It is difficult to know when it is best to carry out the initial fetal blood sampling whatever the plan for further antenatal management; it is necessary to consider the risk of fetal blood sampling and the risk of antenatal haemorrhage without treatment. More information is needed about the frequency and time of occurrence of intracranial haemorrhage in order to determine the optimal timing of the initial fetal blood sample. As already discussed, there is no reliable noninvasive method for assessing the severity of thrombocytopenia. The majority of intracranial haemorrhages occur from 30 weeks' gestation until delivery, but a significant number occur from 16 weeks onwards. If treatment is commenced only from 30 weeks then potentially avoidable haemorrhage will occur, and, because of this uncertainty, fetal blood sampling is usually carried out at 20–22 weeks' gestation.

It has been suggested that antenatal treatment with maternal IVIG be given 'blind', without fetal blood sampling, to determine the fetal platelet count.[49] However, it is important to recognize the problems with 'blind therapy' without an initial blood sample,[50] which include the following:

- The fetal platelet count is difficult to predict unless there is a history of antenatal intracranial haemorrhage in a previous pregnancy.[23] Fetal blood sampling is required to establish the severity of thrombocytopenia, which determines the approach to antenatal management. If the initial fetal blood sampling is not carried out, treatment will be given unnecessarily in some cases, with its consequent risks to both mother and fetus.
- Treatment is not monitored, and there is no opportunity to change the initial treatment if it is ineffective.
- There is a lost opportunity to learn more about the natural history of alloimmune thrombocytopenia and the effectiveness of different approaches to treatment.

Such a noninvasive strategy is not recommended by the two international groups with most experience in this field,[23,34] or in British Committee for Standards in Haematology (BCSH) guidelines on this topic.[51]

14.3.6 Strategy for the antenatal management of pregnancies at risk of very early intracranial haemorrhage

In cases where a sibling has suffered an intracranial haemorrhage prior to 20 weeks, the optimal management of subsequent pregnancies is unclear. Fetal blood sampling is not feasible until 20 weeks and it seems justifiable to treat the mother with IVIG from around 16 weeks' gestation. One of the problems in assessing the benefit of this approach is the absence of a fetal platelet count before the start of treatment. There have been no formal studies of this approach, but there are some data from individual cases, including the following:

- Patient LM[31] who had five miscarriages at 17–18 weeks' gestation; the last was shown to be associated with hydrops, hydrocephalus and severe thrombocytopenia, and a diagnosis of alloimmune thrombocytopenia due to anti-HPA-1a was subsequently made. The next two pregnancies were managed with steroids alone, and steroids and IVIG from 16 weeks' gestation until the first fetal blood sample at 25–26 weeks' gestation. There was severe fetal thrombocytopenia in both cases, but no haemorrhage.
- Patient SR[31,52] who was treated with steroids and IVIG from 14 weeks' gestation in her third pregnancy, following the finding of hydrocephalus at 19 weeks' gestation in her second pregnancy and the detection of anti-HPA-1a. Severe intracranial haemorrhage occurred at 16 weeks' gestation in the third pregnancy. In the fourth pregnancy, weekly intraperitoneal injections of IVIG were given from 12 to 18 weeks, when fetal blood sampling was carried out and the fetal platelet count was 12×10^9/l. The pregnancy eventually had a successful outcome.
- Patient PS (unreported case managed by Dr Pauline Hurley and one of the authors, MF Murphy) had a history of intracranial haemorrhage in two previous pregnancies at 21 and 30 weeks' gestation, associated with alloimmune thrombocytopenia due to anti-HPA-1a. She was treated with IVIG from 15 to 21 weeks' gestation, and the fetal platelet count at 21 weeks was 11×10^9/l. IVIG was discontinued and the remainder of the pregnancy was managed with weekly fetal platelet transfusions.
- Patient JL (unreported case managed by one of the editors, Peter Soothill) had a pregnancy severely affected by alloimmune thrombocytopenia due to anti-HPA-1a; there was intracranial haemorrhage at 28 weeks resulting in a handicapped child. Her husband was typed as HPA-1a/1b. Her next pregnancy was managed initially with IVIG from 20 weeks; the fetal platelet count was 220×10^9/l at 22 weeks, but fell to 19×10^9/l at 24 weeks. The remainder of the pregnancy was managed with a combination of IVIG and fetal platelet transfusions; fetal blood sampling was technically difficult because the patient was obese. It seemed that IVIG produced an increase in the fetal platelet count, and there was a successful outcome (Figure 14.3). IVIG was started at 17 weeks' gestation in her next

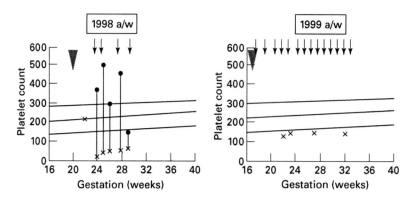

Figure 14.3 Patient JL. Management of pregnancies in 1998 and 1999 (see text). The patient's previous obstetric history included one handicapped child and two terminated pregnancies because of intracranial haemorrhage due to alloimmune thrombocytopenia. There appeared to be a response to IVIG in the 1998 pregnancy, and early use of IVIG in the 1999 pregnancy was only associated with mild thrombocytopenia. Large arrow indicates amniocentesis to obtain fetal DNA for HPA genotyping; small arrows indicate administration of IVIG.

pregnancy, following confirmation of the fetal platelet type as HPA-1a positive, and the fetal platelet count was over $100 \times 10^9/l$ at 22 weeks and remained at that level for the remainder of the pregnancy, suggesting that IVIG had a beneficial effect.

14.4 Preparation of platelet concentrates for transfusion in cases of alloimmune thrombocytopenia

14.4.1 Provision of HPA-typed platelets for neonates with alloimmune thrombocytopenia

In over 90% of cases of alloimmune thrombocytopenia, the maternal antibodies are directed against HPA-1a or HPA-5b[5,6] (see Table 14.2). Approximately 2% of blood donors are negative for both these antigens and the National Blood Service in England has a registry of HPA-1a-negative and HPA-5b-negative platelet donors who donate regularly, and some Blood Centres maintain a constant stock of these platelets. It is a considerable logistical exercise to achieve this, requiring at least 50 plateletpheresis donors to guarantee at least two donations to be available at all times.

14.4.2 Identification and recruitment of HPA-1a-negative and HPA-5b-negative donors

Donors used for the preparation of HPA-1b/1b platelets for fetal and neonatal transfusion undergo extremely stringent selection criteria and, as a result, only one donor in approximately 15000–20000 is suitable (Figure 14.4). These criteria include being tested and found negative for all of the normal microbiological

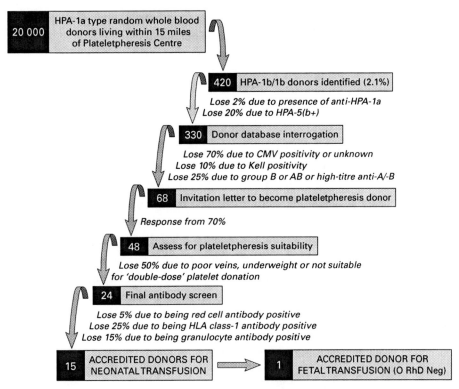

Figure 14.4 Identification and recruitment of HPA-1a-negative and HPA-5b-negative donors suitable for collection of platelet concentrates for fetal and neonatal transfusion in alloimmune thrombocytopenia.

markers (HBsAg, HCV, HIV and syphilis) and, in addition, being negative for cytomegalovirus, platelet-specific antibodies, HLA class-1 antibodies, granulocyte-specific antibodies, irregular red cell antibodies, high-titre anti-A and anti-B, and the antigens D, K, HPA-1a and HPA-5b. They must also be suitable for 'double-dose' plateletpheresis donation and factors such as height, weight, venous access, allergies and platelet count must also be taken into account. HLA typing is normally performed on these donors, as, occasionally, maternal HLA antibodies may result in shortened survival of platelets and, in such cases, the platelets should be prepared from HLA-compatible donors.[52] If not available, maternal platelets should be considered.

14.4.3 Preparation of platelet concentrates for fetal transfusions

The main issues in the preparation of platelet concentrates for fetal transfusions are:

- compatibility with maternal antibodies;
- avoidance of transfusion-transmitted infection;

• avoidance of transfusion-associated graft-versus-host disease; and
• adequate dosage without volume overload.

Concentration of the platelet preparation is essential in order to achieve satisfactory post-transfusion platelet counts without an unacceptably high transfusion volume. 'Hyperconcentrated' platelets are most easily prepared by apheresis using a modified COBE Spectra LRS which allows the collection of both a leukocyte-depleted hyperconcentrated unit of platelets and a normal adult therapeutic dose.[53] Platelets for intrauterine use should be irradiated to prevent graft-versus-host disease; there is no evidence that irradiation causes significant platelet damage.[54]

While there is agreement that the concentration needs to be over $2000 \times 10^9/l$ in order to reduce circulatory overload in the fetus, the precise concentration used varies among fetal medicine units. The COBE LRS product can be tailored to meet these individual requirements as there is a direct relationship between the collection flow rate and the concentration of the final product; thus, the flow rate can be varied to achieve the required concentration. Concentrations in the range $2500–4000 \times 10^9/l$ have been shown to have normal levels of platelet glycoprotein IIb/IIIa and glycoprotein Ib/IX, and have normal levels of activation when compared with normal platelet concentrates, as indicated by surface P-selectin and supernatant Annexin-V.[53]

14.5 Future directions

The current antenatal management of women affected by alloimmune thrombocytopenia, relying on fetal blood sampling and intrauterine transfusions, is invasive and carries significant risks to the fetus. These dangers, combined with the inability to predict the severity of clinical disease have restricted the development of strategies to screen all pregnant women for alloimmune thrombocytopenia and to treat all affected cases. The aim of current research is, therefore, to develop noninvasive methods for the diagnosis of alloimmune thrombocytopenia, for the reliable prediction of disease severity in affected infants and for the effective treatment of alloimmune thrombocytopenia.

Work towards achieving these ambitious goals is helped considerably by the detailed understanding we now have of the molecular basis of the disease. In the majority of cases of alloimmune thrombocytopenia, an antibody response to the HPA-1a platelet antigen is only generated in HPA-1a-negative women who carry the HLA-DR3*0101 allotype. Furthermore, this association permits the identification of the fragments of the HPA-1a antigen that bind to the HLA class II molecule to prime helper T cells.

This knowledge and other modern molecular methods will be crucial in several areas. First, noninvasive fetal genotyping in the first trimester of pregnancy, using the fetal DNA circulating in the maternal circulation, has been possible for the Rh(D) blood group antigen (Section 7.4). Similar noninvasive fetal genotyping for platelet antigens would spare fetal blood sampling of pregnant women with circulating anti-HPA-1a antibodies and a partner who is heterozygous at this locus (HPA-1a/1b).

Prediction of the severity of disease in affected cases would be of considerable value by allowing the reliable targeting of fetal platelet transfusion. Elucidation of the acquired and innate factors that determine disease severity will require cooperative large-scale longitudinal studies and the application of immunological and genetic tests.

Modulation of the disease process by molecular manipulation of the B or T cell and/or effector mechanisms may be possible. In principle, maternal T cells that provide help to the B cells making HPA-1a antibody can be inhibited or tolerised. Tolerisation of T cells requires knowledge of the precise T cell epitope recognized by responding cells. This should be possible to define in most cases of alloimmune thrombocytopenia, as an antibody response to the HPA-1a platelet antigen is nearly always generated by women expressing HLA-DR3*0101 and the T cell epitopes would, therefore, be expected to be similarly highly restricted (Section 1.1.1). In some models of alloimmune disease, the T cells responding to the alloantigen become unresponsive after stimulation with a peptide corresponding to the respective T cell epitope or with the peptide bound to the appropriate HLA class II molecules. It may be possible to use these approaches in alloimmune thrombocytopenia.

Identification of the T cell epitopes in alloimmune thrombocytopenia would permit the use of these peptide sequences to construct HLA class II DR3*0101 molecules bound to the corresponding peptide. When made as tetramers, these conjugates would bind to the pathogenic antigen-specific T cells to allow their isolation and detailed characterization. Furthermore, these class II–peptide conjugates may themselves induce T cell tolerance by binding to T cells in the absence of co-stimulatory signals.

Finally, it may be possible to make 'designer' antibodies that inhibit the binding of harmful maternal HPA-1a antibodies to fetal platelets. It may be possible to block the effector function of antibodies directed against the HPA-1a allotype by combining the variable regions of a monoclonal antibody recognizing HPA-1a with a constant region that will not bind to Fc receptors on phagocytic cells. If these antibodies cross the placenta and do not interfere with platelet or megakaryocyte function then they may block binding of the naturally occurring alloantibodies made by affected women and restore normal platelet function and numbers.

None of these mechanisms of molecular manipulation is yet established in clinical practice. Nevertheless, the highly restricted mechanisms that generate a deleterious HPA-1a antibody response in alloimmune thrombocytopenia suggest that specific molecular treatments may succeed here before more immunologically heterogeneous diseases are tackled.

Acknowledgements

We thank Dr P Hurley and Professor P Soothill for allowing us to report unpublished details on their patients, and Dr W Ouwehand and the staff in the platelet immunology laboratory, National Blood Service, Cambridge, for providing data on the frequencies of antibodies in their cases of alloimmune thrombocytopenia.

14.6 References

1 Blanchette VS, Chen L, de Friedberg ZS, Hogan VA, Trudel E & Decary F (1990). Alloimmunization to the PLA1 platelet antigen: results of a prospective study. *British Journal of Haematology*, **74**, 209–15.

2 Reznikoff-Etievant MF, Kaplan C, Muller JY, Daffos F & Forestier F (1988). Alloimmune thrombocytopenias, definition of group at risk: a prospective study. *Current Studies in Haematology*, **55**, 119–24.

3 Burrows RF & Kelton JG (1993). Fetal thrombocytopenia and its relation to maternal thrombocytopenia. *New England Journal of Medicine*, **329**, 1463–6.

4 Gruel Y, Boizard B, Daffos F, Forestier F, Caen J & Wautier J-L (1986). Determination of platelet antigens and glycoproteins in the human fetus. *Blood*, **68**, 488–92.

5 Mueller-Eckhardt C, Kiefel V, Grubert A et al. (1989). 348 cases of suspected neonatal alloimmune neonatal thrombocytopenia. *Lancet*, **1**, 363–6.

6 Waters A, Murphy M, Hambley H & Nicolaides K (1991). Management of alloimmune thrombocytopenia in the fetus and neonate. In *Clinical and Basic Science Aspects of Immunohaematology*, ed. SJ Nance, pp. 155–77. Arlington, VA: American Association of Blood Banks.

7 Valentin N, Vergracht A, Bignon JD et al. (1990). HLA-DRw52a is involved in alloimmunization against PL-A1 antigen. *Human Immunology*, **27**, 73–9.

8 Decary F, L'Abbe D, Tremblay L & Chartrand P (1991). The immune response to the HPA-1a antigen: association with HLA-DRw52a. *Transfusion Medicine*, **1**, 55–62.

9 Williamson LM, Hackett G, Rennie J et al. (1998). The natural history of fetomaternal alloimmunization to the platelet-specific antigen HPA-1a as determined by antenatal screening. *Blood*, **92**, 2280–7.

10 Prouix C, Filion M, Goldman M et al. (1994). Analysis of immunoglobulin class, IgG subclass and titre of HPA-1a antibodies in alloimmunized mothers giving birth to babies with or without neonatal alloimmune thrombocytopenia. *British Journal of Haematology*, **87**, 813–17.

11 Kaplan C, Daffos F, Forestier F, Morel MC, Chesnel N & Tchernia G (1991). Current trends in neonatal alloimmune thrombocytopenia: diagnosis and therapy. In *Platelet Immunology: Fundamental and Clinical Aspects*, ed. C Kaplan-Gouet, N Schlegel, Ch Salmon & J McGregor, pp. 267–78. Paris: Colloque INSERM/John Libbey Eurotext.

12 Murphy MF, Verjee S & Greaves M (1999). Inadequacies in the postnatal management of fetomaternal alloimmune thrombocytopenia. *British Journal of Haematology*, **105**, 123–6.

13 Blanchette VS, Kuhne T, Hume H & Hellmann I (1985). Platelet transfusion therapy in newborn infants. *Transfusion Medicine Reviews*, **9**, 215–30.

14 Kaplan C, Forestier F, Daffos F, Tchernia G & Waters A (1996). Management of fetal and neonatal alloimmune thrombocytopenia. *Transfusion Medicine Reviews*, **10**, 233–40.

15 Win N (1996). Provision of random-donor platelets (HPA-1a positive) in neonatal alloimmune thrombocytopenia due to anti HPA-1a alloantibodies. *Vox Sanguinis*, **71**, 130–1.

16 Murphy MF & Allen D (1997). Provision of platelets for severe neonatal alloimmune thrombocytopenia. *British Journal of Haematology*, **97**, 931–2.

17 Kaplan C, Daffos F, Forestier F et al. (1988). Management of alloimmune thrombocytopenia: antenatal diagnosis and in utero transfusion of maternal platelets. *Blood*, **72**, 340–3.

18 Letsky EA & Greaves M (1997). Guidelines for the investigation and management of thrombocytopenia in pregnancy and neonatal alloimmune thrombocytopenia. *British Journal of Haematology*, **95**, 21–6.

19 Pietz J, Kiefel V, Sontheimer D, Kobialka B, Linderkamp O & Mueller-Eckhardt C (1991). High-dose intravenous gammaglobulin for neonatal alloimmune thrombocytopenia in twins. *Acta Paediatrica Scandinavica*, **80**, 129–32.

20 Mueller-Eckhardt C, Kiefel V & Grubert A (1989). High dose IgG treatment for neonatal alloimmune thrombocytopenia. *Blut*, **59**, 145–6.

21 Win N, Ouwehand WH & Hurd C (1997). Provision of platelets for severe neonatal alloimmune thrombocytopenia. *British Journal of Haematology*, **97**, 930–1.

22 Shulman NR, Marder VJ, Hiller MC & Collier EM (1964). Platelet and leucocyte isoantigens and their antibodies. *Progress in Hematology*, **4**, 222–304.

23 Bussel JB, Zabusky MR, Berkowitz RL & McFarland JG (1997). Fetal alloimmune thrombocytopenia. *New England Journal of Medicine*, **337**, 22–6.

24 Giovangrandi Y, Daffos F, Kaplan C, Forestier F, MacAleese J & Moirot M (1990). Very early intracranial haemorrhage in alloimmune fetal thrombocytopenia. *Lancet*, **336**, 310.

25 De Vries LS, Connell J, Bydder GM et al. (1988). Recurrent intracranial haemorrhages in utero in an infant with alloimmune thrombocytopenia. Case report. *British Journal of Obstetrics and Gynaecology*, **95**, 299–302.

26 Murphy MF, Hambley H, Nicolaides K & Waters AH (1996). Severe fetomaternal alloimmune thrombocytopenia presenting with fetal hydrocephalus. *Prenatal Diagnosis*, **16**, 1152–5.

27 Daffos F, Capella-Pavlovsky M & Forestier F (1985). Fetal blood sampling during pregnancy with use of a needle guided by ultrasound: a study of 606 consecutive cases. *American Journal of Obstetrics and Gynecology*, **153**, 655–60.

28 Ghidini A, Sepulveda W, Lockwood CJ & Romero R (1993). Complications of fetal blood sampling. *American Journal of Obstetrics and Gynecology*, **168**, 1339–44.

29 Hohlfeld P, Forestier F, Kaplan C, Tissot J-D & Daffos F (1994). Fetal thrombocytopenia: a retrospective survey of 5,194 fetal blood samplings. *Blood*, **84**, 1851–6.

30 Paidas MJ, Berkowitz RL, Lynch L et al. (1995). Alloimmune thrombocytopenia: fetal and neonatal losses related to cordocentesis. *American Journal of Obstetrics and Gynecology*, **172**, 475–9.

31 Murphy MF, Waters AH, Doughty HA et al. (1994). Antenatal management of fetal alloimmune thrombocytopenia: report of 15 affected pregnancies. *Transfusion Medicine*, 4, 281–92.

32 Daffos F, Forestier F & Kaplan C (1988). Prenatal treatment of alloimmune thrombocytopenia. *Lancet*, 2, 910.

33 Bussel JB, Berkowitz RL, Lynch L et al. (1996). Antenatal management of alloimmune thrombocytopenia with intravenous gammaglobulin: a randomized trial of the addition of low dose steroid to IVIg in fifty-five maternal-fetal pairs. *American Journal of Obstetrics and Gynecology*, 174, 1414–23.

34 Kaplan C, Murphy MF, Kroll H & Waters AH (1998). Fetomaternal alloimmune thrombocytopenia: antenatal therapy with IVIgG and steroids – more questions than answers. *British Journal of Haematology*, 100, 62–5.

35 Mir N, Samson D, House MJ & Kovar IZ (1988). Failure of antenatal high-dose immunoglobulin to improve fetal platelet count in neonatal alloimmune thrombocytopenia. *Vox Sanguinis*, 55, 188–9.

36 Lynch L, Bussel JB, McFarland JG, Chitkara U & Berkowitz RL (1992). Antenatal treatment of alloimmune thrombocytopenia. *Obstetrics and Gynecology*, 80, 67–71.

37 Nicolini U, Tannirandorn Y, Gonzalez P et al. (1990). Continuing controversy in alloimmune thrombocytopenia: fetal hyperimmunoglobulinaemia fails to prevent thrombocytopenia. *American Journal of Obstetrics and Gynecology*, 163, 1144–6.

38 Wenstrom KD, Weiner CP & Williamson RA (1992). Antenatal treatment of fetal alloimmune thrombocytopenia. *Obstetrics and Gynecology*, 80, 433–5.

39 Marzusch K, Schnaidt M, Dietl J, Wiest E, Hofstaetter C & Golz R (1992). High dose immunoglobulin in the antenatal treatment of neonatal alloimmune thrombocytopenia: case report and review. *British Journal of Obstetrics and Gynaecology*, 99, 260–2.

40 Kroll H, Kiefel V, Giers G et al. (1994). Maternal intravenous immunoglobulin treatment does not prevent intracranial haemorrhage in fetal alloimmune thrombocytopenia. *Transfusion Medicine*, 4, 293–6.

41 Zimmermann R & Huch A (1992). In utero therapy with immunoglobulin for alloimmune thrombocytopenia. *Lancet*, 340, 606.

42 Bowman J, Harman C, Mentigolou S & Pollock J (1992). Intravenous fetal transfusion of immunoglobulin for alloimmune thrombocytopenia. *Lancet*, 340, 1034–5.

43 Bussel JB, Berkowitz RL, McFarland JG, Lynch L & Chitkara U (1988). Antenatal treatment of neonatal alloimmune thrombocytopenia. *New England Journal of Medicine*, 319, 1374–8.

44 Sainio S, Teramo K & Kekomaki R (1999). Prenatal treatment of severe fetomaternal alloimmune thrombocytopenia. *Transfusion Medicine*, 9, 321–30.

45 Clark AL & Gall SA (1998). Clinical uses of intravenous immunoglobulin in pregnancy. *American Journal of Obstetrics and Gynecology*, 176, 241–53.

46 Daffos F, Forestier F, Muller JY et al. (1984). Prenatal treatment of alloimmune thrombocytopenia. *Lancet*, 2, 632.

47 Nicolini U, Rodeck CH, Kochenour NK et al. (1988). In utero platelet transfusion for alloimmune thrombocytopenia. *Lancet*, ii, 506.

48 Murphy MF, Pullon HWH, Metcalfe P et al. (1990). Management of fetal alloimmune thrombocytopenia by weekly in utero platelet transfusions. *Vox Sanguinis*, 58, 45–9.

49 Summerfield GP, Beeby A, Bosman D & Chapman C (1998). Fetomaternal alloimmune thrombocytopenia: antenatal therapy with IVIgG and steroids. *British Journal of Haematology*, **102**, 1380.

50 Murphy MF, Kaplan C & Kroll H (1998). Fetomaternal alloimmune thrombocytopenia: antenatal therapy with IVIgG and steroids. *British Journal of Haematology*, **102**, 1380–1.

51 British Committee for Standards in Haematology (1997). Guidelines for the investigation and management of thrombocytopenia in pregnancy and neonatal alloimmune thrombocytopenia. *British Journal of Haematology*, **95**, 21–6.

52 Murphy MF, Metcalfe P, Waters AH, Ord J, Hambley H & Nicolaides K (1993). Antenatal management of severe fetomaternal alloimmune thrombocytopenia: HLA incompatibility may affect responses to fetal platelet transfusions. *Blood*, **81**, 2174–9.

53 Dumont LJ, Krailadsiri P, Seghatchian J, Taylor LA, Howell C & Murphy MF (2000). Preparation and storage characteristics of white cell-reduced high concentration platelet concentrates collected by an apheresis system for transfusion in utero. *Transfusion*, **40**, 91–100.

54 British Committee for Standards in Haematology (1996). Guidelines on gamma irradiation of blood components for the prevention of transfusion-associated graft-versus-host disease. *Transfusion Medicine*, **6**, 261–71.

Index

Note: page numbers in bold denote illustrations, those in italics, tables.

279